Pharmacotherapy for Liver Cirrhosis and Its Complications

Xingshun Qi • Yongping Yang
Editors

Pharmacotherapy for Liver Cirrhosis and Its Complications

Springer

Editors
Xingshun Qi
Department of Gastroenterology
General Hospital of Northern
Theater Command
Shenyang, China

Yongping Yang
Faculty of Liver Disease of Chinese
People's Liberation Army General Hospital
The Fifth Medical Center of the Chinese
People's Liberation Army General Hospital
Beijing, China

ISBN 978-981-19-2614-3 ISBN 978-981-19-2615-0 (eBook)
https://doi.org/10.1007/978-981-19-2615-0

This Springer imprint is published by the registered company Springer Nature Singapore Pte Ltd.
The registered company address is: 152 Beach Road, #21-01/04 Gateway East, Singapore 189721, Singapore

Foreword

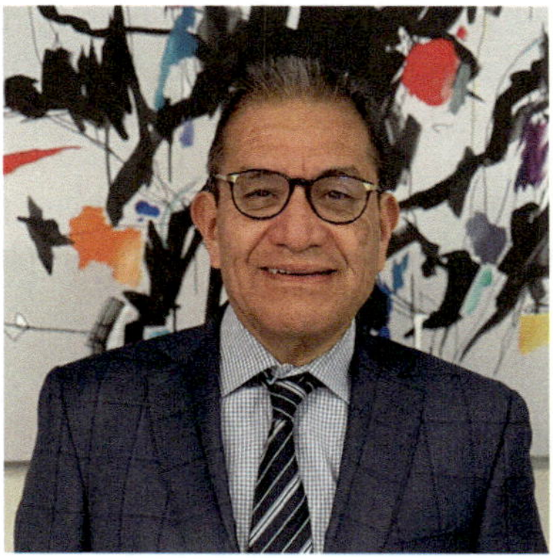

Hepatology is a constantly active and dynamic field, in which a lot of progress has been seen in the last two decades in different areas, such as epidemiology, development of new tools for the diagnosis and assessment of chronic liver disease progression, treatment, and complications. At the present time, it is known that the worldwide morbidity and mortality rates for chronic liver disease and cirrhosis are increasing. The main causes of chronic liver disease are alcohol, viral hepatitis B and C, metabolic dysfunction-associated fatty liver disease (MAFLD), and autoimmune and cholestatic liver disease. In spite of the fact that MAFLD has been considered mainly a problem in Western countries, several studies have reported a growing prevalence of MAFLD in Asia. The increasing prevalence of MAFLD in Asian countries is associated with the growing trend of obesity in this geographical area, which is why it has been reported that the current prevalence of MAFLD in Asia approaches the worldwide MAFLD prevalence of 25% to 30%. Thus, hepatitis B virus and MAFLD are currently the main causes of liver cirrhosis in eastern countries.

Regarding the pathophysiology of liver cirrhosis, initial fibrosis results from chronic damage to the liver in conjunction with the accumulation of extracellular matrix proteins, which is a characteristic of most types of chronic liver diseases.

These alterations in turn distort the hepatic architecture by forming a fibrous scar, with the subsequent development of nodules of regenerating hepatocytes defining cirrhosis. Patients with cirrhosis who experience hepatic decompensation, such as with the development of portal hypertension, ascites, hepatic encephalopathy, portal vein thrombosis, hepatorenal syndrome, and spontaneous bacterial peritonitis are at higher mortality risk. Management should be focused on the prevention of the recurrence of complications, some of which now can be treated specifically.

The Pharmacotherapy for Liver Cirrhosis and Its Complications, edited by Dr. Xingshun Qi, a very recognized young hepatologist, includes 14 chapters written by an international group of experts from seven countries such as China, United States, Argentina, India, Thailand, Austria, and Canada.

This book aims to bring to the readers' attention the latest advances in pharmacotherapy for liver cirrhosis and its complications. The book offers a variety of topics in the field of hepatology such as the use of antiviral drugs for HBV and HCV, anticoagulants, antibiotics, ursodeoxycholic acid, the use of human serum albumin infusion, non-selective beta-blockers, somatostatin and octreotide, terlipressin, diuretics, statins, L-Ornithine L-Aspartate, and lactulose. Each chapter is structured in a clear and comprehensive fashion, in conjunction with the description of practical applications. Undoubtedly, the editor and authors must be congratulated for their far-reaching efforts.

Faculty of Medicine
National Autonomous University of Mexico
Mexico City, Mexico

Nahum Méndez-Sánchez

Preface

Liver cirrhosis, end stage of chronic liver diseases, is one of the leading causes of death worldwide, primarily due to its secondary severe complications, including ascites, acute variceal bleeding, portal vein thrombosis, hepatic encephalopathy, and liver and renal failure. Currently, liver transplantation remains the sole curative treatment option for liver cirrhosis. Besides, the efficacy and safety of "new" drugs for the prevention and treatment of liver cirrhosis related complications have been widely explored, and meanwhile, the indications of "old" drugs are further confirmed and even expanded. Undoubtedly, such advances are potentially effective for the improvement of patients' outcomes. For this reason, Prof. Yongping Yang and I decided to launch this book project to summarize the current status regarding pharmacotherapy for liver cirrhosis and its complications. Finally, a panel of famous experts, who are very skilled at the management of liver cirrhosis and have published high-impact papers related to this topic, have been invited to write a total of 14 chapters regarding etiological treatment of hepatitis B and C infection and cholestasis related liver cirrhosis, prevention and treatment of major liver cirrhosis related complications, and some promising drugs for the improvement of survival of patients with liver cirrhosis.

Shenyang, China
March 18, 2022

Xingshun Qi

Acknowledgement

In the contemporary era, emerging medical knowledge can be rapidly disseminated, which is very helpful for physicians to effectively prevent and treat various diseases and for patients to understand them. Such a great benefit is contributed to a certain extent by the development of publishers. Therefore, I should appreciate this valuable opportunity provided by the Springer Nature publisher for launching and finalizing this current book project. Notably, Miss Joyce Zhou, who is an in-house editor of the Springer, and Mr. Kumar Athiappan, who is a coordinator of the book project, have given me lots of guidance and assistance in the book preparation.

A book cannot be finished without great efforts of authors. It should be acknowledged that all chapter authors have made their contributions to this book project. Notably, some authors have revised their chapters for many times to achieve the publication level, despite their heavy engagement in clinical practice and academic research.

Finally, as I have acknowledged in my first three Springer Nature books, I must be thankful for the life-long support of my wife, Jun Liu, and my family.

Xingshun Qi

Contents

Anti-HBV Drugs in Liver Cirrhosis

1

Qing-Lei Zeng

Abstract

Cirrhosis is one of the severe consequences of chronic hepatitis B, and it is more likely to progress to decompensated form and hepatocellular carcinoma without antiviral treatment. Currently, the preferred first-line antiviral agents for compensated cirrhosis include peginterferon α, entecavir, tenofovir disoproxil fumarate, and tenofovir alafenamide. Notably, in patients with decompensated cirrhosis, peginterferon α is contraindicated due to its safety concerns, and tenofovir alafenamide is not officially recommended due to limited administration data. The oral antiviral treatment duration for compensated cirrhosis is indefinitely long-term, and lifelong antiviral treatment is recommended for all patients with decompensated cirrhosis. Recent studies have demonstrated that high rates of compensated cirrhosis can be regressed, and high rates of decompensated cirrhosis can be recompensated after long-term antiviral therapy, accompanying with the decreasing risk of liver transplantation and hepatocellular carcinoma.

Keywords

Compensated cirrhosis · Decompensated cirrhosis · Antiviral treatment Peginterferon α · Entecavir · Tenofovir disoproxil fumarate · Tenofovir alafenamide

Q.-L. Zeng (✉)
Department of Infectious Diseases and Hepatology, The First Affiliated Hospital of Zhengzhou University, Zhengzhou, Henan Province, China

X. Qi, Y. Yang (eds.), *Pharmacotherapy for Liver Cirrhosis and Its Complications*, https://doi.org/10.1007/978-981-19-2615-0_1

Table 1.1 Approved antiviral agents in adults with HBV-related cirrhosis

Drug	Dose in adults	C-cirrhosis	D-cirrhosis	Treatment duration	Potential side effects
Peg-IFN α[a]	α-2a 180 μg, α-2b 100 μg, weekly	Yes[b]	No	48 weeks	Flu-like symptoms, fatigue, mood disturbances, cytopenia, autoimmune disorders, anorexia, weight loss
ETV	0.5 mg daily[b]	Yes	Yes	Indefinite or lifelong	Lactic acidosis (D-cirrhosis only)
TDF	300 mg daily	Yes	Yes	Indefinite or lifelong	Nephropathy, Fanconi syndrome, osteomalacia
TAF	25 mg daily	Yes	Yes[c]	Indefinite or lifelong	Lactic acidosis

[a] Peg-IFN α can be used in patients with well-compensated cirrhosis. [b] Entecavir of 1.0 mg daily for decompensated cirrhosis. [c] Not officially approved but it is reasonable to be used. *C-cirrhosis* compensated cirrhosis; *D-cirrhosis* decompensated cirrhosis

Hepatitis B virus (HBV)-related cirrhosis is the severe stage of chronic hepatitis B (CHB) and has higher risk of developing hepatocellular carcinoma (HCC) than non-cirrhotic patients, although HBV can cause HCC even in patients who do not have cirrhosis. In general, cirrhosis can be divided into two forms, i.e., compensated and decompensated cirrhosis, and the latter is commonly characterized by the presence of one or more complications of ascites, bleeding from the esophageal and gastric varices, and hepatic encephalopathy. Antiviral treatment should be initiated in all patients with compensated cirrhosis with detectable HBV DNA and any alanine aminotransferase (ALT) level. Meanwhile, all hepatitis B surface antigen (HBsAg) positive patients with decompensated cirrhosis should be treated with nucleos(t)ide analogs (NA) with high barrier to resistance, irrespective of HBV DNA and ALT levels. Additionally, patients with decompensated cirrhosis should be treated in specialized liver units or inpatient departments to achieve the clinical recompensation. Encouragingly, more and more clinical studies demonstrated that HBV-related cirrhosis can be reversed or alleviated by long-term anti-HBV therapy, especially the Lancet "Regression of Cirrhosis Study" published online at the end of 2012 by Marcellin et al. [1]. Given that the current first-line antiviral agents are peginterferon α (Peg-IFN α), entecavir (ETV), tenofovir disoproxil fumarate (TDF), and tenofovir alafenamide (TAF) (Table 1.1) [2–4], this chapter mainly focuses on the role of these drugs for the treatment of HBV-related cirrhosis.

1.1 Anti-HBV Drugs in Compensated Cirrhosis

1.1.1 Pegylated-Interferon α

Peg-IFN α in regimens similar to those administered in CHB can be considered for the treatment of compensated cirrhosis, especially for patients who require short-term treatment and high probability of sustained off-therapy response, although adverse events like thrombocytopenia are more obvious and need more careful management. The standard treatment duration is 48 weeks, and the extension of the duration of peg-IFN α therapy beyond 48 weeks may be beneficial in selected patients, therefore, response-guided therapy can be considered for cirrhotic patients. Notably, the potential benefit from peg-IFN α treatment on the HCC incidence seems to be superior to that of NA therapy, especially in Asian patients [5], although HCC may still develop after sustained off-treatment responses based on peg-IFN α treatment, particularly in cirrhotic patients [3].

In a previous study, 70 advanced fibrotic (Ishak fibrosis score 4–6) CHB patients underwent peg-IFN α-2b; meanwhile, 169 patients without advanced fibrosis who received peg-IFN α-2b plus lamivudine combination therapy were the control group, with the treatment duration of 48 weeks; and the virologic response was defined as hepatitis e antigen (HBeAg) seroconversion plus HBV DNA < 10,000 copies/ml at week 78 [6]. It is found that the virological response occurred significantly more often in advanced fibrotic patients than in those without (25% vs. 12%, respectively; $P = 0.02$), thereinto, the HBeAg seroconversion rates were 36% and 29%, and the rates of HBV DNA < 10,000 copies/ml were 30% and 17%, respectively. Notably, improvement in liver fibrosis occurred more frequently in advanced fibrotic patients (66% vs. 26%, $P < 0.001$). The adverse events were observed equally as frequently in advanced fibrotic patients and those without, and thrombocytopenia occurred more often in advanced fibrotic patients than in those without ($P < 0.01$).

1.1.2 Entecavir

Given the potency and minimal risk of resistance, ETV is the preferred monotherapy for HBV-related compensated cirrhosis, and the treatment duration is indefinitely long-term or even lifelong [2–4]. The optimal effect is reversal of cirrhosis, and suboptimal outcome is the stabilization and prevention of progression to decompensated cirrhosis [7, 8], furthermore, long-term ETV treatment can decrease the risk of HCC to some extent. During ETV treatment, long-term monitoring of the HBV DNA, ALT, and HCC is warranted, because ETV cannot completely exclude the risk of exacerbation of hepatitis B and the risk of HCC. Additionally, recent studies found that the low-level viremia (LLV), which is defined as either persistent or intermittent episodes of <2000 IU/ml detectable HBV DNA during NA therapy, can be observed in long-term ETV-treated patients, including patients with fibrosis and cirrhosis, which may lead to poor outcomes like progression to cirrhosis or even HCC [9, 10]. Therefore, the carefully long-term monitoring is applicable and helpful for the early detection of LLV and subsequent adjustment of treatment regimens in cirrhotic patients.

An important but small study included 57 ETV-treated patients who had adequate baseline liver biopsy samples as well as adequate long-term liver biopsy samples [7]. The median time of ETV treatment was 280 weeks. Thereinto, 10 of the 57 patients had advanced fibrosis or cirrhosis (Ishak score > 4) at the baseline. With long-term ETV treatment, all ten patients demonstrated at least a 1-point improvement or reduction in the Ishak fibrosis score with a median reduction from the baseline of 1.5 points. Notably, four of the ten patients had cirrhosis at the baseline (Ishak fibrosis score > 5), and all the four patients demonstrated an improvement in the Ishak fibrosis score with a median drop of 3 points, which indicated the reversal of the cirrhosis after the long-term ETV treatment.

1.1.3 Tenofovir Disoproxil Fumarate

Given the potency and no resistance, TDF is also the preferred monotherapy for HBV-related compensated cirrhosis, and the treatment duration is indefinitely long-term or even lifelong [2–4]. For the effectiveness, TDF is comparable with or even better than ETV because of the 0% resistance to date. However, patients with the following three conditions were not to be recommended for the TDF regimen, i.e., (1) aged more than 60 years, (2) bone disease, and (3) renal alteration [3]. Additionally, long-term monitoring of the HBV DNA, ALT, HCC, kidney impairment, and bone toxicity is also warranted during treatment.

Just because of the TDF, hepatologists widely learned that cirrhosis can be reversed after long-term antiviral therapy. In December 2012, the groundbreaking findings were presented by Prof. Marcellin et al. in the Lancet [1]. This study enrolled CHB patients receiving TDF treatment for 5 years, and liver biopsies were performed at baseline, 1 year, and 5 years of treatment. Thereinto, 96 patients with HBV-related cirrhosis (Ishak score 5 or 6) at baseline, notably and encouragingly, 71 (74%) of them no longer had cirrhosis (≥1 unit decrease in score) after 5 years of TDF treatment. In this relatively large study, the liver biopsy-proved regression of cirrhosis changed our knowledge of "cirrhosis is irreversible" and opened up a new field for future research.

Cirrhosis is an independent risk factor of HCC development. Currently, ETV and TDF are equally recommended as the first-line therapy for treatment-naïve CHB patients. However, Choi et al. showed a better HCC chemoprevention effect of TDF over ETV in a Korean nationwide historical population cohort of 24,156 patients and a validation hospital cohort of 2701 patients [11, 12]. Meanwhile, a similar conclusion was found in a Hong Kong cohort [13]. However, another multicenter study, also from South Korea, had a different conclusion [14], and a recent study with a relatively small sample size also supports the "no differences of ETV and TDF for HCC development" conclusion [15]. Therefore, the final conclusion is confusing to date.

1.1.4 Tenofovir Alafenamide

TAF is newly preferred monotherapy for HBV-related compensated cirrhosis, and the treatment duration is indefinitely long-term or even lifelong. As updated version of TDF, TAF is a unique nucleotide analog that inhibits reverse transcription of pregenomic RNA to HBV DNA [4]. TAF is more stable than TDF in plasma and delivers the active metabolite to hepatocytes more efficiently, allowing a lower dose to be used with similar antiviral activity, less systemic exposure, and thus decreased renal and bone toxicity [4]. Because of similar efficacy, no resistance, and lower renal and bone toxicity compared with TDF, TAF is probably the successor of TDF in the future [16–18]. However, TAF is not recommended in patients with estimated glomerular filtration rate (eGFR) < 15 mL/min/1.73m^2 or those on dialysis [4], but notably, the latest drug instructions indicate that dialysis patients with eGFR <15 mL/min/1.73m^2 do not need to adjust the dosage, i.e., 25 mg per day.

The GS-US-320-0108 and GS-US-320-0110 studies are randomized, double-blind, international phase III trials designed to compare the efficacy and safety of TAF with that of TDF in patients with CHB including 65 (about 10% of 636 cases with known the cirrhosis status) cases with known compensated cirrhosis in TAF group [19–21]. After 48 weeks of treatment, TAF was shown in both studies to be statistically non-inferior to TDF in antiviral efficacy, as measured by rates of HBV DNA < 29 IU/ml [19, 20]. Moreover, patients receiving TAF in both trials had significantly smaller decreases in bone mineral density, smaller increases in serum creatinine, as well as other biomarkers of bone and renal safety than TDF. At 96 weeks of treatment, TAF continues to be as effective as TDF with continued improved renal and bone safety profiles [21]. In addition, a recent study, including 32 (about 14% of 233 cases with known the cirrhosis status) compensated cirrhotic patients switched from TDF to TAF therapy for 48 weeks, showed favorable safety and efficacy profiles after switchover, which suggests that TAF can be substituted for TDF for improved safety without a loss of the efficacy [17].

Notably, in a retrospective study, 285 and 285 matched CHB patients treated with TAF and TDF were enrolled, 96 (34%) and 94 (33%) of those were compensated cirrhosis, and the risk of HCC development was not significantly different between TDF and TAF groups of CHB patients after a median follow-up duration of 45.2 months (interquartile range 26.8–62.4) and 27.9 months (interquartile range 21.8–52.4), respectively [22]. Meanwhile, other studies indicated that ETV, TDF, and TAF are similarly safe and effective antiviral agents for cirrhosis-related complications and annual HCC incidence rates [15, 23].

1.2 Anti-HBV Drugs in Decompensated Cirrhosis

1.2.1 Pegylated-Interferon α

The risk of hepatic decompensation in patients with HBV-related compensated cirrhosis is around 3–5% annually. In general, a Child–Turcotte–Pugh (CTP) score of equal to or more than 7 is considered as liver decompensation, and the 2015 guideline by Asian Pacific Association for the Study of the Liver defined liver decompensation as a serum bilirubin >2.5 times the upper limit of normal and prothrombin time by more than 3 seconds (or international normalized ratio > 1.5) or occurrence of complications related to decompensation, such as ascites or hepatic encephalopathy [2]. In this setting, the peg-IFN α is contraindicated in those patients with decompensated cirrhosis because of the poor tolerance and safety concerns [2–4].

1.2.2 Entecavir

HBV-related decompensated cirrhosis should be treated in inpatients department or unit of liver diseases, and liver transplantation can be considered by the patients and their family. Meanwhile, NA with high barrier to resistance should be initiated immediately, including first-line antiviral agent, the ETV. The licensed ETV dose for patients with decompensated cirrhosis is 1 mg (instead of 0.5 mg for patients with compensated cirrhosis) once daily [2–4]. The treatment duration was indefinite, commonly, lifelong treatment is recommended. The main goal of NA treatment in patients with decompensated liver disease is to achieve clinical recompensation and to avoid liver transplantation, although other symptomatic therapies are also needed to work together to realize this goal in this setting [2–4]. Lactic acidosis has been reported in advanced decompensated cirrhotic patients treated with NA, particularly ETV, however, it is rarely reported among Asian patients with decompensated cirrhosis [2, 24]. Although it is likely to be a rare event, clinical vigilance must be adopted for this potentially fatal complication. Meanwhile, it is important to note that even the decompensated cirrhotic patients under effective NA therapy, the risk of developing HCC is still high in these patients, and therefore careful long-term HCC surveillance is mandatory [2–4, 25].

A previous large study indicated that ETV (0.5 mg daily) treatment for 12 months were well tolerated and resulted in improved CTP and model for end-stage liver disease (MELD) scores, and the cumulative transplantation-free survival was 87.1% at 1 year [24]. Meanwhile, the 1-year cumulative rates of HBV DNA negativity (<51 copies/ml) and HBeAg loss were 92.3% and 54.0%, respectively [24]. In another study including 22 HBV-related decompensated cirrhosis treated with ETV for 48 weeks, it is found that ETV was well tolerated during treatment, and tolerability failure was infrequent and occurred in only 9.1% of patients [26]. The adverse event and laboratory profiles were consistent with advanced liver disease, with no unexpected safety signals. At week 48, HBV DNA < 400 copies/ml (69 IU/ml) was obtained in 72.7% of patients, and the ALT normalization occurred in 55% of patients, however, no one achieved HBeAg loss or seroconversion. In addition, the CTP and MELD scores improved during treatment.

1.2.3 Tenofovir Disoproxil Fumarate

TDF is another first-line antiviral agent recommended by guidelines for patients with HBV-related decompensated cirrhosis [2–4]. The indication, safety, efficacy, and treatment duration are similar to ETV in decompensated cirrhotic patients. Although TDF has more favorable efficacy than ETV, the close monitoring of potential adverse events, such as kidney and bone toxicities, lactic acidosis, and HCC development, in decompensated cirrhosis treated with TDF are still needed.

In a previous study including 45 HBV-related decompensated cirrhosis treated with TDF for 48 weeks, it is found that TDF was well tolerated during treatment, and tolerability failure was infrequent and occurred in only 6.7% of patients [26]. At week 48, HBV DNA < 400 copies/ml (69 IU/ml) was observed in 70.5% of patients, the normal ALT proportion was 57%, and HBeAg loss or seroconversion was obtained in 21% of patients. Furthermore, the CTP and MELD scores improved during treatment. In a prospective study of 57 patients with decompensated cirrhosis treated with TDF for 12 months, TDF was effective for decreasing HBV DNA levels and improving hepatic function with relatively lower complete virological response (HBV DNA < 116 copies/ml) than in compensated cirrhosis, and 49% of those improved their CTP score by 2 points [27]. In another retrospective study including 52 patients with decompensated cirrhosis, 20 and 32 of those were treated with TDF and ETV, respectively, and the results showed similar renal safety of TDF to that of ETV over a 2-year period [28].

1.2.4 Tenofovir Alafenamide

Data on TAF for the treatment of decompensated cirrhosis are limited, but the use of TAF would be reasonable in patients, when TDF adverse effects are a concern and ETV is not an option, especially if patients have comorbidities of renal dysfunction and/or bone disease. The 2018 Indian National Association for Study of the Liver (INASL) guidelines strongly recommend lifelong NA therapy (including TAF) with high barrier to resistance in patients with decompensated cirrhosis, irrespective of HBV replication [29, 30]. It is well known that TAF is potentially the safest anti-HBV drug to date, however, severe lactic acidosis due to acute intoxication by TAF and emtricitabine has been reported [31]. Therefore, the close monitoring of potential adverse events, including lactic acidosis and HCC development, in decompensated cirrhosis treated with TAF is also required.

In a small study concerning TAF to treat the HBV-related acute on chronic liver failure (ACLF) for 48 weeks, 7 of 10 patients were decompensated cirrhosis during treatment [32]. The TAF showed favorable safety and effectiveness in short-term and long-term treatment of HBV-ACLF. At 48 weeks of treatment, 8 (80%) patients in TAF group, 6 (60%) patients in TDF group, and 17 (85%) patients in ETV group survived without liver transplantation ($P = 0.251$). Another Chinese study included 23 HBV-ACLF patients who underwent TAF treatment for 48 weeks, thereinto, 9 of 14 patients had known cirrhosis before the TAF initiation, and some patients experienced episodes of decompensation during treatment [33]. At 48 weeks of treatment, the HBV DNA undetectable rates in TAF group (80%) were comparable with TDF group (75%). Compared with the TDF group, TAF group had a greater decrease in serum creatinine and an increase in eGFR at week 12 of treatment. In addition, a total of 13 patients survived at 48 weeks of treatment, the survival rates in TAF group were comparable with TDF group during treatment.

1.3 Conclusions

Numerous studies and clinical practice have demonstrated that HBV-associated cirrhosis can be reversed by long-term oral antiviral therapy. To date, TAF is not officially approved for treatment of decompensated cirrhosis, but the usage is reasonable. Considering the excellent safety profiles and favorable efficacy/effectiveness with no resistance, TAF may be "the first-line of the first-line oral antiviral agents" for patients with CHB as well as compensated and decompensated cirrhosis in the future. Meanwhile, peg-IFN α can be used in well-compensated HBV-related cirrhosis, but is contraindicated for decompensated cirrhosis. Notably, both oral anti-HBV agents and peg-IFN α can decrease the risk of HCC, however, close monitoring of HCC development and side effects are still warranted during any type of antiviral treatment.

References

1. Marcellin P, Gane E, Buti M, Afdhal N, Sievert W, Jacobson IM, et al. Regression of cirrhosis during treatment with tenofovir disoproxil fumarate for chronic hepatitis B: a 5-year open-label follow-up study. Lancet. 2013;381:468–75.
2. Sarin SK, Kumar M, Lau GK, Abbas Z, Chan HL, Chen CJ, et al. Asian-Pacific clinical practice guidelines on the management of hepatitis B: a 2015 update. Hepatol Int. 2016;10:1–98.
3. Lampertico P, Agarwal K, Berg T, Buti M, Janssen HLA, Papatheodoridis G, et al. EASL 2017 clinical practice guidelines on the management of hepatitis B virus infection. J Hepatol. 2017;67:370–98.
4. Terrault NA, Lok ASF, McMahon BJ, Chang KM, Hwang JP, Jonas MM, et al. Update on prevention, diagnosis, and treatment of chronic hepatitis B: AASLD 2018 hepatitis B guidance. Hepatology. 2018;67:1560–99.
5. Liang KH, Hsu CW, Chang ML, Chen YC, Lai MW, Yeh CT. Peginterferon is superior to Nucleos(t)ide analogues for prevention of hepatocellular carcinoma in chronic hepatitis B. J Infect Dis. 2016;213:966–74.
6. Buster EH, Hansen BE, Buti M, Delwaide J, Niederau C, Michielsen PP, et al. Peginterferon alpha-2b is safe and effective in HBeAg-positive chronic hepatitis B patients with advanced fibrosis. Hepatology. 2007;46:388–94.
7. Chang TT, Liaw YF, Wu SS, Schiff E, Han KH, Lai CL, et al. Long-term entecavir therapy results in the reversal of fibrosis/cirrhosis and continued histological improvement in patients with chronic hepatitis B. Hepatology. 2010;52:886–93.
8. Schiff ER, Lee SS, Chao YC, Kew Yoon S, Bessone F, Wu SS, et al. Long-term treatment with entecavir induces reversal of advanced fibrosis or cirrhosis in patients with chronic hepatitis B. Clin Gastroenterol Hepatol. 2011;9:274–6.
9. Kim JH, Sinn DH, Kang W, Gwak GY, Paik YH, Choi MS, et al. Low-level viremia and the increased risk of hepatocellular carcinoma in patients receiving entecavir treatment. Hepatology. 2017;66:335–43.
10. Sun Y, Wu X, Zhou J, Meng T, Wang B, Chen S, et al. Persistent low level of hepatitis. B virus promotes fibrosis progression during therapy. Clin Gastroenterol Hepatol. 2020;18:2582–91. e6
11. Choi J, Kim HJ, Lee J, Cho S, Ko MJ, Lim YS. Risk of hepatocellular carcinoma in patients treated with Entecavir vs Tenofovir for chronic hepatitis B: a Korean Nationwide cohort study. JAMA Oncol. 2019;5:30–6.

12. Yip TC, Lai JC, Wong GL. Secondary prevention for hepatocellular carcinoma in patients with chronic hepatitis B: are all the nucleos(t)ide analogues the same? J Gastroenterol. 2020;55:1023–36.
13. Yip TC, Wong VW. Chan HL, Tse YK, Lui GC, Wong GL. Tenofovir is associated with lower risk of hepatocellular carcinoma than Entecavir in patients with chronic HBV infection in China. Gastroenterology. 2020;158:215–25 e6.
14. Kim SU, Seo YS, Lee HA, Kim MN, Lee YR, Lee HW, et al. A multicenter study of entecavir vs. tenofovir on prognosis of treatment-naive chronic hepatitis B in South Korea. J Hepatol. 2019;71:456–64.
15. Jeong S, Shin HP, Kim HI. Real-world single-center comparison of the safety and efficacy of Entecavir, Tenofovir Disoproxil fumarate, and Tenofovir Alafenamide in patients with chronic hepatitis B. Intervirology. 2021;1-10
16. Cathcart AL, Chan HL, Bhardwaj N, Liu Y, Marcellin P, Pan CQ, et al. No resistance to Tenofovir Alafenamide detected through 96 weeks of treatment in patients with chronic hepatitis B infection. Antimicrob Agents Chemother. 2018;62:e01064–18.
17. Lampertico P, Buti M, Fung S, Ahn SH, Chuang WL, Tak WY, et al. Switching from tenofovir disoproxil fumarate to tenofovir alafenamide in virologically suppressed patients with chronic hepatitis B: a randomised, double-blind, phase 3, multicentre non-inferiority study. Lancet Gastroenterol Hepatol. 2020;5:441–53.
18. Roade L, Loglio A, Borghi M, Riveiro-Barciela M, Soffredini R, Facchetti F, et al. Application of EASL 2017 criteria for switching hepatitis B patients from tenofovir disoproxil to entecavir or tenofovir alafenamide. Dig Liver Dis. 2020;52:1164–9.
19. Buti M, Gane E, Seto WK, Chan HL, Chuang WL, Stepanova T, et al. Tenofovir alafenamide versus tenofovir disoproxil fumarate for the treatment of patients with HBeAg-negative chronic hepatitis B virus infection: a randomised, double-blind, phase 3, non-inferiority trial. Lancet Gastroenterol Hepatol. 2016;1:196–206.
20. Chan HL, Fung S, Seto WK, Chuang WL, Chen CY, Kim HJ, et al. Tenofovir alafenamide versus tenofovir disoproxil fumarate for the treatment of HBeAg-positive chronic hepatitis B virus infection: a randomised, double-blind, phase 3, non-inferiority trial. Lancet Gastroenterol Hepatol. 2016;1:185–95.
21. Agarwal K, Brunetto M, Seto WK, Lim YS, Fung S, Marcellin P, et al. 96 weeks treatment of tenofovir alafenamide vs. tenofovir disoproxil fumarate for hepatitis B virus infection. J Hepatol. 2018;68:672–81.
22. Lee HW, Cho YY, Lee H, Lee JS, Kim SU, Park JY, et al. Effect of tenofovir alafenamide vs. tenofovir disoproxil fumarate on hepatocellular carcinoma risk in chronic hepatitis B. J Viral Hepat. 2021;28:1570–8.
23. Lee HW, Cho YY, Lee H, Lee JS, Kim SU, Park JY, et al. Impact of tenofovir alafenamide vs. entecavir on hepatocellular carcinoma risk in patients with chronic hepatitis B. Hepatol Int. 2021;15:1083–92.
24. Shim JH, Lee HC, Kim KM, Lim YS, Chung YH, Lee YS, et al. Efficacy of entecavir in treatment-naive patients with hepatitis B virus-related decompensated cirrhosis. J Hepatol. 2010;52:176–82.
25. Kim SS, Hwang JC, Lim SG, Ahn SJ, Cheong JY, Cho SW. Effect of virological response to entecavir on the development of hepatocellular carcinoma in hepatitis B viral cirrhotic patients: comparison between compensated and decompensated cirrhosis. Am J Gastroenterol. 2014;109:1223–33.
26. Liaw YF, Sheen IS, Lee CM, Akarca US, Papatheodoridis GV, Suet-Hing Wong F, et al. Tenofovir disoproxil fumarate (TDF), emtricitabine/TDF, and entecavir in patients with decompensated chronic hepatitis B liver disease. Hepatology. 2011;53:62–72.
27. Lee SK, Song MJ, Kim SH, Lee BS, Lee TH, Kang YW, et al. Safety and efficacy of tenofovir in chronic hepatitis B-related decompensated cirrhosis. World J Gastroenterol. 2017;23:2396–403.

28. Park J, Jung KS, Lee HW, Kim BK, Kim SU, Kim DY, et al. Effects of Entecavir and Tenofovir on renal function in patients with hepatitis B virus-related compensated and decompensated cirrhosis. Gut and liver. 2017;11:828–34.
29. Arora A, Anand AC, Kumar A, Singh SP, Aggarwal R, Dhiman RK, et al. INASL guidelines on Management of Hepatitis B Virus Infection in patients receiving chemotherapy, biologicals, Immunosuppressants, or corticosteroids. J Clin Exp Hepatol. 2018;8:403–31.
30. Charlton MR, Alam A, Shukla A, Dashtseren B, Lesmana CRA, Duger D, et al. An expert review on the use of tenofovir alafenamide for the treatment of chronic hepatitis B virus infection in Asia. J Gastroenterol. 2020;55:811–23.
31. Chaparala S, Da Silva RC, Papadopoulos JP. Severe lactic acidosis due to acute intoxication by Emtricitabine/Tenofovir Alafenamide. Cureus. 2021;13:e19008.
32. Li J, Hu C, Chen Y, Zhang R, Fu S, Zhou M, et al. Short-term and long-term safety and efficacy of tenofovir alafenamide, tenofovir disoproxil fumarate and entecavir treatment of acute-on-chronic liver failure associated with hepatitis B. BMC Infect Dis. 2021;21:567.
33. Zhang Y, Xu W, Zhu X, Li X, Li J, Shu X, et al. The 48-week safety and therapeutic effects of tenofovir alafenamide in hbv-related acute-on-chronic liver failure: a prospective cohort study. J Viral Hepat. 2021;28:592–600.

2 Antiviral Therapy for Hepatitis C Virus Infection in Cirrhosis

Yunyu Zhao, Xinyuan He, and Fanpu Ji

Abstract

The advent of direct-acting antivirals (DAAs) has made a cure for hepatitis C virus (HCV) a reality, while the WHO has set a goal of eliminating HCV worldwide by 2030. DAA-based interferon-free therapies for chronic hepatitis C are highly effective, achieving a more than 90% sustained virologic response (SVR) including patients with advanced chronic liver disease. Studies have demonstrated that elimination of HCV improves the prognosis of patients with cirrhosis, reduces the risk of liver decompensation, and reduces, but does not completely eliminate, the risk of hepatocellular carcinoma (HCC). Based on the current guidelines, this paper discussed the goal, indication, assessment before treatment, and endpoint of antiviral therapy for patients with cirrhosis and HCV infection. We also discussed the treatment for special population of patients with cirrhosis, including children and adolescents, patients with renal insufficiency, coinfection with human immunodeficiency virus or hepatitis B virus, or patients with HCC. Finally, the monitoring strategy of cirrhotic patients during DAA treatment and after SVR was presented.

Keywords

HCV · DAAs · DDIs · Cirrhosis · aCLD · HCC

Y. Zhao · X. He · F. Ji (✉)
Department of Infectious Diseases, The Second Affiliated Hospital of Xi'an Jiaotong University, Xi'an, China
e-mail: infection@xjtu.edu.cn

X. Qi, Y. Yang (eds.), *Pharmacotherapy for Liver Cirrhosis and Its Complications*, https://doi.org/10.1007/978-981-19-2615-0_2

Abbreviations

aCLD	advanced chronic liver disease
ALT	alanine aminotransferase
CKD	chronic kidney disease
DAA	direct-acting antiviral
DDI	drug–drug interaction
EBR	elbasvir
eGFR	glomerular filtration rate
GLE	glecaprevir
GT	genotype
GZR	grazoprevir
HCC	hepatocellular carcinoma
HCV	hepatitis C virus
IFN	interferon
MELD	model for end-stage disease
PIB	pibrentasvir
RAS	resistance associated substitution
RBV	ribavirin
SOF	sofosbuvir
SVR	sustained virological response
UNL	upper normal limit
VEL	velpatasvir
VOX	voxilaprevir

The advent of new direct-acting antivirals (DAAs) has revolutionized the treatment of patients with hepatitis C virus (HCV) infection in recent years, making a cure for HCV infection a reality [1]. Before the era of DAAs, pegylated-interferon (IFN) combined with ribavirin was the standard of care for HCV infection; unfortunately, this therapy not only required a long treatment cycle but also triggered many adverse reactions, including but not limited to influenza-like symptoms, bone marrow suppression, neurological and psychiatric symptoms, and the possible induction of autoimmune diseases. For advanced chronic liver diseases (aCLDs), including compensated or decompensated cirrhosis, when splenomegaly and hypersplenism occur, IFN-based therapy can further aggravate the related hemocytopenia, leading to interruption of the treatment, ultimately hindering HCV elimination, and allowing progression of the aCLD [2, 3]. Compared with IFN-based treatment, IFN-free DAA treatments are well tolerated, effectively overcome the abovementioned disadvantages, and greatly improve patient compliance. They also result in high cure rates of more than 94% for different genotypes (GTs) of HCV in patients suffering from different stages of liver disease [1, 4].

2.1 Indication, Goal, and Endpoint of HCV Therapy for Patients with Cirrhosis

For cirrhotic patients with HCV infection, including compensated (Child–Pugh grade A) and decompensated (Child–Pugh grade B or C) cirrhosis, the liver fibrotic condition should be treated without delay; the key exception is patients with limited life expectancy, because of non-liver-related comorbidities. The paramount goal of antiviral therapy is to eliminate the HCV itself, which will eliminate or alleviate HCV-related liver damage and extrahepatic manifestations, prevent progression to decompensated cirrhosis, liver failure or hepatocellular carcinoma (HCC), improve long-term survival and quality of life, and prevent transmission of the virus. The elimination of HCV in patients with cirrhosis can also reduce the risk of liver decompensation as well as occurrence of HCC, although the latter may not be completely avoided [5, 6]. Antiviral therapy before a liver transplantation can improve liver function, resulting in removal of some patients from the wait list, and prevent reinfection after the transplantation; antiviral therapy administered after the transplantation can improve survival rate [7, 8].

Treatment endpoints are defined as undetectable serum or plasma HCV RNA at 12 or 24 weeks after the end of treatment, using a sensitive test (detection limit ≤15 IU/mL), yielding a sustained virological response (SVR), known as SVR12 or SVR24. Failure to detect HCV core antigen at 12 or 24 weeks after completion of treatment can be used as an alternative treatment endpoint for patients who were classified as HCV core antigen-positive prior to treatment.

2.2 Assessment before DAA Treatment

Quantitative detection of HCV RNA in serum or plasma is preferably performed with a sensitive detection method. If the high-sensitivity HCV RNA test is not feasible at the time, a non-high-sensitivity HCV RNA test can be used; however, upon a result of undetectable HCV RNA, a subsequent confirmation by the high-sensitivity method is recommended [5].

The severity of liver disease should be evaluated before beginning any antiviral therapy in patients with cirrhosis. In those with decompensated cirrhosis or previous episodes of decompensation, regimens containing NS3/4A protease inhibitors, such as grazoprevir (GZR), glecaprevir (GLE), and voxilaprevir (VOX), are not recommended.

Markers of renal function, including creatinine level and glomerular filtration rate (eGFR), should also be assessed before treatment initiation. For patients with a chronic kidney disease (CKD) and showing an eGFR of less than 30 mL/min/1.73m^2, the use of a treatment regimen containing sofosbuvir (SOF) should be avoided; meanwhile, for patients with decompensated cirrhosis and severe CKD, a regimen containing SOF should be applied with caution [6].

The cure rate of pan-GT DAA regimens is high. Another advantage is that DAAs may be initiated without knowledge of the virus GT or subtype. Identification of HCV GTs and subtypes can help identify patients who will benefit most from individualized treatment, and it will also help to determine an optimal monitoring program after SVR is achieved.

Presence of hepatitis B surface antigen (HBsAg) and anti-human immunodeficiency virus (HIV) should be tested before DAA treatment to exclude the complicating factor of coinfection with the hepatitis B virus (HBV) or HIV. Comorbidities, including HCV extrahepatic manifestations and concurrent intake of other medications, should also be evaluated before treatment—for the latter, performing a focused evaluation on the potential drug–drug interactions (DDIs) that may occur with the DAAs (www.hepdruginteractions.org will be regularly updated with recommendations). It is important to note that all DAA regimens are contraindicated when specific cytochrome enzyme P450/P glycoprotein inducers (e.g., carbamazepine, phenytoin, and phenobarbital) will not be converted to other drug substitutes, as these drugs are known to significantly reduce the plasma concentration of DAAs.

2.3 DAAs Classification

DAAs are small molecule drugs, whose main targets (at present) are the viral nonstructural proteins of NS3/4A, NS5A, and NS5B. The NS3/4A serine protease participates in the cleavage and shearing of HCV virus polypeptide chains, at multiple sites. NS5B encodes RNA polymerase during HCV replication, and the NS5A complex protein plays an important role in viral replication and assembly. DAAs play an antiviral role by inhibiting these important viral proteins during the HCV life cycle, thereby blocking the intrahepatic replication at various stages. Table 2.1 provides an overview of DAAs currently approved for use as HCV therapeutics in Europe.

Table 2.1 HCV DAAs approved for clinical use in Europe [5]

Category	Medicine	Specification	Dosage
Pan-genotypic			
NS5B nucleoside polymerase inhibitors	SOF	400 mg	One tablet once daily
NS5B nucleoside polymerase inhibitors/NS5A inhibitors	SOF/VEL	400 mg SOF/100 mg VEL	One tablet once daily
NS3/4A protease inhibitor/NS5A inhibitors	GLE/PIB	100 mg GLE/40 mg PIB	Three tablets once daily with food
NS5B nucleoside polymerase inhibitors/NS5A inhibitors/NS3/4A protease inhibitors	SOF/VEL/VOX	400 mg SOF/100 mg VEL/100 mg VOX	One tablet once daily with food
GT-specific			
NS5A inhibitors/NS3/4A protease inhibitor	EBR/GZR	50 mg EBR/100 mg GZR	One tablet once daily

2.4 Treatment of Patients with Compensated Cirrhosis

Pan-genotypic DAAs are recommended for patients with compensated cirrhosis due to their well-demonstrated effectiveness, safety, tolerability, and simple application; they are indicated for both treatment-naive and treatment-experienced patients (Table 2.2).

2.4.1 SOF/Velpatasvir (VEL)

SOF/VEL is a first-line treatment for patients with chronic HCV infection. In a clinical trial involving an Asian population of patients with HCV GT1–6 and non-cirrhotic or compensated cirrhosis, SOF/VEL treatment for 12 weeks yielded a 97% rate of SVR12. Among the 42 patients infected with GT3b, in particular, the SVR12 rates were 89% in the non-cirrhotic patients and 50% in the compensated cirrhosis patients [9]. In another study, administration of SOF/VEL plus ribavirin (RBV) at 900–1200 mg for 12 weeks as treatment for GT3 cirrhosis and for any GT decompensated cirrhosis achieved 100% SVR12 (among 74 cirrhosis patients); headache, fatigue, and nausea were the most commonly reported adverse events [10].

2.4.2 GLE/Pibrentasvir (PIB)

In a phase 3 clinical trial involving an Asian population of patients with GT1–6 compensated cirrhosis, treatment with GLE/PIB (for 12 weeks, or 16 weeks in treatment-experienced patients with GT3a) yielded an SVR12 rate of 99.4% [11]. In

Table 2.2 GT-based DAA treatment recommendations for patients with compensated HCV cirrhosis [5]

GT	Treatment experience	SOF/VEL	GLE/PIB	SOF/VEL/VOX	EBR/GZR
GT 1a	Naive	12 weeks	8 weeks	NR	NR
	Experienced	12 weeks	12 weeks	NR	NR
GT 1b	Naive	12 weeks	8 weeks	NR	12 weeks
	Experienced	12 weeks	12 weeks	NR	12 weeks
GT 2	Naive	12 weeks	8 weeks	NR	NR
	Experienced	12 weeks	12 weeks	NR	NR
GT 3	Naive	12 weeks + RBV	12 weeks	12 weeks	NR
	Experienced	12 weeks + RBV	16 weeks	12 weeks	NR
GT 4	Naive	12 weeks	8 weeks	NR	NR
	Experienced	12 weeks	12 weeks	NR	NR
GT 5	Naive	12 weeks	8 weeks	NR	NR
	Experienced	12 weeks	12 weeks	NR	NR
GT 6	Naive	12 weeks	8 weeks	NR	NR
	Experienced	12 weeks	12 weeks	NR	NR

NR not recommended

another clinical trial, 8 weeks of the GLE/PIB regimen in treatment-naive compensated cirrhosis patients with GT1–6 achieved SVR12 rates of 97.7%–99.7%; the treatment was generally well tolerated and common adverse reactions were fatigue, pruritus, headache, and nausea [12]. Considering the relatively high risk of treatment failure in GT3 patients, the European Association for the Study of the Liver (EASL) guideline recommended 12 weeks of the GLE/PIB regimen for treatment-naive GT3 patients with compensated cirrhosis, and extended this to 16 weeks for treatment-experienced patients with compensated cirrhosis. Therefore, GT testing is recommended to identify GT3 in areas where the GT3 prevalence exceeds 5% [5].

2.4.3 SOF/VEL/VOX

The SOF/VEL/VOX DAAs combination is a pan-GT regimen designed to re-treat patients who have failed DAA treatment. In a phase 3 clinical trial, the SOF/VEL/VOX combination was applied for 12 weeks in patients who had failed an NS5A inhibitor regimen, and the overall SVR12 was 93% for the compensated cirrhosis patients [13]. In a UK cohort study including 38% GT3 patients and 10% HCC patients, the SVR12 achieved by 12 weeks of SOF/VEL/VOX in cirrhosis patients who had previously failed DAA therapies was 81%, with GT3 infection, baseline cirrhosis, and prior use of SOF/VEL identified as patient factors significantly associated with risk of re-treatment failure; moreover, the most common adverse events were headache, fatigue, diarrhea, and nausea, but the rate of treatment discontinuation owing to adverse events was 1% or lower [14].

2.4.4 Elbasvir (EBR)/GZR

In a multicenter clinical study, a 12-week regimen of EBR/GZR achieved SVR12 rates of 92%, 99%, 100%, and 80% in patients infected with GT1a, GT1b, GT4, and GT6, respectively, reaching as high as 97% in HCV-infected patients (all GTs) with compensated cirrhosis. In general, the EBR/GZR treatment was well tolerated, with the most common adverse events being headache, fatigue, and nausea [15].

2.5 Treatment of Patients with Decompensated Cirrhosis

Patients with decompensated cirrhosis should receive antiviral therapy at a treatment center with appreciable experience in such; all patients should remain under close monitoring during the treatment period, with discontinuation occurring upon worsening of the decompensation. NS3/4A protease inhibitors and IFN should not be used in patients with decompensated cirrhosis or those with current compensated cirrhosis but history of prior decompensation episodes. These patients should be treated with a 12-week regimen of SOF/VEL in combination with RBV (1000 mg/d for body weight < 75 kg and 1200 mg/d for ≥75 kg); the RBV can be started at a dose of 600 mg/d and then gradually adjusted, according to tolerance. If RBV is contraindicated or is found to be intolerable, an RBV-free SOF/VEL 24-week regimen should be used [5].

In a clinical trial, patients with GT1–6 decompensated cirrhosis received either SOF/VEL for 12 weeks, SOF/VEL + RBV for 12 weeks, or SOF/VEL for 24 weeks, yielding SVR12 rates of 83%, 94%, and 86%, respectively [16]. As is typical, the most common adverse reactions were fatigue, nausea, and headache; however, anemia was the most common adverse reaction in the patients who received the RBV combination treatment. In a real-world study that had used old DAA regimens, SVR12 was achieved in 329 out of 406 patients (81.0%) and generally led to prolonged improvement in liver function [17]. A recent study showed that DAA-induced SVR was not associated with a reduced risk of clinical disease progression in patients with Child–Pugh B/C cirrhosis, and a more than 2-point decline in model for end-stage disease (MELD) score after treatment did not translate into improved clinical outcome [18].

Patients with decompensated cirrhosis who are not on the liver transplant wait list and have no life-threatening complications should be treated as soon as possible. Patients with decompensated cirrhosis, no HCC, waiting for liver transplantation and with a MELD score of less than 18–20 points should receive antiviral treatment (i.e., DAAs) before transplantation; however, if their MELD score is more than 18–20 points, the transplantation should be performed first, with antiviral therapy following [5].

2.6 Treatment and Management of Special Population of Patients with Cirrhosis

2.6.1 Children or Adolescents

Although cirrhosis is rare in children or adolescents, individuals with thalassemia, iron overload, HIV coinfection, or hematological or solid tumors who are receiving chemotherapy may develop advanced liver fibrosis or cirrhosis. Adolescent (12–17 years old) patients with compensated cirrhosis should be treated according to the general recommendations for adult patients (see Table 2.2). Child patients (3–11 years old) with compensated cirrhosis, regardless of prior treatment history, can be treated with fixed-dose (according to body weight) combinations of SOF and VEL or GLE and PIB, administered once daily for 12 weeks [5].

2.6.2 Patients with Renal Insufficiency

Compared to the general population, cirrhosis patients with HCV infection have a much higher rate of CKD. In addition, the rate of HCV antibody positivity is also significantly higher among patients with CKD. DAA treatment can allow patients with CKD complicated with HCV to achieve SVR, providing a remarkable clinical benefit. Therefore, it is generally considered that all patients with CKD combined with compensated or decompensated cirrhosis should receive antiviral therapy immediately.

NS3/4A protease inhibitors, NS5A inhibitors, and NS5B non-nucleoside polymerase inhibitors, most of which are mainly metabolized by the liver, can be used in patients with CKD. The main metabolite of the NS5B nucleoside polymerase inhibitor SOF is metabolized through the kidney. Therefore, for patients with compensated cirrhosis and mild-to-moderate renal insufficiency (eGFR of $\geq$30 mL/min/1.73m^2), the choice of DAA can be made by referring to the treatment regimen otherwise provided to the general population and without need for dose adjustment. In contrast, patients with severe renal dysfunction (eGFR of <30 mL/min/1.73m^2) and end-stage renal disease who have begun hemodialysis are advised to receive an RBV-free, SOF-free DAA regimen based upon their particular HCV GTs, such as GLE/PIB (for pan-GT), ELB/GZR (for GT1), etc. However, 12 weeks of treatment with SOF/VEL was safe and effective in dialysis patients with compensated cirrhosis and end-stage renal disease [19]. Patients with severe renal impairment (eGFR <30 mL/min/1.73m^2) and decompensated cirrhosis remain a challenge for application of DAA-based therapies, although the EASL guideline recommends a 24-week fixed-dose combination of SOF and VEL without RBV [5].

2.6.3 Coinfection with HIV or HBV

HCV patients coinfected with HIV should receive the same DAA treatment regimen as HCV single-infection patients, as it provides the same SVR rates to both groups. If the DAAs administered are predicted to interact with the patient's antiretrovirals, the treatment regimen(s) and dosage(s) need to be adjusted. The SOF/VEL/VOX combination is not recommended for use with the HIV drugs efavirenz, etravirine, and nevirapine, nor with the protease inhibitors atazanavir/ritonavir and lopinavir/ritonavir. Also, GLE/PIB is contraindicated by atazanavir-containing regimens and is not recommended with other HIV protease inhibitors.

Patients coinfected with HBV and compensated or decompensated cirrhosis who fulfill the standard criteria for HBV treatment should receive nucleoside/nucleotide analog treatment according to local guidelines for HBV infection. Patients with compensated cirrhosis who are HBsAg-positive but have undetectable HBV DNA should receive nucleoside/nucleotide analog prophylaxis, at least until week 12 after the anti-HCV therapy, with monthly monitoring being conducted if the HBV treatment is stopped. In patients that are HBsAg-negative but HBcAb-positive, serum alanine aminotransferase (ALT) levels should be monitored monthly to detect possible reactivation [5].

2.6.4 Patients with Cirrhosis and HCC

Real-world studies and meta-analyses have shown lower SVR rates to be achieved with IFN-free DAA treatments for HCV-related HCC, though the response occurred primarily among patients with active HCC—a finding that was recently confirmed in well-controlled studies [20–23]. The HCC tumor cells, serving as HCV reservoirs, and the tumor microenvironment, which interferes with drug distribution, can cause lower treatment response rates. Studies from both the East and West have also shown that DAA achievement of SVR is significantly associated with a more than 60% improvement in both overall and liver-related survivals [24, 25]. For early-stage HCC patients, HCC treatment should be considered prior to the initiation of any DAA therapy, whenever possible. Indeed, HCC patients who underwent liver transplantation achieved a higher SVR rate, but the optimal timing of HCV treatment for HCC patients awaiting liver transplantation will have to be individualized [20].

Limited data has been published for DAA treatment of HCV in patients with advanced HCC. On the one hand, given the safety records of DAAs and their wide availability with low-cost generics, it is reasonable to expand the application of DAA therapy to advanced HCC patients [26, 27]. On the other hand, the lack of evidence supporting the benefits of DAAs in advanced HCC means that DAA treatment should be determined on a case-by-case basis, and patients should be informed of the potential risks (in addition to the benefits) of this antiviral therapeutic approach [28].

2.7 Treatment Monitoring and Follow-Up

Patients should be monitored to track the DAAs' efficacy and safety throughout the treatment course. It is recommended to detect HCV RNA at baseline, at the 4th week of treatment, at the end of treatment, and at 12 or 24 weeks after treatment cessation.

Patients with cirrhosis receiving a DAA regimen should be evaluated at each visit for clinical adverse effects, along with monitoring of ALT, bilirubin and international normalized ratio levels at baseline and at the 4th, 12th, and 24th weeks of treatment or at any-symptom onset; this is especially important for patients with decompensated cirrhosis. For patients with reduced eGFR, renal function markers should be monitored monthly during SOF treatment. Markers of efficacy and potential DDIs, as well as safety, should be monitored during treatment. For patients receiving RBV therapy, if hemoglobin levels drop to 100 g/L, the RBV should be reduced in a 200-mg stepwise manner; if hemoglobin levels drop to 85 g/L, the RBV should be discontinued.

After achievement of SVR, HCC should be monitored by ultrasound every 6 months, because the risk of HCC occurrence or recurrence is reduced but not completely eliminated after SVR in patients with cirrhosis. Alcohol intake and hepatic decompensation are independent risk factors for HCC development, and baseline non-characterized nodules are associated with a 2.83-fold increased risk of HCC compared to patients without non-characterized nodules [29]. Fortunately, predictive models for HCC development in patients with compensated cirrhosis with or without non-characterized liver nodules show good predictive performance [30, 31]. A vigilant monitoring of HCC development in patients with compensated and decompensated cirrhosis should be mandatory after SVR, especially for patients stratified as a high-risk population.

2.8 Conclusions

Viral hepatitis and related mortality remain a serious global public burden, and continuous efforts are needed to achieve the goal of eliminating viral hepatitis by 2030. For patients with cirrhosis and HCV infection, DAA-based IFN-free therapies can achieve a high SVR rate with good safety and tolerability. The elimination of HCV can improve the prognosis of patients with cirrhosis and reduce the risk of liver decompensation and HCC. Therefore, patients with aCLD should receive anti-HCV treatment as early as possible. It is necessary to classify and identify the risk of developing HCC in this population, so as to develop individualized monitoring after SVR to achieve more optimized cost-effectiveness.

References

1. Carrat F, Fontaine H, Dorival C, et al. Clinical outcomes in patients with chronic hepatitis C after direct-acting antiviral treatment: a prospective cohort study. Lancet. 2019;393:1453–64.
2. Ji F, Dang S, Cai Z, Xue H, Huang N, Liu L, Zhang S, Guo Y, Jia X, Wang Y, Li Z, Deng H. Antiviral treatment and long-term clinical outcome of decompensated cirrhotic patients with hepatitis C virus infection. Zhonghua Gan Zang Bing Za Zhi. 2015;23:647–52.
3. Ji F, Zhang S, Deng H, Li Z. Efficacy of interferon-based antiviral therapy on the risk of hepatocellular carcinoma of patients with chronic hepatitis C: further evidence in decompensation cirrhosis. J Hepatol. 2013;58:1262–4.
4. Ji F, Li J, Liu L, et al. High hepatitis C virus cure rates with approved interferon-free direct-acting antivirals among diverse mainland Chinese patients including genotypes 3a and 3b. J Gastroenterol Hepatol. 2021;36:767–74.
5. European Association for the Study of the Liver. EASL recommendations on treatment of hepatitis C: final update of the series. J Hepatol. 2020;73:1170–218.
6. Chinese Society of Hepatology; Chinese Society of Infectious Diseases, Chinese Medical Association. [Guidelines for the prevention and treatment of hepatitis C (2019 version)]. Zhonghua Gan Zang Bing Za Zhi. 2019;27:962–79.
7. Pascasio JM, Vinaixa C, Ferrer MT, et al. Clinical outcomes of patients undergoing antiviral therapy while awaiting liver transplantation. J Hepatol. 2017;67:1168–76.
8. Jung J, Kwon JH, Song GW, et al. Pre-emptive treatment of HCV after living donor liver transplantation with direct-acting antiviral agents. J Gastrointest Surg. 2018;22:1334–42.

9. Wei L, Lim SG, Xie Q, et al. Sofosbuvir-velpatasvir for treatment of chronic hepatitis C virus infection in Asia: a single-arm, open-label, phase 3 trial. Lancet Gastroenterol Hepatol. 2019;4:127–34.
10. Xu Q, Zhang W, Ma Y, et al. 12-week sofosbuvir/velpatasvir for patients with chronic hepatitis C in Northwest China, a real-world multicenter study. Zhonghua Gan Zang Bing Za Zhi. 2021;29:1046–52.
11. Wei L, Wang G, Alami NN, et al. Glecaprevir-pibrentasvir to treat chronic hepatitis C virus infection in Asia: two multicentre, phase 3 studies- a randomised, double-blind study (VOYAGE-1) and an open-label, single-arm study (VOYAGE-2). Lancet Gastroenterol Hepatol. 2020;5:839–49.
12. Brown RS Jr, Buti M, Rodrigues L, et al. Glecaprevir/pibrentasvir for 8 weeks in treatment-naïve patients with chronic HCV genotypes 1-6 and compensated cirrhosis: the EXPEDITION-8 trial. J Hepatol. 2020;72:441–9.
13. Bourlière M, Gordon SC, Flamm SL, et al. Sofosbuvir, Velpatasvir, and Voxilaprevir for previously treated HCV infection. N Engl J Med. 2017;376:2134–46.
14. Smith DA, Bradshaw D, Mbisa JL, et al. Real world SOF/VEL/VOX retreatment outcomes and viral resistance analysis for HCV patients with prior failure to DAA therapy. J Viral Hepat. 2021;28:1256–64.
15. Zeuzem S, Ghalib R, Reddy KR, et al. Grazoprevir-Elbasvir combination therapy for treatment-naive cirrhotic and noncirrhotic patients with chronic hepatitis C virus genotype 1, 4, or 6 infection: a randomized trial. Ann Intern Med. 2015;163:1–13.
16. Curry MP, O'Leary JG, Bzowej N, et al. Sofosbuvir and Velpatasvir for HCV in patients with decompensated cirrhosis. N Engl J Med. 2015;373:2618–28.
17. Cheung MCM, Walker AJ, Hudson BE, et al. Outcomes after successful direct-acting antiviral therapy for patients with chronic hepatitis C and decompensated cirrhosis. J Hepatol. 2016;65:741–7.
18. Krassenburg LAP, Maan R, Ramji A, et al. Clinical outcomes following DAA therapy in patients with HCV-related cirrhosis depend on disease severity. J Hepatol. 2021;74:1053–63.
19. Borgia SM, Dearden J, Yoshida EM, et al. Sofosbuvir/velpatasvir for 12 weeks in hepatitis C virus-infected patients with end-stage renal disease undergoing dialysis. J Hepatol. 2019;71:660–5.
20. Ji F, Yeo YH, Wei M, et al. Sustained virologic response to direct-acting antiviral therapy in patients with chronic hepatitis C and hepatocellular carcinoma: a systematic review and meta-analysis. J Hepatol. 2019;71:473–85.
21. Prenner SB, VanWagner LB, Flamm SL, et al. Hepatocellular carcinoma decreases the chance of successful hepatitis C virus therapy with direct-acting antivirals. J Hepatol. 2017;66:1173–81.
22. Ji F, Wei B, Yeo YH, et al. Systematic review with meta-analysis: effectiveness and tolerability of interferon-free direct-acting antiviral regimens for chronic hepatitis C genotype 1 in routine clinical practice in Asia. Aliment Pharmacol Ther. 2018;4:550–62.
23. Ogawa E, Toyoda H, Iio E, et al. Hepatitis C virus cure rates are reduced in patients with active but not inactive hepatocellular carcinoma: a practice implication. Clin Infect Dis. 2020;71:2840–8.
24. Singal AG, Rick NE, Mehta N, et al. Direct-acting antiviral therapy for hepatitis C virus infection is associated with increased survival in patients with a history of hepatocellular carcinoma. Gastroenterology. 2019;157:1253–1263e2.
25. Dang H, Yeo Y, Yasuda S, et al. Cure with interferon-free DAA is associated with increased survival in patients with HCV related HCC from both east and west. Hepatology. 2020;71:1910–22.
26. Mocan T, Nenu I, Crăciun R, Spârchez Z. Treatment of hepatitis C virus infection in patients with hepatocellular carcinoma: truth or dare? J Gastroenterol Hepatol. 2021;36:1518–28.
27. Ji F, Li T, Nguyen MH. Improved survival and high sustained virologic response with DAA therapy in patients with HCV-related HCC: a call for expanded use. J Gastroenterol Hepatol. 2021;36:1721–2.

28. Reig M, Cabibbo G. Antiviral therapy in the palliative setting of HCC (BCLC-B and -C). J Hepatol. 2021;74:1225–33.
29. Mariño Z, Darnell A, Lens S, et al. Time association between hepatitis C therapy and hepatocellular carcinoma emergence in cirrhosis: relevance of non-characterized nodules. J Hepatol. 2019;70:874–84.
30. Sanduzzi-Zamparelli M, Mariño Z, Lens S, et al. Liver cancer risk after HCV cure in patients with advanced liver disease without non-characterized nodules. J Hepatol. 2021;S0168-8278:02228–5.
31. Semmler G, Meyer EL, Kozbial K, et al. HCC risk stratification after cure of hepatitis C in patients with compensated advanced chronic liver disease. J Hepatol. 2021;S0168-8278:02234–0.

Anticoagulants and Antiplatelet Agents in Cirrhosis

3

Feng Su and Patrick G. Northup

Abstract

Anticoagulants and antiplatelet agents are increasingly used to treat or prevent thromboembolic conditions in patients with cirrhosis. In this chapter, we discuss common indications for anticoagulants and antiplatelet agents in patients with cirrhosis. We will review individual agents, including aspirin, thienopyridines, heparin, vitamin K antagonists, and direct oral anticoagulants. We focus on the unique challenges of using these agents in the setting of altered hemostasis and impaired liver function, and review evidence regarding the safety and efficacy of each agent in patients with cirrhosis.

Keywords

Aspirin · Warfarin · Direct oral anticoagulant · Coagulopathy · Atrial fibrillation Portal vein thrombosis · Liver disease

F. Su (✉) · P. G. Northup
Division of Gastroenterology and Hepatology, University of Virginia, Charlottesville, VA, USA
e-mail: vcf7ch@virginia.edu

X. Qi, Y. Yang (eds.), *Pharmacotherapy for Liver Cirrhosis and Its Complications*, https://doi.org/10.1007/978-981-19-2615-0_3

Abbreviations

AF	atrial fibrillation
aPTT	activated partial thromboplastin time
CTP	Child-Turcotte-Pugh
DOAC	direct oral anticoagulant
INR	international normalized ratio
LMWH	low molecular weight heparin
NAFLD	nonalcoholic fatty liver disease
NASH	nonalcoholic steatohepatitis
PAI-1	plasminogen activator inhibitor 1
PT	prothrombin time
PVT	portal vein thrombosis
TAFI	thrombin-activatable fibrinolysis inhibitor
tPA	tissue-plasminogen activator
UFH	unfractionated heparin
VKA	vitamin K antagonists
VTE	venous thromboembolism
vWF	von Willebrand Factor

3.1 Introduction

In patients with cirrhosis, anticoagulants and antiplatelet agents are used to treat venous and splanchnic thrombosis and to prevent thromboembolic complications of cardiovascular disease. The aging population of patients with cirrhosis, combined with the rising prevalence of nonalcoholic fatty liver disease (NAFLD), which is strongly associated with comorbid cardiovascular disease, means that an increasing number of patients with cirrhosis have indications for these agents. The use of anticoagulants and antiplatelet agents in patients with cirrhosis presents several challenges. First, complex alterations in hemostatic pathways occur in cirrhosis. While cirrhosis has historically been considered a state of impaired hemostasis due to deviations in traditional laboratory markers of coagulation, it is now recognized that cirrhosis is more accurately considered a state of rebalanced hemostasis. In addition to having reduced levels of procoagulants, patients with cirrhosis also have reduced levels of natural anticoagulants. This balance is tenuous, and small perturbations easily tip the patient toward excessive clotting or bleeding. Moreover, coagulation parameters traditionally relied upon for therapeutic drug monitoring are often altered in cirrhosis due to impaired liver synthetic function. In addition, some anticoagulants undergo hepatic metabolism, which may be impaired in individuals with cirrhosis. And lastly, patients with cirrhosis are at risk of portal hypertension-related bleeding, and there is an understandable reluctance to aggravate bleeding risk in such patients.

In the following sections, we will review disruptions in hemostatic pathways in cirrhosis to establish a basic understanding of the milieu in which anticoagulants are used in these patients. We also review indications for anticoagulation and antiplatelet agents among patients with cirrhosis, and lastly, we provide an overview of the safety and efficacy of different classes of antiplatelet agents and anticoagulants in the setting of cirrhosis.

3.2 Hemostatic Pathways in Cirrhosis

Hemostasis can be separated into primary hemostasis, secondary hemostasis, and fibrinolysis [1]. Primary hemostasis refers to platelet activation, aggregation, and plug formation at the site of injury. Damage to the blood vessel wall results in platelet adhesion through binding to exposed collagen and von Willebrand Factor (vWF). Secondary hemostasis refers to activation and propagation of the coagulation pathway, beginning with tissue factor and resulting in thrombin generation and deposition of crosslinked fibrin polymers. Unchecked coagulation is prevented by natural inhibitors of coagulation, including antithrombin as well as protein C and its cofactor, protein S. In fibrinolysis, fibrin clots are dissolved into soluble fragments by plasmin. Cirrhosis is characterized by alterations of components of all stages of hemostasis. Changes that favor bleeding and changes that favor clotting occur simultaneously, resulting in a precariously "rebalanced" state of hemostasis [2].

3.2.1 Alterations in Primary Hemostasis Associated with Cirrhosis

Alterations in primary hemostasis that favor bleeding include thrombocytopenia and platelet dysfunction. Thrombocytopenia is a common finding in patients with cirrhosis and is due to both reduced platelet production and increased platelet clearance [3]. Reduced platelet production is due to reduced thrombopoietin levels, which is synthesized by hepatocytes and is the key regulator of platelet production [4]. Additionally, bone marrow suppression in the setting of viral hepatitis or alcohol-related liver disease may play a role in reduced platelet production in some patients. Increased platelet clearance is related to hypersplenism, which leads to platelet sequestration and increased platelet destruction. There is also suggestion of antiplatelet autoantibodies in cirrhosis that can enhance platelet removal [3]. The decrease in platelet level and function is counterbalanced by elevated levels of vWF [5], which favors clotting. vWF is a large, multimeric glycoprotein synthesized by endothelial cells and megakaryocytes that bridges platelets to sites of endothelial injury, serves as a vehicle for platelet aggregation, and promotes fibrin formation by binding to and stabilizing factor VIII [6]. vWF levels have been shown to be significantly higher in patients with cirrhosis compared to healthy volunteers, and in vitro tests showed superior platelet adhesion when platelets were mixed with plasma from patients with cirrhosis [5]. There have also been studies reporting decreased levels of the vWF cleaving protein, ADAMTS13, in cirrhosis [7, 8], resulting in large vWF multimers. However, this has not been a consistent finding in all studies [5] and its effect on the hemostatic state of patients with cirrhosis remains unsettled [1].

3.2.2 Alterations in Coagulation Associated with Cirrhosis

Secondary hemostasis is impaired in cirrhosis due to decreased levels of clotting factors, such as II, V, VII, IX, and X, which are all produced in the liver. Offsetting the reduced levels of procoagulants are increased levels of factor VIII, which is produced by sinusoidal endothelial cells, and decreased levels of naturally occurring anticoagulants, including protein C, protein S, and antithrombin [9]. Indeed, while thrombin generation appears lower in patients with cirrhosis compared to healthy controls in vitro when considering only coagulation protein levels, when physiologic conditions are mimicked through the addition of thrombomodulin—the protein C activator—thrombin generation is similar between patients with cirrhosis and healthy controls [9]. Moreover, plasma from patients with cirrhosis has been shown to be more resistant to the effect of thrombomodulin, theoretically resulting in less natural anticoagulation [10]. This may be due to a net excess of procoagulant factors, such as factor VIII, or a deficiency of naturally occurring anticoagulants, such as protein C [10].

3.2.3 Alterations in Tertiary Hemostasis

In tertiary hemostasis, fibrin clots are dissolved by plasmin. Plasminogen is activated to plasmin by tissue-plasminogen activator (tPA). Inhibitors of fibrinolysis include plasminogen activator inhibitor 1 (PAI-1), which inhibits tPA, thrombin-activatable fibrinolysis inhibitor (TAFI), and plasmin inhibitors [1]. Patients with cirrhosis have alterations that make them susceptible to hyperfibrinolysis, including increased tPA levels and activity [1]. They may also be predisposed to hypofibrinolysis through reduced plasminogen levels [1]. Increased PAI-1 and decreased TAFI levels additionally occur in cirrhosis, but the impact of these changes on their activity is unclear [1]. In addition, while studies have shown potentially impaired fibrin polymerization in cirrhosis due to increased sialic acid content of fibrinogen, clot permeability is decreased in cirrhosis [11], suggesting resistance to fibrinolysis. Finally, fibrinogen is produced in the liver and lower fibrinogen levels are a reflection of decreased protein synthesis and correlate with severity of liver disease [12].

3.2.4 External Factors Impacting Hemostasis in Cirrhosis

The net result of these complex alterations in hemostatic pathways is a state of tenuous balance between pro- and anti-hemostatic forces. However, this balance is easily perturbed by external factors, such as sepsis, renal dysfunction, or acute portal hypertension bleeding events. A study of patients hospitalized with acute decompensation of cirrhosis or acute-on-chronic liver failure, for instance, showed a tendency toward hypofibrinolysis in patients with sepsis compared to patients without sepsis [13]. The same study demonstrated substantial individual variation in fibrinolytic status, with some individuals showing marked hyperfibrinolysis and others hypofibrinolysis [13], perhaps driven by variations in etiology of liver disease, severity of liver dysfunction, trigger for decompensation, and presence of extrahepatic organ dysfunction. A common extrahepatic organ dysfunction in those with cirrhosis is renal injury. Renal dysfunction has been shown to be an independent predictor of procedural bleeding among patients with decompensated cirrhosis [14], presumably due to impaired platelet function, although alterations in coagulation factors and fibrinolysis have also been described among patients with cirrhosis and acute kidney injury [15, 16]. Therefore, despite a generally rebalanced hemostatic system, patients with cirrhosis have little reserve and acute insults may readily precipitate thrombosis or bleeding.

Faced with a precarious hemostatic system, a propensity to develop portal hypertensive bleeding (which is not dependent on the baseline hemostatic system), and abnormal routine tests of coagulation, clinicians providing care to patients with cirrhosis may be reluctant to initiate anticoagulants or antiplatelet agents for fear of precipitating bleeding. There is also a paucity of evidence to guide clinicians in these settings. However, patients with cirrhosis are increasingly faced with clinical situations where anticoagulation would otherwise be indicated based on acute thrombosis or high cardiovascular risk. The prothrombotic changes in the hemostatic system of patients with cirrhosis may also elevate their risk of thrombosis compared to the general population. In the next sections, we will review common indications for anticoagulants and antiplatelet agents among patients with cirrhosis, and discuss the different classes of medications.

3.3 Indications for Anticoagulants and Antiplatelet Agents in Cirrhosis

Patients with cirrhosis have benefitted from increased lifespan due to improved understanding of portal hypertension and advances in medical care and technology [17]. As patients with cirrhosis age, they are not immune to medical conditions that afflict the general population. With the rising prevalence of NAFLD in Western societies, the average level of comorbidity of a typical patient with cirrhosis is also more advanced than in previous eras [18]. Therefore, patients with cirrhosis now have indications for anticoagulation and antiplatelet therapy at rates similar to the general medical population. In general, there is a steadily increasing prevalence of outpatient anticoagulant use [19]. Despite this, most pivotal clinical trials of modern anticoagulants and antiplatelet agents exclude patients with known cirrhosis. Thus, the use of these agents in patients with cirrhosis has not been evaluated in prospective, randomized studies. Below we will discuss the general indications and safety considerations for anticoagulants and antiplatelet agents in cirrhosis.

3.3.1 Cardiovascular Disease

The most frequent indication for anticoagulation in Western society is atrial fibrillation (AF), which in 2010 affected more than 5.2 million people in the USA and is projected to affect more than 12 million by 2030 [20]. Although there is no definite etiologic link between advanced liver disease and cardiovascular disease, patients with nonalcoholic steatohepatitis (NASH) may have an increased predilection for atherosclerotic disease through an unknown mechanism suspected to be related to endothelial dysfunction [21]. Retrospective studies have suggested an increased risk for AF in patients with NAFLD [22]. Despite this high burden of cardiovascular disease, patients with cirrhosis are often not offered anticoagulation for AF presumably due to thrombocytopenia, elevated INR, and fear of bleeding complications. While prospective studies of anticoagulation in patients with cirrhosis and AF are lacking, there are many detailed retrospective analyses and meta-analyses of this topic in large patient populations [23–25]. For instance, a recent retrospective population-based analysis of 2694 patients with AF and cirrhosis found that all-cause mortality was lower with warfarin (HR 0.65, 95% CI 0.55–0.76) and with direct oral anticoagulants (DOACs) (HR 0.68, 95% CI 0.50–0.93) versus no anticoagulation with no differences found in major bleeding events between anticoagulated and not anticoagulated patients [25]. Although hampered by retrospective design, selection bias, and other flaws inherent to administrative database studies, the consensus from such studies is that anticoagulants in patients with cirrhosis and AF are associated with reduced all-cause mortality and similar bleeding complications compared to the general population.

Typical indications for antiplatelet agents in patients with cirrhosis include coronary artery disease and secondary prevention of myocardial infarction, ischemic stroke, and prevention of coronary stent thrombosis. Prospective studies on these agents are generally lacking in this population, and the literature is limited to retrospective cohorts [26–28] or database analyses [29]. There has been one prospective study of clopidogrel in patients with cirrhosis undergoing percutaneous coronary intervention prior to liver transplantation [30]. While published only in letter format and containing only 11 patients, this study found that despite impaired hepatic function, clopidogrel showed appropriate inhibition of platelet aggregation and did not cause excess bleeding. Because of the proven benefit of these agents for the above indications, until more useful data regarding safety and efficacy in the population with cirrhosis are published, it would be reasonable to use the antiplatelet agents as indicated in the general population.

3.3.2 Venous Thromboembolism

Patients with cirrhosis are at high risk of hospitalization as their disease process progresses, which places them at high risk for non-splanchnic venous thromboembolism (VTE), such as deep vein thrombosis and pulmonary embolism. Furthermore, the rebalance of hemostasis in patients with cirrhosis can result in some patients having a hypercoagulable phenotype [10]. As a result, patients with cirrhosis are thought to have at least similar risk of peripheral VTE compared to the general medical population, and some studies suggest an increased risk [31–33]. Over recent years, VTE risk stratification calculators, such as the Padua [34] and IMPROVE [35] scores, have been developed to identify patients at the highest risk for VTE, while sparing patients at low risk of VTE from the potential harms of pharmacologic prophylaxis. Patients with advanced cirrhosis were excluded from the patient cohort used to derive the Padua score; however, the IMPROVE score derivation cohort did include patients with cirrhosis. A single retrospective series [36] found that only 19% of hospitalized patients with cirrhosis would warrant VTE prophylaxis with application of the IMPROVE score. Prospective validation of a broader range of VTE risk stratification scores would be helpful in deciding which patients would benefit the most from VTE prophylaxis.

Once non-splanchnic VTE occurs in patients with cirrhosis, there is little guidance regarding the use of therapeutic anticoagulation and safety, and efficacy data are often extrapolated from more common indications (see below). Until more definitive data are published, given the life-threatening nature of non-splanchnic VTE, it is clinically prudent to use therapeutic anticoagulation in patients with cirrhosis unless there is a strong contraindication.

3.3.3 Portal Vein Thrombosis

Thrombosis of the portal vein (PVT) or branches of the mesenteric veins are common in the natural history of chronic liver disease. Clinical presentation can range from intestinal venous outflow obstruction with life-threatening bowel ischemia to symptoms of increased portal hypertension to a complete absence of symptoms. Complete review and discussion of PVT is beyond the scope of this text and has been covered extensively elsewhere [37–39]. PVT is often of uncertain significance in patients with cirrhosis who are asymptomatic or minimally symptomatic. For example, a large prospective observational study [40] showed no correlation between the development of PVT and hepatic decompensation or overall survival, implying that PVT treatment may not be beneficial for the underlying disease process. Conversely, a small randomized controlled trial using low molecular weight heparin (LMWH) for prevention of PVT in patients with cirrhosis [41] demonstrated a lower rate of PVT, a delay in hepatic decompensation, and improved overall survival in subjects randomized to LMWH. These results suggest that PVT prevention, or perhaps LMWH itself, can significantly modify the disease history of patients with cirrhosis. Furthermore, a patent portal vein offers technical benefits at the time of liver transplantation and is associated with improved post-transplant survival [42].

Given the uncertain prognostic importance of PVT, the benefit of anticoagulation for PVT is unclear in most patients with cirrhosis, except in the case of patients awaiting liver transplant. To further complicate treatment decisions, consistent and widely accepted definitions of extent, location, and percent of obstruction of the main portal vein are lacking, making it difficult to compare studies on this subject. Because of the uncertainties outlined above, treatment recommendations are varied (Table 3.1) and usually best made on a case-by-case basis for an individual patient.

3.4 Antiplatelet Agents

Pathologic platelet aggregation is a well-known trigger of arterial thrombotic diseases, such as myocardial and cerebrovascular infarction. Inhibition of platelet aggregation is also highly desirable in the setting of intra-arterial stent placement to prevent stent thrombosis. There are no prospective randomized studies supporting the safety or efficacy of antiplatelet agents in patients with cirrhosis. The specific use and benefit of these agents in vascular disease are beyond the scope of this

Table 3.1 Various society recommendations on the anticoagulant treatment of portal vein thrombosis. All guidelines recommend treatment in patients without cirrhosis and in patients with ongoing bowel ischemia barring an absolute contraindication

	Treat	Observe
American Association for the Study of Liver Disease [37]	• More than 50% obstruction of the lumen of the main portal vein. • Progression of main portal vein thrombosis during observation.	• Chronic complete occlusion of the main portal vein with cavernous transformation. • Less than 50% of the lumen of the main portal vein.
American College of Gastroenterology [38]	• Evidence of inherited or acquired thrombophilia. • Progression into mesenteric veins. • Complete main portal vein thrombosis. • Patients awaiting liver transplantation (consider).	• No specific recommendations for patients who may be observed.
European Society for the Study of the Liver [43]	• Superior mesenteric vein thrombosis. • Liver transplant candidates.	• Decision should be individualized by institution.
American Gastroenterology Association [44]	• Cirrhosis with acute and subacute nontumoral portal vein thrombosis.	• No specific recommendations for patients who may be observed.

chapter, but we will discuss issues with the most commonly used agents in the context of cirrhosis.

A frequent concern when considering antiplatelet agents in patients with cirrhosis is the presence of thrombocytopenia. It is not known what level of thrombocytopenia provides innate protection against thrombosis and would therefore obviate the use of antiplatelet therapy in the presence of an otherwise solid indication for these drugs. In vitro data using platelets and plasma from patients with cirrhosis suggest that thrombin generation, and presumably the ability to synthesize clots, persists at low normal levels in patients with cirrhosis who have platelet counts above $55 \times 10^9/L$ [45]. In patients with platelet counts below this level, it is unknown if the benefits of antiplatelet therapy for proven indications outweigh the risks. Further study is needed in this area.

3.4.1 Aspirin

Naturally occurring salicylates have long been used for antipyretic and analgesic effects, but medicinal aspirin (acetylsalicylic acid) was first produced in the 1890s for treatment of various inflammatory conditions [46]. Aspirin inhibits platelet aggregation inhibition through permanent acetylation of a protein serine moiety in the cyclooxygenase pathway, thereby inhibiting conversion of arachidonic acid to prostaglandin H_2. This results in a decrease in production of thromboxane A_2, which is a key component in the induction of platelet aggregation [46, 47]. Importantly, platelet inhibition is optimized at concentrations ten times lower than the doses required for antipyretic or analgesic effect, thus enabling the use of low-dose aspirin as an effective antithrombotic agent [47]. The active metabolite of aspirin is processed primarily by the liver via several different pathways mostly through glucuronidation and conjugation. Aspirin is heavily albumin bound so in hypoalbuminemic states, higher serum levels can be expected. In all but the most advanced liver disease, however, metabolic pathways are generally preserved sufficiently that low-dose aspirin pharmacokinetics are essentially unchanged [48].

Data on bleeding events with aspirin use, especially gastrointestinal bleeding, are widely available in the general medical population [49]. In contrast, the data on aspirin safety and tolerability in patients with cirrhosis are less robust. A case series of 84 patients with decompensated cirrhosis and coronary artery disease—30 of whom received low-dose aspirin therapy—showed a modest drop in mean platelet count in the treated patients ($125 \times 10^9/L$ to $95 \times 10^9/L$, $p = 0.004$) but no excess bleeding events including variceal bleeding [50]. A retrospective database analysis of 1180 patients with cirrhosis who suffered from a primary stroke included 170 patients treated for at least 2 years with aspirin therapy [29]. Patients treated with aspirin had no excess gastrointestinal (GI) bleeding compared to those who were untreated (9.2% versus 7.6%, $p = 0.930$). Treated patients also showed improved all-cause mortality and fewer recurrent strokes. There are no known laboratory methods for monitoring patients on aspirin therapy, and the routine clinical use of platelet function assays or other platelet analyzers has not been extensively tested or validated in patients with cirrhosis. Many of these assays depend heavily on circulating platelet count as a measure of platelet function, but the thrombocytopenia of chronic liver disease is not a good measure of clotting capacity due to the rebalance of hemostasis. In summary, given the benefit of aspirin in the setting of coronary and cerebrovascular disease in the general population and the circumstantial safety data in the cirrhosis population, aspirin should not be withheld based purely on the presence of liver disease.

3.4.2 Thienopyridines

The thienopyridines are now commonly used either alone or with aspirin to further inhibit platelet aggregation in the setting of acute coronary syndrome or to prevent thrombosis after coronary stent placement, amongst other indications. The most common of the thienopyridines include clopidogrel, ticlopidine, and prasugrel. These drugs inhibit the glycoprotein IIb/IIIa receptor, which is pivotal in crosslinking fibrin [51]. This is accomplished through the irreversible inhibition of the $P2Y_{12}$ receptor, thus preventing release of adenosine diphosphate from the dense granules of the platelet. Clopidogrel is an inactive prodrug and requires metabolism by hepatic cytochrome P450 (CYP3A4/5 and CYP2C19) [52] to its activated form to effectively inhibit platelet aggregation [53]. Caution must be exercised in using clopidogrel with drugs that inhibit the P450 enzymes as they could potentially decrease its antiplatelet effect. The most common drug interaction is with the proton pump inhibitor omeprazole; however, a landmark randomized controlled trial [54] showed no significant worsening of cardiovascular event endpoints when these two drugs were used together in the general medical population. Despite the dependence on hepatic metabolism, patients with severe hepatic impairment on clopidogrel inhibit platelet aggregation to a similar degree as healthy subjects, and no dose adjustment is recommended based on liver disease [53].

Safety data specific to the population with liver cirrhosis is sparse with the thienopyridines. In the same study mentioned previously examining the efficacy of aspirin in cirrhosis patients after stroke, 70 patients were treated with clopidogrel alone. No differences were observed between treated and non-treated patients with respect to GI bleeding, but the sample size prevented definitive safety conclusions [29]. A large retrospective database analysis of more than 914 patients with well-compensated cirrhosis receiving either single agent or dual agent antiplatelet therapy, including aspirin and clopidogrel, showed no difference in gastrointestinal bleeding or major bleeding with the addition of clopidogrel to aspirin [55]. During clinical trials of clopidogrel, abnormal liver chemistries were not different than placebo. However, there are post-approval case reports of rare hepatotoxicity, sometimes severe, attributed to the drug [56].

3.5 Heparin

The heparins are used as an adjunct when treating arterial thrombi to prevent extension of clot from fibrin deposition, and are also used in the treatment or prevention of venous thrombi, which tend to be less platelet rich and more stasis dependent [57]. The anticoagulation effect of heparin molecules was first discovered in the early 1900s when they were initially isolated from canine liver cells, hence the name "heparin". Commercial unfractionated heparin (UFH) is still derived from animal mucosa [58] and contains a complex collection of polysaccharides that have broad effect, mainly through augmentation of the anticoagulant effect of the antithrombin molecule. Antithrombin inhibits several innate coagulation proteins, including factors IIa, Xa, IXa, Xia, and XIIa [57] and thereby inhibits thrombin formation. The low molecular weight molecules in UFH are degraded more slowly and show more affinity for inhibition of factor Xa compared to UFH. These beneficial properties prompted the development of techniques for isolation of LMWH molecules as a separate pharmacologic agent.

Therapeutic monitoring of heparins has traditionally relied upon the activated partial thromboplastin time (aPTT). However, the aPTT is subject to inter-lab variability, in part because aPTT reagents are not standardized. There is also a lack of correlation of aPTT with clinical outcomes in randomized trials of UFH [59, 60]. In patients with cirrhosis, the aPTT is inaccurate due to lower baseline factor levels and resultant elevation in PT and aPTT [10]. These concerns have led to routine use of the anti-factor Xa assay for therapeutic monitoring of heparins, which better reflects the actual concentration of circulating heparin. In patients with cirrhosis and impaired synthetic function, however, the anti-factor Xa assay can also be misleading, as these patients tend to have decreased levels of antithrombin which artificially decreases results of anti-factor Xa assays. This is most pronounced in patients with Child-Turcotte-Pugh (CTP) C cirrhosis, and a direct correlation between antithrombin levels and anti-factor Xa values with LMWH therapy has been described [61, 62]. This correlation can lead to falsely decreased anti-factor Xa levels in patients with cirrhosis compared to controls with the same level of circulating UFH or LMWH and has been shown to underestimate anticoagulant levels in vitro by as much as 50% [63]. Thus, monitoring patients with cirrhosis receiving UFH or LMWH using anti-factor Xa assays could lead to excessively high doses of anticoagulant agents and predispose to bleeding complications [64]. There is no guidance on more appropriate monitoring of these agents in the setting of cirrhosis, but caution should be used in patients with significantly low baseline antithrombin activity. There are no published reports of the reversal agent protamine specifically in patients with cirrhosis.

Safety data relating to the therapeutic and prophylactic use of heparins in patients with cirrhosis are sparse. Traditional contraindications to LMWH, such as renal dysfunction, are particularly relevant to patients with cirrhosis, as kidney disease is highly prevalent in this population. The incidence of heparin-induced thrombocytopenia in patients with cirrhosis appears to occur at rates comparable to the general population [65]. General safety data are limited to retrospective cohort analyses or uncontrolled case series. The use of prophylactic doses of UFH and LMWH in patients with cirrhosis to prevent in-hospital VTE was evaluated in two retrospective cohort studies. One study showed an increased risk of in-hospital bleeding in patients receiving VTE prophylaxis (OR 2.36, 95% CI 1.12–4.97, $p = 0.023$) but no statistical difference in blood transfusion requirement or in-hospital death [66]. In contrast, a smaller study showed no difference between groups in bleeding events or survival [65]. Studies examining the safety of therapeutic doses of heparins are more abundant, but only one was a prospective randomized controlled trial. In a study of 70 outpatients with cirrhosis at risk for PVT, 34 were randomized and treated in a non-blinded fashion to prophylaxis with enoxaparin 4000 IU/day for 48 weeks and 36 were randomized to no anticoagulation [41]. In this study, one patient stopped LMWH due to thrombocytopenia, and there were three bleeding episodes from esophageal varices, including two in the treated group and one in the control group (p = ns). There were no significant differences in overall bleeding events between the treated and untreated populations. A single-center prospective observational study treated 91 patients with PVT using weight-based LMWH for up to 6 months [67]. During this study, two patients died due to hemorrhage, including one from a duodenal varix and another from an intracranial hemorrhage. Another prospective cohort of 33 patients treated with LMWH for PVT compared bleeding outcomes to 21 untreated controls [68]. All patients in this study had aggressive control of esophageal varices with non-selective beta-blockers and/or endoscopic variceal band ligation. At the end of the study, there were three major hemorrhage events, including one epistaxis, one hematuria, and one intracranial hemorrhage with residual deficits. There was also one case of heparin-induced thrombocytopenia. There was no statistical difference in esophageal variceal bleeding between groups. Finally, a prospective study of 65 patients with cirrhosis and PVT treated with weight-based enoxaparin either 1 mg/kg every 12 hours versus 1.5 mg/kg every 24 hours [69] showed no variceal bleeding events but increased general bleeding in the once daily group compared to the twice daily group (23.5% versus 6.4%). Other studies have shown bleeding rates between 5.2% and 9% for long-term use of LMWH in cirrhosis [70–74], but the studies involve heterogeneous patient populations and in some cases, poorly defined bleeding events, often grouping mild bleeding and severe bleeding events.

There are many retrospective studies examining bleeding rates in patients with cirrhosis on UFH or LMWH, but all are hampered by selection bias, indication bias, and other limitations. Many are limited to inpatient therapy only. A recent meta-analysis of 8 studies using anticoagulation for PVT in patients with cirrhosis [75] concluded that the use of LMWH offered protection from variceal bleeding versus untreated patients (pooled OR 0.103, 95% CI 0.040–0.264, $p = 0.041$) but there was no difference from those treated with warfarin ($p = 0.545$). In summary, although the quality of data is not strong, the safety profile of the heparins in patients with cirrhosis appears to result in bleeding rates between 5% and 9% per year. Aggressive control of esophageal varices is recommended as per practice guidelines and, until further data are published, avoidance of once daily 1.5 mg/kg of enoxaparin is advised (Table 3.2).

Table 3.2 Mechanism of action and clinical data of antiplatelet agents and anticoagulants in cirrhosis

Agent	Clinical Use	Mechanism of Action	Monitoring	Clinically Significant Bleeding Risk	Reversal Agent
Aspirin	Permanent (life of the platelet) inhibition of platelet aggregation	Inhibition of cyclooxygenase pathway resulting in a decrease in production of thromboxane A2, which is a key component of platelet aggregation induction	No routine monitoring recommended	About 2% per year of GI bleeding and peptic ulcer disease, diminished with the use of concurrent PPI. Comparable to general population	None specific other than platelet transfusion
Clopidogrel (Plavix)	Permanent (life of the platelet) inhibition of platelet aggregation	Inhibition of the glycoprotein IIb/IIIa receptor through the inhibition of the P2Y12 receptor	No routine monitoring recommended	Similar to aspirin with no increase in bleeding with dual therapy. Comparable to the general population	None specific other than platelet transfusion
Unfractionated heparin	Anticoagulant	Inhibition several of the innate coagulation proteins, including factors IIa, Xa, IXa, Xia, and XIIa, and therefore preventing thrombin formation	aPTT unproven and not correlated with outcome. Anti-factor Xa can falsely underestimate anticoagulant dose in patients with advanced cirrhosis	Poorly defined since used exclusively as inpatient therapy. Prophylaxis dose 5–8%. Therapeutic intravenous infusion 11–19%.	Protamine

(continued)

Table 3.2 (continued)

Agent	Clinical Use	Mechanism of Action	Monitoring	Clinically Significant Bleeding Risk	Reversal Agent
Low molecular weight heparin (enoxaparin and others)	Anticoagulant	Similar to unfractionated heparin with more specificity to inhibition of factor X	Not routinely recommended when weight based but similar issues with unfractionated heparin	Prophylaxis dose 3–5% per year. Treatment dose 5–9% per year with twice daily administration	Protamine reportedly less effective than in unfractionated heparin but no data specific to cirrhosis
Vitamin K antagonists	Anticoagulant	Inhibit vitamin K epoxide reductase, leading to formation of biologically inactive coagulation factors II, VII, IX, and X	PT/INR, although not validated in patients with cirrhosis and therapeutic target is unclear with baseline INR elevations	2.6% per year [76] 5.7% per year [25]	Vitamin K Transfusion (prothrombin complex concentrate, fresh frozen plasma)
Direct oral anticoagulants	Anticoagulant	Directly inhibit thrombin (dabigatran) or factor Xa (rivaroxaban, apixaban, edoxaban, betrixaban)	No routine monitoring recommended	1.8–2.9% per year [76] 3.4% per year [25]	Idarucizumab (dabigatran) Adexanet alfa (rivaroxaban, apixaban, edoxaban)

3.6 Vitamin K Antagonists

Warfarin and other vitamin K antagonists (VKA) (phenprocoumon, acenocoumarol, and fluindione) exert their anticoagulant effect by decreasing levels of vitamin K-dependent procoagulant proteins (factors II, VII, IX, and X) through post-translational modification [6]. VKAs inhibit vitamin K epoxide reductase, an enzyme that converts dietary vitamin K to the form that serves as a cofactor for vitamin K carboxylase. Vitamin K carboxylase is the enzyme that catalyzes gamma carboxylation of the vitamin K-dependent clotting factors in the liver, a step necessary for clotting factors to bind to phospholipid membranes. By inhibiting vitamin K epoxide reductase, VKAs lead to the formation of biologically inactive clotting factors. They also reduce levels of anticoagulant proteins C and S, leading to a paradoxical procoagulant effect when VKAs are first initiated. The full anticoagulant activity of VKAs is realized when functional clotting factors are cleared and replaced by nonfunctional clotting factors, which may take up to 1 week.

VKAs have a narrow therapeutic window, and their anticoagulant activity is influenced by a number of factors, including dietary intake of vitamin K, genetics, and drug interactions. As such, they require intensive monitoring by frequent measurement of prothrombin time (PT) and the international normalized ratio (INR). Target INR values have been established for various indications, and time in therapeutic range is known to correlate with clinical outcomes. Because there is a delay between VKA initiation and full anticoagulant effect, there is often a need to "bridge" with a second anticoagulant during the first several days of treatment. In the event of active bleeding or other indication for reversal of anticoagulation, vitamin K can be used or factor replacement therapy if more rapid reversal is required.

Monitoring VKAs in patients with cirrhosis presents several challenges. VKAs undergo extensive hepatic metabolism by cytochrome P450 enzymes, therefore making drug activity unpredictable in any individual patient. In addition, although the INR was developed to standardize PT measurements among patients on VKA therapy, it was not calibrated to patients with cirrhosis. And since the INR is usually prolonged in cirrhosis, the target INR is not clear. Moreover, due to the complex alterations in coagulation factors and hemostatic pathways among patients with cirrhosis, a prolonged INR in patients with cirrhosis does not necessarily correlate with hemostatic capacity. Further complicating the use of VKAs in cirrhosis is significant interlaboratory variability in INR measurements among patients with cirrhosis [77–79]. In a study examining laboratory variability in INR, blood samples from patients with cirrhosis were sent to 13 different laboratories in the USA. There was substantial interlaboratory variability in INR measurements, with greater variability at samples with higher INR values [78]. In a similar study of laboratories in Europe, agreement between laboratories was worse among patients with cirrhosis than non-cirrhotic controls who had elevated INRs from anticoagulant therapy [77]. Variability of measured INRs can be reduced by calibrating to patients with cirrhosis, known as INR(liver) [80], but this technique is not widely available and has not been adopted by most clinical laboratories.

Studies evaluating the safety and efficacy of VKAs in patients with cirrhosis have shown mixed results. While some have demonstrated acceptable risk of bleeding among patients with cirrhosis treated with VKAs [23, 70, 72, 75, 81–84], other studies show higher bleeding rates among patients treated with VKAs compared to no anticoagulation [25, 85–87] or other types of anticoagulants [24, 76, 88–91]. The two major categories of studies are those evaluating anticoagulation in patients with PVT, and those evaluating anticoagulation in patients with AF. Studies of patients receiving VKAs for PVT have generally shown favorable outcomes when compared to no anticoagulation. A meta-analysis of 8 studies compared patients who were anticoagulated for PVTs and patients who remained untreated [75]. Rates of bleeding were similar in anticoagulated versus untreated patients (11% in both groups), with a higher rate of variceal bleeding among untreated patients (12% versus 2%). Not surprisingly, the proportion of patients who had recanalization of their PVT was higher among those receiving anticoagulation (71% versus 42%). The favorable result of these studies is most likely because anticoagulation is effective for recanalization of the portal vein, which reduces the risk of portal hypertensive complications, such as variceal bleeding, and the risk of hepatic decompensation.

Several large population-based cohort studies have evaluated the safety and efficacy of VKAs in the treatment of patients with cirrhosis and AF. In one study utilizing a national health insurance database in Taiwan, patients with cirrhosis and AF who were treated with warfarin had a similar risk of intracranial bleeding as patients not on anticoagulation, and a lower risk of ischemic stroke [23]. In contrast, another study utilizing US Veterans Affairs Health Administration data found that warfarin was associated with a higher risk of bleeding compared to no anticoagulation (HR 1.5, 95% CI 1.10–2.06), but lower risk of stroke and all-cause mortality [25]. VKAs have also been compared to DOACs in several studies. While studies differ regarding the efficacy of VKAs versus DOACs for stroke prevention, they consistently show that VKAs are associated with a higher risk of bleeding than DOACs among patients with cirrhosis [25, 76, 90].

Existing data regarding the safety and efficacy of VKAs in patients with cirrhosis are hampered by biases inherent to retrospective, observational studies, and most include only small numbers of patients from single centers. In addition, definitions of cirrhosis and bleeding endpoints are highly variable. As such, specific recommendations on the use of VKAs in patients with cirrhosis are not evidence based. What is clear is that VKA use in cirrhosis is problematic from a drug monitoring perspective. Moreover, newer DOACs may have equivalent efficacy for treatment and prevention of thrombotic complications while potentially being less likely to cause clinically significant bleeding. A rational approach to the use of VKAs may be to carefully consider the indication for anticoagulation as well as the ability to use newer forms of anticoagulants that do not rely on therapeutic monitoring for proper dosing. In situations where other agents are unavailable or contraindicated, VKA use may be justifiable on the basis of superior outcomes compared to no anticoagulation when there is a strong clinical indication for anticoagulation. However, patients should be made aware of the possibility of increased bleeding risk, and in particular the unproven nature of INR as a means of drug monitoring in this population.

3.7 Direct Oral Anticoagulants

DOACs achieve their anticoagulant effect by binding to and directly inhibiting the action of thrombin (dabigatran) or factor Xa (rivaroxaban, apixaban, edoxaban, and betrixaban). Unlike traditional anticoagulants, such as heparin or VKAs, they have the advantage of oral administration, quick onset of action, and do not require therapeutic drug monitoring. DOACs have been shown to be effective for the prevention and treatment of VTE, stroke prevention in patients with AF, and in patients with ischemic heart disease. However, clinical trials of these agents excluded patients with known liver disease. Consequently, current package inserts recommend cautious use or overtly advise against use in patients with impaired liver function (Table 3.3). The clinical experience with DOACs among patients with cirrhosis is therefore limited.

Due to predictable drug levels for a given dose, routine monitoring of coagulation parameters is not required for DOACs. While routine tests of coagulation are variably responsive to certain DOACs, they are not equally responsive to all agents and not adequate to determine the level of anticoagulation [92]. Drug calibrated chromogenic anti-Xa assays may have some utility in quantifying anticoagulation by direct factor Xa inhibitors [92], but are not currently in widespread use or calibrated for use in patients with liver disease. It is possible to obtain drug concentrations for each agent, but there are no established therapeutic concentrations, and these methods are not widely available. A challenge with DOACs in the setting of cirrhosis is that each agent undergoes a variable degree of hepatobiliary clearance and is variably susceptible to hepatic metabolism by the cytochrome P450 system [93], which may be altered in the setting of impaired liver function. Of note, whether the altered pharmacokinetics of DOACs in patients with liver disease have clinically meaningful effects on drug safety and efficacy is unclear. Patients with cirrhosis also have a high prevalence of renal dysfunction, and all DOACs undergo renal clearance and require some level of dose adjustment in the setting of kidney dysfunction. Generally, current FDA recommendations do not advise dose adjustment,

Table 3.3 Current Food and Drug Administration package recommendations regarding direct oral anticoagulant use in patients with liver disease

		FDA recommendations in liver disease		
	Mechanism	CTP A	CTP B	CTP C
Dabigatran	Direct thrombin inhibitor	No restrictions	No restrictions	No restrictions
Rivaroxaban	Direct factor Xa inhibitor	No restrictions	Not recommended	Not recommended
Apixaban	Direct factor Xa inhibitor	No restrictions	No restrictions	Not recommended
Edoxaban	Direct factor Xa inhibitor	No restrictions	Not recommended	Not recommended
Betrixaban	Direct factor Xa inhibitor	No restrictions	Not recommended	Not recommended

nor do they restrict the use of any DOACs in patients with compensated, CTP class A cirrhosis. In contrast, with the exception of dabigatran, the FDA recommends avoidance of all DOACs in patients with CTP B or C cirrhosis, although apixaban is only labeled against CTP C cirrhosis.

Dabigatran is a direct thrombin inhibitor approved in the USA for stroke prevention in patients with nonvalvular AF and for the treatment and prevention of VTE. In a single oral dose study, 12 patients with CTP B cirrhosis and 12 healthy age, weight, and sex-matched volunteers were given a single dose of dabigatran, after which blood was drawn to measure pharmacokinetic and pharmacodynamic parameters [94]. Drug exposure was very similar between patients with CTP B cirrhosis and healthy volunteers, and the effect of dabigatran on coagulation parameters, including INR and thrombin time, was similar [94]. These results are not surprising as dabigatran is primarily cleared by the kidneys (80%) rather than the liver (20%), and does not undergo cytochrome P450 metabolism [95].

Rivaroxaban is an oral direct factor Xa inhibitor approved in the USA for stroke prevention in patients with nonvalvular AF, the treatment and prevention of VTE, and secondary prophylaxis of cardiovascular events in combination with aspirin in patients with cardiovascular disease or PAD. Rivaroxaban is cleared by the kidney (66%) and liver (34%), and is metabolized by the liver to inactive metabolites via cytochrome P450 enzymes and by CYP-independent mechanisms [96]. In patients with CTP A cirrhosis, the pharmacokinetics of rivaroxaban are similar to those of healthy subjects, however, significant increases in rivaroxaban exposure are seen in patients with CTP B cirrhosis [97]. Moreover, inhibition of factor Xa activity is greater in patients with CTP B cirrhosis [97]. In general, while the risk of drug-induced liver injury resulting from DOACs is very low and idiosyncratic, there are post-marketing reports of rare cases of liver injury attributed to rivaroxaban [98].

Apixaban is also an oral direct factor Xa inhibitor approved in the USA for stroke prevention in patients with nonvalvular AF and for the treatment and prevention of VTE. Of the DOACs, apixaban relies the most on hepatic clearance (75%) and is primarily metabolized by CYP3A4 but is also a P-glycoprotein substrate [95]. Patients with CTP A and B cirrhosis have been shown to have slightly higher apixaban exposure compared to healthy subjects [95].

Edoxaban is an oral direct factor Xa inhibitor approved in the USA for stroke prevention in the setting of nonvalvular AF and for the treatment and prevention of VTE. It is partially cleared by the liver (65%) and undergoes minimal cytochrome P450 metabolism [95]. In a single oral dose study, drug concentrations of edoxaban were slightly lower among patients with CTP A and B cirrhosis compared to healthy controls [95].

Betrixaban is the newest oral direct factor Xa inhibitor and is approved in the USA for the prevention of VTE in hospitalized patients. It does not undergo P450 metabolism, but is a P-glycoprotein substrate [99]. It is unique among DOACs in that it undergoes very little renal clearance, instead relying primarily on biliary excretion. The current package label advises against use in patients with moderate to severe liver disease.

Studies evaluating the safety and efficacy of DOACs in patients with cirrhosis are limited to small cohort studies or retrospective population-based studies. Collectively, currently available data suggest that DOACs are efficacious and may result in similar, if not lower, incidence of bleeding compared to traditional anticoagulants [100]. The initial study that described outcomes of patients with cirrhosis who received DOACs included 20 patients with CTP A or B cirrhosis who received DOACs and 19 who received LMWH or warfarin [101]. Indications for anticoagulation were splanchnic or non-splanchnic VTE and stroke prevention in the setting of AF. Major bleeding occurred in one patient in the DOAC group (5%) and two patients in the traditional anticoagulant group (11%). The difference between the two groups was not statistically significant. There were no independent predictors of bleeding in multivariable analysis. Other observational studies either concur that DOACs do not result in significantly different bleeding risk compared to traditional anticoagulants [83, 102, 103] or are associated with lower risk of bleeding compared to traditional anticoagulants [88, 89]. Large population-based cohort studies of patients receiving DOACs for stroke prevention in AF have also suggested that DOACs are associated with a lower risk of bleeding compared to VKAs [25, 76, 90]. Observational studies are hampered by similar limitations as studies of traditional anticoagulants. Most are retrospective, contain small sample sizes, use variable inclusion criteria, and use variable definitions of bleeding endpoints. Moreover, a large proportion of patients on DOACs in these studies received doses lower than labeled recommendations. A retrospective multicenter consortium study revealed that only 36% of patients with cirrhosis received full-dose anticoagulation, compared to 71% of patients without cirrhosis [104].

The only randomized trial examining DOAC use in the setting of cirrhosis included 80 patients with compensated hepatitis C-related cirrhosis who developed acute PVT [105]. Patients were randomized to rivaroxaban or warfarin after initially receiving enoxaparin. There were no bleeding events in the rivaroxaban group, whereas 17 (43%) patients in the warfarin-treated group experienced GI bleeding. Of note, patients in this study were not representative of the general population of patients with cirrhosis and PVT, in that most had undergone recent splenectomy or developed acute PVT in the setting of abdominal infection. A meta-analysis of seven studies comparing DOACs to traditional anticoagulants in patients with cirrhosis concluded that there was no difference in risk of major bleeds, all bleeding events, or GI bleeds between the two groups [106].

Notably, studies of DOACs in cirrhosis include predominantly patients with well-compensated or asymptomatic liver disease. Data evaluating DOACs in patients with more advanced cirrhosis are sparse. A single-center analysis of 138 patients with cirrhosis who received DOACs for a variety of indications contained 93 (66.7%) patients with CTP B or C cirrhosis [107]. Bleeding occurred in 32.6% of the overall population, while major bleeding occurred in 8.0%. Bleeding rates were not significantly different in CTP classes (CTP A 28.9%, CTP B 34.3%, CTP C 34.8%), although baseline CTP score was higher in subjects with a major bleed. Another single-center study of 133 patients with chronic liver disease included 55 patients with CTP B or C cirrhosis [108]. All patients received DOACs for a variety of indications. The 12-month cumulative incidence of spontaneous bleeding was higher in CTP B and C patients compared to CTP A (36.9% versus 15.9%). The cumulative incidence of major bleeds was also higher in CTP B and C patients compared to CTP A (22.0% versus 5%). Neither of these studies included a control group of patients receiving traditional anticoagulants. Another study of 101 patients with CTP B or C cirrhosis did compare bleeding events between patients on DOACs and traditional anticoagulants [109]. A greater proportion of patients in the DOAC group experienced a bleed (36%) than the traditional anticoagulant group (22%), but this difference was not statistically significant. A higher rate of bleeding was also observed among CTP C patients (70%) compared to CTP B (31%). Collectively, these results highlight the need for additional controlled studies with larger sample sizes to evaluate the use of DOACs in patients with decompensated cirrhosis.

In summary, there is limited guidance regarding the safety, efficacy, and appropriate dosage of DOACs among patients with cirrhosis, and available studies are largely observational and hampered by a number of limitations. Despite this, results of these studies are reasonably consistent and show that patients with cirrhosis who are treated with DOACs appear to have similar or lower risk of bleeding compared to patients treated with traditional anticoagulants. Based on these results, DOACs can be considered in patients with compensated cirrhosis if there is an appropriate clinical indication. Additional studies are needed to guide DOACs use in patients with decompensated cirrhosis. Until those data are available, these patients should be considered cautiously on a case-by-case basis.

3.8 Conclusion

Clinicians caring for patients with cirrhosis are increasingly faced with clinical scenarios where antiplatelet agents or anticoagulants must be considered. These decisions are challenging due to the complex hemostatic alterations and impaired synthetic function seen in cirrhosis, which affect the safety, efficacy, and monitoring of each agent. Apart from PVT, the indications for antiplatelet and anticoagulants are similar in patients with cirrhosis as in the general population. Although existing studies have numerous limitations, they generally support the use of these agents in patients with cirrhosis when clinically appropriate. Failure to initiate appropriate anticoagulant or antiplatelet therapy may in fact result in poor outcomes, and the use of these agents should not be avoided purely due to fear of precipitating bleeding events. Indeed, many studies suggest that anticoagulants and antiplatelet agents do not necessarily lead to a higher rate of bleeding events in patients with cirrhosis, although there should be caution particularly when using agents requiring therapeutic drug monitoring as traditional means of drug monitoring may be unreliable in the setting of cirrhosis. DOACs appear to be reasonable choices for many patients with cirrhosis who have an indication for anticoagulation, but have not been studied extensively in patients with decompensated liver function. Patients and clinicians will benefit from additional high-quality data to elucidate the risks, benefits, and complexities of anticoagulant and antiplatelet use in all subgroups of patients with chronic liver disease.

Declaration of Funding Sources None.

Declaration of Personal Interests None.

References

1. Zermatten MG, Fraga M, Moradpour D, Bertaggia Calderara D, Aliotta A, Stirnimann G, et al. Hemostatic alterations in patients with cirrhosis: from primary hemostasis to fibrinolysis. Hepatology. 2020;71:2135–48.
2. Tripodi A, Mannucci PM. The coagulopathy of chronic liver disease. N Engl J Med. 2011;365:147–56.
3. Violi F, Basili S, Raparelli V, Chowdary P, Gatt A, Burroughs AK. Patients with liver cirrhosis suffer from primary haemostatic defects? Fact or fiction? J Hepatol. 2011;55:1415–27.
4. Rios R, Sangro B, Herrero I, Quiroga J, Prieto J. The role of thrombopoietin in the thrombocytopenia of patients with liver cirrhosis. Am J Gastroenterol. 2005;100:1311–6.
5. Lisman T, Bongers TN, Adelmeijer J, Janssen HL, de Maat MP, de Groot PG, et al. Elevated levels of von Willebrand factor in cirrhosis support platelet adhesion despite reduced functional capacity. Hepatology. 2006;44:53–61.
6. Hoffman R, ClinicalKey Flex. Hematology basic principles and practice. Philadelphia, PA: Elsevier; 2018. Available from: http://RE5QY4SB7X.search.serialssolutions.com/?V=1.0&L=RE5QY4SB7X&S=JCs&C=TC0001833407&T=marc
7. Mannucci PM, Canciani MT, Forza I, Lussana F, Lattuada A, Rossi E. Changes in health and disease of the metalloprotease that cleaves von Willebrand factor. Blood. 2001;98:2730–5.
8. Uemura M, Fujimura Y, Matsumoto M, Ishizashi H, Kato S, Matsuyama T, et al. Comprehensive analysis of ADAMTS13 in patients with liver cirrhosis. Thromb Haemost. 2008;99:1019–29.
9. Tripodi A, Salerno F, Chantarangkul V, Clerici M, Cazzaniga M, Primignani M, et al. Evidence of normal thrombin generation in cirrhosis despite abnormal conventional coagulation tests. Hepatology. 2005;41:553–8.
10. Tripodi A, Primignani M, Chantarangkul V, Dell'Era A, Clerici M, de Franchis R, et al. An imbalance of pro- vs anti-coagulation factors in plasma from patients with cirrhosis. Gastroenterology. 2009;137:2105–11.
11. Hugenholtz GC, Macrae F, Adelmeijer J, Dulfer S, Porte RJ, Lisman T, et al. Procoagulant changes in fibrin clot structure in patients with cirrhosis are associated with oxidative modifications of fibrinogen. J Thromb Haemost. 2016;14:1054–66.
12. Weisel JW. Fibrinogen and fibrin. Adv Protein Chem. 2005;70:247–99.
13. Blasi A, Patel VC, Adelmeijer J, Azarian S, Hernandez Tejero M, Calvo A, et al. Mixed fibrinolytic phenotypes in decompensated cirrhosis and acute-on-chronic liver failure with Hypofibrinolysis in those with complications and poor survival. Hepatology. 2020;71:1381–90.
14. Hung A, Garcia-Tsao G. Acute kidney injury, but not sepsis, is associated with higher procedure-related bleeding in patients with decompensated cirrhosis. Liver Int. 2018;38:1437–41.
15. Zanetto A, Rinder HM, Campello E, Saggiorato G, Deng Y, Ciarleglio M, et al. Acute kidney injury in decompensated cirrhosis is associated with both hypo-coagulable and hyper-coagulable features. Hepatology. 2020;72:1327–40.

16. Intagliata NM, Davis JPE, Lafond J, Erdbruegger U, Greenberg CS, Northup PG, et al. Acute kidney injury is associated with low factor XIII in decompensated cirrhosis. Dig Liver Dis. 2019;51:1409–15.
17. D'Amico G, Garcia-Tsao G, Pagliaro L. Natural history and prognostic indicators of survival in cirrhosis: a systematic review of 118 studies. J Hepatol. 2006;44:217–31.
18. Vaz J, Eriksson B, Strömberg U, Buchebner D, Midlöv P. Incidence, aetiology and related comorbidities of cirrhosis: a Swedish population-based cohort study. BMC Gastroenterol. 2020;20:84.
19. Barnes GD, Lucas E, Alexander GC, Goldberger ZD. National Trends in ambulatory Oral anticoagulant use. Am J Med. 2015;128:1300–5.e2.
20. Virani SS, Alonso A, Aparicio HJ, Benjamin EJ, Bittencourt MS, Callaway CW, et al. Heart disease and stroke statistics–2021 update. Circulation. 2021;143:e254–743.
21. Villanova N, Moscatiello S, Ramilli S, Bugianesi E, Magalotti D, Vanni E, et al. Endothelial dysfunction and cardiovascular risk profile in nonalcoholic fatty liver disease. Hepatology. 2005;42:473–80.
22. Käräjämäki AJ, Pätsi O-P, Savolainen M, Kesäniemi YA, Huikuri H, Ukkola O. Non-alcoholic fatty liver disease as a predictor of atrial fibrillation in middle-aged population (OPERA study). PLoS One. 2015;10:e0142937.
23. Kuo L, Chao TF, Liu CJ, Lin YJ, Chang SL, Lo LW, et al. Liver cirrhosis in patients with atrial fibrillation: would oral anticoagulation have a net clinical benefit for stroke prevention? J Am Heart Assoc 2017;6:e005307.
24. Chokesuwattanaskul R, Thongprayoon C, Bathini T, Torres-Ortiz A, O'Corragain OA, Watthanasuntorn K, et al. Efficacy and safety of anticoagulation for atrial fibrillation in patients with cirrhosis: a systematic review and meta-analysis. Dig Liver Dis. 2019;51:489–95.
25. Serper M, Weinberg EM, Cohen JB, Reese PP, Taddei TH, Kaplan DE. Mortality and hepatic decompensation in patients with cirrhosis and atrial fibrillation treated with anticoagulation. Hepatology. 2021;73:219–32.
26. Russo MW, Pierson J, Narang T, Montegudo A, Eskind L, Gulati S. Coronary artery stents and antiplatelet therapy in patients with cirrhosis. J Clin Gastroenterol. 2012;46:339–44.
27. Krill T, Brown G, Weideman RA, Cipher DJ, Spechler SJ, Brilakis E, et al. Patients with cirrhosis who have coronary artery disease treated with cardiac stents have high rates of gastrointestinal bleeding, but no increased mortality. Aliment Pharmacol Ther. 2017;46:183–92.
28. Shin S, Lee SH, Lee M, Kim JH, Lee W, Lee HW, et al. Aspirin and the risk of hepatocellular carcinoma development in patients with alcoholic cirrhosis. Medicine (Baltimore). 2020;99:e19008.
29. Chen CY, Lee KT, Lee CT, Lai WT, Huang YB. Effectiveness and safety of antiplatelet therapy in stroke recurrence prevention in patients with liver cirrhosis: a 2-year follow-up study. Pharmacoepidemiol Drug Saf. 2012;21:1334–43.
30. Trankle CR, Vo C, Martin E, Puckett L, Siddiqui MS, Brophy DF, et al. Clopidogrel responsiveness in patients with decompensated cirrhosis of the liver undergoing pre-transplant PCI. JACC Cardiovasc Interv. 2020;13:661–3.
31. Northup PG, McMahon MM, Ruhl AP, Altschuler SE, Volk-Bednarz A, Caldwell SH, et al. Coagulopathy does not fully protect hospitalized cirrhosis patients from peripheral venous thromboembolism. Am J Gastroenterol. 2006;101:1524–8. quiz 680
32. Sogaard KK, Horvath-Puho E, Montomoli J, Vilstrup H, Sorensen HT. Cirrhosis is associated with an increased 30-day mortality after venous thromboembolism. Clin Transl Gastroenterol. 2015;6:e97.
33. Ambrosino P, Tarantino L, Di Minno G, Paternoster M, Graziano V, Petitto M, et al. The risk of venous thromboembolism in patients with cirrhosis. A systematic review and meta-analysis. Thromb Haemost. 2017;117:139–48.
34. Barbar S, Noventa F, Rossetto V, Ferrari A, Brandolin B, Perlati M, et al. A risk assessment model for the identification of hospitalized medical patients at risk for venous thromboembolism: the Padua prediction score. J Thromb Haemost. 2010;8:2450–7.

35. Decousus H, Tapson VF, Bergmann JF, Chong BH, Froehlich JB, Kakkar AK, et al. Factors at admission associated with bleeding risk in medical patients: findings from the IMPROVE investigators. Chest. 2011;139:69–79.
36. Davis JPE, O'Leary KE, Intagliata NM. Overuse of venous thromboembolism prophylaxis among hospitalized patients with liver disease. Eur J Haematol. 2020;104:223–9.
37. Northup PG, Garcia-Pagan JC, Garcia-Tsao G, Intagliata NM, Superina RA, Roberts LN, et al. Vascular liver disorders, portal vein thrombosis, and procedural bleeding in patients with liver disease: 2020 practice guidance by the American Association for the Study of Liver Diseases. Hepatology. 2021;73:366–413.
38. Simonetto DA, Singal AK, Garcia-Tsao G, Caldwell SH, Ahn J, Kamath PS. ACG clinical guideline: disorders of the hepatic and mesenteric circulation. Am J Gastroenterol. 2020;115:18–40.
39. European Association for the Study of the Liver. EASL clinical practice guidelines: vascular diseases of the liver. J Hepatol. 2016;64:179–202.
40. Nery F, Chevret S, Condat B, de Raucourt E, Boudaoud L, Rautou PE, et al. Causes and consequences of portal vein thrombosis in 1,243 patients with cirrhosis: results of a longitudinal study. Hepatology. 2015;61:660–7.
41. Villa E, Camma C, Marietta M, Luongo M, Critelli R, Colopi S, et al. Enoxaparin prevents portal vein thrombosis and liver decompensation in patients with advanced cirrhosis. Gastroenterology. 2012;143:1253–60 e4.
42. Englesbe MJ, Schaubel DE, Cai S, Guidinger MK, Merion RM. Portal vein thrombosis and liver transplant survival benefit. Liver Transpl. 2010;16:999–1005.
43. EASL Clinical Practice Guidelines. Vascular diseases of the liver. J Hepatol. 2016;64:179–202.
44. O'Shea RS, Davitkov P, Ko CW, Rajasekhar A, Su GL, Sultan S, et al. AGA clinical practice guideline on the Management of Coagulation Disorders in patients with cirrhosis. Gastroenterology. 2021;161:1615–27 e1.
45. Tripodi A, Primignani M, Chantarangkul V, Clerici M, Dell'Era A, Fabris F, et al. Thrombin generation in patients with cirrhosis: the role of platelets. Hepatology. 2006;44:440–5.
46. Awtry EH, Loscalzo J. Aspirin. Circulation. 2000;101:1206–18.
47. Roth GJ, Majerus PW. The mechanism of the effect of aspirin on human platelets. I. Acetylation of a particulate fraction protein. J Clin Invest. 1975;56:624–32.
48. Needs CJ, Brooks PM. Clinical pharmacokinetics of the salicylates. Clin Pharmacokinet. 1985;10:164–77.
49. Lanas A, Wu P, Medin J, Mills EJ. Low doses of acetylsalicylic acid increase risk of gastrointestinal bleeding in a meta-analysis. Clin Gastroenterol Hepatol. 2011;9:762–8.e6.
50. Patel SS, Guzman LA, Lin F-P, Pence T, Reichman T, John B, et al. Utilization of aspirin and statin in management of coronary artery disease in patients with cirrhosis undergoing liver transplant evaluation. Liver Transpl. 2018;24:872–80.
51. Dorsam RT, Kunapuli SP. Central role of the P2Y12 receptor in platelet activation. J Clin Invest. 2004;113:340–5.
52. Ford NF. The metabolism of Clopidogrel: CYP2C19 is a minor pathway. J Clin Pharmacol. 2016;56:1474–83.
53. Plavix [package insert]. 1997:Bridgewater, NJ: Bristol-Myers Squibb/Sanofi Pharmaceuticals Partnership.
54. Bhatt DL, Cryer BL, Contant CF, Cohen M, Lanas A, Schnitzer TJ, et al. Clopidogrel with or without omeprazole in coronary artery disease. N Engl J Med. 2010;363:1909–17.
55. Wu VC-C, Chen S-W, Chou A-H, Ting P-C, Chang C-H, Wu M, et al. Dual antiplatelet therapy in patients with cirrhosis and acute myocardial infarction–a 13-year nationwide cohort study. PLoS One. 2019;14:e0223380.
56. Keshmiri H, Behal A, Shroff S, Berkelhammer C. Clopidogrel-induced severe hepatitis: a case report and literature review. Case Reports Hepatol. 2016;2016:8068276.
57. Hirsh J, Anand SS, Halperin JL, Fuster V. Guide to anticoagulant therapy: heparin. Circulation. 2001;103:2994–3018.

58. van der Meer J-Y, Kellenbach E, van den Bos LJ. From farm to pharma: an overview of industrial heparin manufacturing methods. Molecules. 2017;22:1025.
59. Levine MN, Hirsh J, Gent M, Turpie AG, Cruickshank M, Weitz J, et al. A randomized trial comparing activated thromboplastin time with heparin assay in patients with acute venous thromboembolism requiring large daily doses of heparin. Arch Intern Med. 1994;154:49–56.
60. An International Randomized Trial Comparing Four Thrombolytic Strategies for Acute Myocardial Infarction. N Engl J Med. 1993;329:673–82.
61. Bechmann LP, Sichau M, Wichert M, Gerken G, Kroger K, Hilgard P. Low-molecular-weight heparin in patients with advanced cirrhosis. Liver Int. 2011;31:75–82.
62. Senzolo M, Rodriguez-Castro KI, Rossetto V, Radu C, Gavasso S, Carraro P, et al. Increased anticoagulant response to low-molecular-weight heparin in plasma from patients with advanced cirrhosis. J Thromb Haemost. 2012;10:1823–9.
63. Potze W, Arshad F, Adelmeijer J, Blokzijl H, van den Berg AP, Porte RJ, et al. Routine coagulation assays underestimate levels of antithrombin-dependent drugs but not of direct anticoagulant drugs in plasma from patients with cirrhosis. Br J Haematol. 2013;163:666–73.
64. Fuentes A, Gordon-Burroughs S, Hall JB, Putney DR, Monsour HP, Jr. Comparison of anti-Xa and activated partial thromboplastin time monitoring for heparin dosing in patients with cirrhosis. Ther Drug Monit 2015;37:40–4.
65. Intagliata NM, Henry ZH, Shah N, Lisman T, Caldwell SH, Northup PG. Prophylactic anticoagulation for venous thromboembolism in hospitalized cirrhosis patients is not associated with high rates of gastrointestinal bleeding. Liver Int. 2014;34:26–32.
66. Shatzel J, Dulai PS, Harbin D, Cheung H, Reid TN, Kim J, et al. Safety and efficacy of pharmacological thromboprophylaxis for hospitalized patients with cirrhosis: a single-center retrospective cohort study. J Thromb Haemost. 2015;13:1245–53.
67. Kwon J, Koh Y, Yu SJ, Yoon JH. Low-molecular-weight heparin treatment for portal vein thrombosis in liver cirrhosis: efficacy and the risk of hemorrhagic complications. Thromb Res. 2018;163:71–6.
68. Senzolo M, Sartori TM, Rossetto V, Burra P, Cillo U, Boccagni P, et al. Prospective evaluation of anticoagulation and transjugular intrahepatic portosystemic shunt for the management of portal vein thrombosis in cirrhosis. Liver Int. 2012;32:919–27.
69. Cui SB, Shu RH, Yan SP, Wu H, Chen Y, Wang L, et al. Efficacy and safety of anticoagulation therapy with different doses of enoxaparin for portal vein thrombosis in cirrhotic patients with hepatitis B. Eur J Gastroenterol Hepatol. 2015;27:914–9.
70. Delgado MG, Seijo S, Yepes I, Achecar L, Catalina MV, Garcia-Criado A, et al. Efficacy and safety of anticoagulation on patients with cirrhosis and portal vein thrombosis. Clin Gastroenterol Hepatol. 2012;10:776–83.
71. Amitrano L, Guardascione MA, Menchise A, Martino R, Scaglione M, Giovine S, et al. Safety and efficacy of anticoagulation therapy with low molecular weight heparin for portal vein thrombosis in patients with liver cirrhosis. J Clin Gastroenterol. 2010;44:448–51.
72. Chen H, Liu L, Qi X, He C, Wu F, Fan D, et al. Efficacy and safety of anticoagulation in more advanced portal vein thrombosis in patients with liver cirrhosis. Eur J Gastroenterol Hepatol. 2016;28:82–9.
73. Pettinari I, Vukotic R, Stefanescu H, Pecorelli A, Morelli M, Grigoras C, et al. Clinical impact and safety of anticoagulants for portal vein thrombosis in cirrhosis. Am J Gastroenterol 2019;114:258–66.
74. Francoz C, Belghiti J, Vilgrain V, Sommacale D, Paradis V, Condat B, et al. Splanchnic vein thrombosis in candidates for liver transplantation: usefulness of screening and anticoagulation. Gut. 2005;54:691–7.
75. Loffredo L, Pastori D, Farcomeni A, Violi F. Effects of anticoagulants in patients with cirrhosis and portal vein thrombosis: a systematic review and meta-analysis. Gastroenterology. 2017;153:480–7 e1.
76. Lee SR, Lee HJ, Choi EK, Han KD, Jung JH, Cha MJ, et al. Direct Oral anticoagulants in patients with atrial fibrillation and liver disease. J Am Coll Cardiol. 2019;73:3295–308.

77. Lisman T, van Leeuwen Y, Adelmeijer J, Pereboom IT, Haagsma EB, van den Berg AP, et al. Interlaboratory variability in assessment of the model of end-stage liver disease score. Liver Int. 2008;28:1344–51.
78. Trotter JF, Olson J, Lefkowitz J, Smith AD, Arjal R, Kenison J. Changes in international normalized ratio (INR) and model for endstage liver disease (MELD) based on selection of clinical laboratory. Am J Transplant. 2007;7:1624–8.
79. Porte RJ, Lisman T, Tripodi A, Caldwell SH, Trotter JF. Coagulation in liver disease study G. the international normalized ratio (INR) in the MELD score: problems and solutions. Am J Transplant. 2010;10:1349–53.
80. Tripodi A, Chantarangkul V, Primignani M, Fabris F, Dell'Era A, Sei C, et al. The international normalized ratio calibrated for cirrhosis (INR(liver)) normalizes prothrombin time results for model for end-stage liver disease calculation. Hepatology. 2007;46:520–7.
81. Werner KT, Sando S, Carey EJ, Vargas HE, Byrne TJ, Douglas DD, et al. Portal vein thrombosis in patients with end stage liver disease awaiting liver transplantation: outcome of anticoagulation. Dig Dis Sci. 2013;58:1776–80.
82. Chung JW, Kim GH, Lee JH, Ok KS, Jang ES, Jeong SH, et al. Safety, efficacy, and response predictors of anticoagulation for the treatment of nonmalignant portal-vein thrombosis in patients with cirrhosis: a propensity score matching analysis. Clin Mol Hepatol. 2014;20:384–91.
83. Goriacko P, Veltri KT. Safety of direct oral anticoagulants vs warfarin in patients with chronic liver disease and atrial fibrillation. Eur J Haematol. 2018;100:488–93.
84. La Mura V, Braham S, Tosetti G, Branchi F, Bitto N, Moia M, et al. Harmful and beneficial effects of anticoagulants in patients with cirrhosis and portal vein thrombosis. Clin Gastroenterol Hepatol. 2018;16:1146–52 e4.
85. Cerini F, Gonzalez JM, Torres F, Puente A, Casas M, Vinaixa C, et al. Impact of anticoagulation on upper-gastrointestinal bleeding in cirrhosis. Hepatology. 2015;62:575–83.
86. Lee SJ, Uhm JS, Kim JY, Pak HN, Lee MH, Joung B. The safety and efficacy of vitamin K antagonist in patients with atrial fibrillation and liver cirrhosis. Int J Cardiol. 2015;180:185–91.
87. Choi J, Kim J, Shim JH, Kim M, Nam GB. Risks versus benefits of anticoagulation for atrial fibrillation in cirrhotic patients. J Cardiovasc Pharmacol. 2017;70:255–62.
88. Hum J, Shatzel JJ, Jou JH, Deloughery TG. The efficacy and safety of direct oral anticoagulants vs traditional anticoagulants in cirrhosis. Eur J Haematol. 2017;98:393–7.
89. Pastori D, Lip GYH, Farcomeni A, Del Sole F, Sciacqua A, Perticone F, et al. Incidence of bleeding in patients with atrial fibrillation and advanced liver fibrosis on treatment with vitamin K or non-vitamin K antagonist oral anticoagulants. Int J Cardiol. 2018;264:58–63.
90. Lee HF, Chan YH, Chang SH, Tu HT, Chen SW, Yeh YH, et al. Effectiveness and safety of non-vitamin K antagonist Oral anticoagulant and warfarin in cirrhotic patients with Nonvalvular atrial fibrillation. J Am Heart Assoc. 2019;8:e011112.
91. Violi F, Vestri A, Menichelli D, Di Rocco A, Pastori D, Pignatelli P. Direct Oral anticoagulants in patients with atrial fibrillation and advanced liver disease: an exploratory meta-analysis. Hepatol Commun. 2020;4:1034–40.
92. Douxfils J, Gosselin RC. Laboratory assessment of direct oral anticoagulants. Semin Thromb Hemost. 2017;43:277–90.
93. Qamar A, Vaduganathan M, Greenberger NJ, Giugliano RP. Oral anticoagulation in patients with liver disease. J Am Coll Cardiol. 2018;71:2162–75.
94. Stangier J, Stahle H, Rathgen K, Roth W, Shakeri-Nejad K. Pharmacokinetics and pharmacodynamics of dabigatran etexilate, an oral direct thrombin inhibitor, are not affected by moderate hepatic impairment. J Clin Pharmacol. 2008;48:1411–9.
95. Graff J, Harder S. Anticoagulant therapy with the oral direct factor Xa inhibitors rivaroxaban, apixaban and edoxaban and the thrombin inhibitor dabigatran etexilate in patients with hepatic impairment. Clin Pharmacokinet. 2013;52:243–54.
96. Lisman T, Kamphuisen PW, Northup PG, Porte RJ. Established and new-generation antithrombotic drugs in patients with cirrhosis - possibilities and caveats. J Hepatol. 2013;59:358–66.

97. Kubitza D, Roth A, Becka M, Alatrach A, Halabi A, Hinrichsen H, et al. Effect of hepatic impairment on the pharmacokinetics and pharmacodynamics of a single dose of rivaroxaban, an oral, direct factor Xa inhibitor. Br J Clin Pharmacol. 2013;76:89–98.
98. Russmann S, Niedrig DF, Budmiger M, Schmidt C, Stieger B, Hurlimann S, et al. Rivaroxaban postmarketing risk of liver injury. J Hepatol. 2014;61:293–300.
99. Connolly SJ, Eikelboom J, Dorian P, Hohnloser SH, Gretler DD, Sinha U, et al. Betrixaban compared with warfarin in patients with atrial fibrillation: results of a phase 2, randomized, dose-ranging study (explore-Xa). Eur Heart J. 2013;34:1498–505.
100. Steuber TD, Howard ML, Nisly SA. Direct oral anticoagulants in chronic liver disease. Ann Pharmacother. 2019;53:1042–9.
101. Intagliata NM, Henry ZH, Maitland H, Shah NL, Argo CK, Northup PG, et al. Direct oral anticoagulants in cirrhosis patients pose similar risks of bleeding when compared to traditional anticoagulation. Dig Dis Sci. 2016;61:1721–7.
102. Davis KA, Puleo CR, Kovalic AJ, Nisly SA. Efficacy and safety of direct oral anticoagulant therapy for the treatment of venous thromboembolism in patients with chronic liver disease. Thromb Res. 2019;176:27–9.
103. Davis KA, Joseph J, Nisly SA. Direct oral anticoagulants and warfarin in patients with cirrhosis: a comparison of outcomes. J Thromb Thrombolysis. 2020;50:457–61.
104. De Gottardi A, Trebicka J, Klinger C, Plessier A, Seijo S, Terziroli B, et al. Antithrombotic treatment with direct-acting oral anticoagulants in patients with splanchnic vein thrombosis and cirrhosis. Liver Int. 2017;37:694–9.
105. Hanafy AS, Abd-Elsalam S, Dawoud MM. Randomized controlled trial of rivaroxaban versus warfarin in the management of acute non-neoplastic portal vein thrombosis. Vasc Pharmacol. 2019;113:86–91.
106. Nisly SA, Mihm AE, Gillette C, Davis KA, Tillett J. Safety of direct oral anticoagulants in patients with mild to moderate cirrhosis: a systematic review and meta-analysis. J Thromb Thrombolysis. 2021;52:817–27.
107. Mort JF, Davis JPE, Mahoro G, Stotts MJ, Intagliata NM, Northup PG. Rates of bleeding and discontinuation of direct Oral anticoagulants in patients with decompensated cirrhosis. Clin Gastroenterol Hepatol. 2021;19:1436–42.
108. Semmler G, Pomej K, Bauer DJM, Balcar L, Simbrunner B, Binter T, et al. Safety of direct oral anticoagulants in patients with advanced liver disease. Liver Int 2021;41:2159–70.
109. Oldham M, Palkimas S, Hedrick A. Safety and efficacy of direct oral anticoagulants in patients with moderate to severe cirrhosis. Ann Pharmacother. 2022;56:782–90.

Antibiotics in Liver Cirrhosis

4

Swati Chouhan, Prajna Anirvan,
and Shivaram Prasad Singh

Abstract

Patients with cirrhosis are susceptible to a wide variety of infections. Sepsis is an established precipitant of acute on chronic liver failure (ACLF). The occurrence of sepsis in cirrhosis is associated with high morbidity and mortality and warrants early recognition and prompt treatment. Antibiotics are widely used in patients with cirrhosis both prophylactically and as a part of treatment to control sepsis. However, since a majority of the antibiotics used are metabolized through the liver, it is important to take note of the altered pharmacodynamics and pharmacokinetics in cirrhosis while prescribing antibiotics. Drugs and medications can cause hepatic injury and exacerbate pre-existing liver disease, leading to decompensations and ACLF. Besides, patients with cirrhosis often have underlying renal dysfunction. This can be further potentiated by the use of nephrotoxic antibiotics. Antibiotics can also cause cytopenias, neurotoxicity, and skin injury. The emergence of drug-resistant bacteria is also a challenge in the setting of cirrhosis. Judicious and rational use of antibiotics, early de-escalation, and implementation of antibiotic stewardship programmes are essential to tackle the problem of drug resistance. Careful selection of antibiotics, knowledge of pharmacological profiles of antibiotics used, awareness of antibiotic-associated toxicities, and strategies to tackle drug resistance are important while prescribing antibiotics in patients with cirrhosis.

S. Chouhan
Bharati Vidyapeeth (deemed to be University) Medical College, Pune, Maharashtra, India

P. Anirvan · S. P. Singh (✉)
Department of Gastroenterology, S.C.B. Medical College, Cuttack, Odisha, India

X. Qi, Y. Yang (eds.), *Pharmacotherapy for Liver Cirrhosis and Its Complications*, https://doi.org/10.1007/978-981-19-2615-0_4

Keywords

Cirrhosis · Acute on chronic liver failure (ACLF) · Antibiotics · Antibiotic stewardship programme · Bacterial infections · Multidrug-resistant (MDR) infections · Sepsis · Spontaneous bacterial peritonitis (SBP)

4.1 Introduction

It is well known that patients with cirrhosis have a high risk of a wide variety of bacterial infections, and these bacterial infections by the way of inducing widespread systemic inflammation and subsequent alteration of haemodynamics can cause decompensation in compensated cirrhosis and in already decompensated cases can lead to sepsis and further decompensation by way of hepatic and extra hepatic organ failure (involving kidney, circulation/heart, lung) causing a syndrome called acute on chronic liver failure (ACLF) resulting in increased morbidity and mortality [1–3]. Thus, bacterial infections frequently precipitate ACLF [1, 4, 5] and are responsible for increased in-hospital mortality (four-fold to five-fold) [6]. Early diagnosis and timely initiation of appropriate antibiotic therapy in such cases will help in reducing the morbidity and mortality and improve the overall prognosis of the patient. This also includes prophylactic antibiotic therapy in selected cases. However, the burgeoning menace of multidrug-resistant (MDR) bacteria has complicated the situation by reducing the efficacy of commonly used antibiotics like third-generation cephalosporins. Prompt initiation of empirical broad-spectrum antibiotics as per local antibiogram has shown to improve prognosis of patients who are at high risk of MDR infections, such as those with nosocomial infections. However, early de-escalation of antibiotics is recommended to tackle further drug resistance. Strategies to prevent renal injury and other organ damage must be adopted.

Prophylactic antibiotic therapy should only be restricted to carefully selected cases who are at a very high risk of bacterial infections, where the benefit outweighs the risks so as not to escalate MDR. Antibiotics should be used judiciously, keeping in mind their pharmacokinetics, pharmacodynamics and adverse effect profile, so as to ensure effective and safe use and limit toxicities, especially hepatotoxicity and nephrotoxicity, which could further lead to decompensation in cirrhosis.

4.2 Bacterial Infections in Cirrhosis: An Overview

Bacterial infections are the leading cause of hospitalization in cirrhosis with a prevalence of 25–45% in patients admitted with decompensation. Patients with cirrhosis are 2.6 times more likely to develop sepsis than those without. The probability of death of patients with decompensated cirrhosis increases 3.75-fold because of bacterial infections, amounting to 30% at one month and 63% at one year, thus significantly increasing both short-term and long-term mortality [6, 7].

The higher risk of infections in cirrhosis is multifactorial and includes genetic predisposition in patients who carry NOD2, TLR 2, TLR 4, and FXR risk variants of genes [8–11].

Intestinal bacterial overgrowth (IBO) or intestinal dysbiosis (ID) is a major contributor to increased infection burden in cirrhosis [12–15]. Intestinal barrier dysfunction involving reduced secretion of protective IgA [16], biliary lipids [17], antimicrobial peptides (AMPs) [18] and impaired cellular tight junctions (TJ) [19, 20] further aid in infection pathogenesis by increasing pathological bacterial translocation (BT). Finally, cirrhosis-associated immune dysfunction (CAID), which comprises both innate and adaptive immune dysfunction along with persistent immune activation leading to immune paralysis, is the main underlying risk factor responsible for increased susceptibility to bacterial infections in cirrhosis [21–23].

Clinical factors which are associated with increased risk of infections are poor liver function, variceal haemorrhage (VH), low ascitic fluid protein level, prior spontaneous bacterial peritonitis (SBP), and hospitalization [24, 25]. Patients hospitalized with cirrhosis and infections are at high risk for subsequent infections, mostly at different sites, within 6 months of index infection resolution. Those at highest risk include previously infected older patients receiving proton pump inhibitors (PPIs) and/or SBP prophylaxis, although these associations do not prove that these factors are directly responsible for the infections [26].

SBP and urinary tract infections (UTI) are the most frequently reported infections followed by pneumonia, skin and soft tissue infections and bacteraemia [2, 24, 27]. Enterobacteriaceae and non-enterococcal streptococci cause the majority of infections in cirrhosis. Hence, beta-lactams and fluoroquinolones have been extensively used for treatment and prophylaxis. However, this has contributed to selection of resistant strains and altered the epidemiology of bacterial infections in cirrhosis [3, 25]. Spontaneous and secondary infections due to atypical pathogens or MDR bacteria are being increasingly reported and currently pose a major challenge in the management of cirrhosis of liver [2, 25]. The different MDR bacterial infections reported from several areas around the world include those caused by ESBL producing Enterobacteriaceae, which accounts for the majority of MDR infection burden. Others include *Pseudomonas aeruginosa, Acinetobacter baumannii*, vancomycin-susceptible enterococci (VSE), vancomycin-resistant enterococci (VRE) and methicillin-resistant *Staphylococcus aureus* (MRSA) [2, 8, 28].

The pathophysiology and manifestations of infection-induced organ failure are incompletely understood [3]. However, it has been demonstrated that these infections trigger an exaggerated host inflammatory response in a setting of pre-existing circulatory dysfunction due to splanchnic vasodilatation and cardiac dysfunction in cirrhosis. The inflammation causes rapid worsening of cardiovascular function and organ perfusion leading to acute kidney injury (AKI) and hepatorenal syndrome (HRS type-1). On the other hand, direct inflammatory organ damage due to endothelial dysfunction, oxidative stress, etc., leads to worsening of liver function, manifesting as jaundice and coagulopathy, and affects other organs, like brain, adrenal glands and gut, causing encephalopathy, adrenal insufficiency and increased translocation of bacteria and endotoxins. Thus ensues a clinical syndrome of hepatic and extra hepatic multi organ failure called ACLF, which is responsible for tremendously increasing mortality in cirrhosis [8, 29].

4.3 Antibiotic Pharmacology: Pharmacokinetics and Pharmacodynamics

Administration of routine antibiotics can sometimes pose a challenge in the special setting of cirrhosis and requires prior knowledge about their pharmacokinetics, pharmacodynamics, and adverse effects profile. A majority of antibiotics from several classes have predominant hepatic metabolism. Drug handling is impaired in patients with liver cirrhosis due to multiple causes, which include: (i) liver cell necrosis, (ii) shunting of the blood through portosystemic collaterals, (iii) reduction in the concentration of drug-binding proteins, (iv) abnormal drug pharmacokinetics, including altered volume distribution, drug elimination and metabolism, (v) altered pharmacodynamics, (vi) associated renal dysfunction, and (vii) drug–drug interaction. The impairment of drug metabolism is proportional to the liver dysfunction [30, 31]. Drug dosing should be individualized depending on a number of factors like nutritional status, renal function, adherence, and drug–drug interaction. Monitoring of the liver function at frequent intervals is a must [32, 33].

A thorough review of literature was performed to identify the antibiotics that need dosage alteration in patients with liver cirrhosis. Macrolide antibiotics, like erythromycin, azithromycin, clarithromycin, and others, like chloramphenicol and clindamycin, which are excreted and detoxified by liver, should be used with caution in these patients. Tetracycline, isoniazid, and rifampicin have prolonged half-life in patients with liver cirrhosis. Metronidazole, ketoconazole, miconazole, fluconazole, itraconazole, nitrofurantoin, and pyrazinamide are best avoided and should be used with great caution only if really necessary. Beta-lactam antibiotics can cause leukopenia, while amino glycosides can increase susceptibility to renal failure. Vancomycin can cause increased toxicity in patients with liver failure. Antibiotics which can produce hepatitis or cholestasis, like chloramphenicol, clindamycin, trimethoprim-sulfamethoxazole, and macrolides, should be avoided or used with great caution. Metronidazole dose should be reduced by 50% in patients with severe cirrhosis and/or associated renal insufficiency. There is no precise information on the safe use of nitrofurantoin, chloramphenicol, sodium fusidate, and pyrazinamide. But they are potentially toxic and hence their use is best avoided in liver disease [32, 34].

Reduction in fungal diversity or dysbiosis of mycobiota in cirrhosis patients has been linked to antibiotic use (rifaximin and SBP prophylaxis) and current practice of antibiotic therapy in culture-negative infections, thereby necessitating a low threshold for antifungal therapy in these patients [35]. Antifungal drugs, like ketoconazole, fluconazole, itraconazole, and miconazole, are hepatotoxic and should be used in patients with cirrhosis only when really necessary, but with monitoring of serum drug concentration and serial liver function tests. Compared with older generations of antifungals (i.e., amphotericin B, itraconazole, fluconazole, and voriconazole), echinocandins have been shown to have more favourable safety profiles, while having similar efficacy profiles [36–39]. According to a study, among the echinocandins, anidulafungin, caspofungin, and micafungin have shown similar risk profiles for severe hepatotoxicity. However, anidulafungin is a better choice for patients who are sicker or who have a poorer prognosis and comorbidities [40], as according to pharmacokinetic data, anidulafungin is the only echinocandin that undergoes elimination by chemical degradation [8] and non-specific peptidases in the plasma, instead of being metabolized by the liver [41].

4.4 Antibiotic Therapy in Cirrhosis: Indications

Antibiotic therapy in cirrhosis is broadly classified as prophylactic and therapeutic. Prophylaxis is restricted to a highly selective group of patients who are at very high risk of infections, such as those with prior history of SBP, cases of variceal bleed, and those with a very low level of ascitic fluid protein along with poor liver function and/or renal dysfunction (Table 4.1) [8]. The most commonly used drug is norfloxacin 400 mg once daily or twice daily. Since norfloxacin is not available in the USA, ciprofloxacin can be used as an alternative, although it has systemic side effects and a higher chance of selection of MDR organism strains.

Selective Intestinal Decontamination (SID), commonly performed using oral fluoroquinolones, a strategy to reduce infection rates, especially that of SBP in

Table 4.1 Antibiotic prophylaxis in cirrhosis: current indications[a]

Indication	Antibiotic and dose	Duration
Primary prophylaxis of SBP in patients with low-protein ascites (<1.5 g/dL) and advanced cirrhosis[b]	Norfloxacin 400 mg/day *or* ciprofloxacin 500 mg/day PO	Until liver transplantation or death
Secondary prophylaxis of SBP	Norfloxacin 400 mg/day *or* ciprofloxacin 500 mg/day PO	Until liver transplantation or death
Gastrointestinal bleeding	• Norfloxacin 400 mg/12 h *or* ciprofloxacin 500 mg/12 h PO. • Intravenous ceftriaxone 1 g/day in patients with advanced cirrhosis (presence of at least two of the following: Ascites, jaundice, hepatic encephalopathy and malnutrition).	5–7 days

Abbreviation: PO-by mouth (per os)

"Modified from J Hepatol. 2014;60(6), Jalan R, Fernandez J, Wiest R, Schnabl B, Moreau R, Angeli P, et al., Bacterial infections in cirrhosis: a position statement based on the EASL Special Conference 2013, Pages 1310–24, Copyright (2014), with permission from European Association for the Study of the Liver"

[a] These recommendations are supported by a good level of evidence (grade A1) according to the Grading of Recommendations Assessment, Development and Evaluation system

[b] Child–Pugh score ≥ 9 points with serum bilirubin ≥3 mg/dL and/or impaired renal function (serum creatinine ≥1.2 mg/dL, blood urea nitrogen ≥25 mg/dL, or serum sodium ≤130 mEq/L)

patients with advanced cirrhosis and variceal bleed, has been found to be effective in several randomized studies. However, it is not recommended as it significantly escalates the problem of MDR infections without any significant overall mortality or survival benefit. Rifaximin is a non-absorbed antibiotic recommended for the prevention of recurrent hepatic encephalopathy that has a broad spectrum of activity against Gram-negative and Gram-positive aerobes and anaerobes. Rather than having a bactericidal effect, rifaximin seems to have direct effects on bacterial function and virulence (e.g., bacterial adherence to intestinal cells). It causes very little disturbance of the normal stool microbiome, as confirmed in patients with cirrhosis [42]. A case–control study found a significant benefit with rifaximin for prophylaxis of SBP when used in patients with hepatic encephalopathy, without concomitant increase in the risk of MDR bacterial infections or *Clostridium difficile* infection because of its low bioavailability in blood after oral administration and bacterial virulence reducing effects [43]. Non-randomized data suggest that this is an effective yet balanced antibiotic strategy to reduce infections in cirrhosis, especially SBP, while also reducing complications like hepatic encephalopathy, VH, and HRS, without increasing risk of development of MDR [42, 44, 45]. The jury is still out on recommending its routine prophylactic use in cirrhosis as more robust evidence is necessary.

In case of patients who are hospitalized with infection, early initiation of appropriate broad-spectrum antibiotics is advocated. According to the EASL position paper, C-reactive protein (CRP) $\geq$10 ng/ml is a useful marker to predict the likelihood of clinically significant bacterial infections in patients with cirrhosis without overt infections, while the combination of CRP and procalcitonin (PCT) with cut-off values of $\geq$24.7 ng/ml and $\geq$ 0.49, respectively, has proven to be extremely useful in diagnosis of sepsis, in addition to clinical and other parameters [8]. The choice of antibiotics used is based on the site and severity of infection, whether it is community acquired, health care associated or nosocomial and the local prevalence of MDR organism, in consultation with the overall local antibiogram of the institute (Table 4.2). Blood and body fluid culture and sensitivity carried out prior to initiation of antibiotics are an important tool to guide antibiotic usage, especially to narrow down and de-escalate antibiotics as per the isolate detected, so as to reduce the emergence of MDR organisms.

For patients with severe sepsis or septic shock or those requiring critical care with APACHE II score $\geq$ 15 or SOFA score $\geq$ 8, empirical antibiotic therapy should be initiated early as per a Spanish National stewardship programme with a regimen of meropenem + glycopeptides with or without addition of ciprofloxacin, amikacin and/or colistin and ± echinocandin for antifungal coverage (Fig. 4.1). However, for less critical patients not fulfilling the above criteria, third-generation cephalosporins, like ceftriaxone, can be started if MDR bacteria risk is low, while ertapenem ± glycopeptides must be started if MDR bacteria risk is high as per the local epidemiological data (Fig. 4.1). It is extremely important to re-evaluate the antibiotic treatment at 48–72 h, based on the culture and susceptibility pattern of isolated strain and the clinical outcome of patient. Suitable modification and de-escalation of antibiotics should be done according to the above parameters, and treatment

Table 4.2 Recommended empirical antibiotic treatment for community-acquired and nosocomial bacterial infections in cirrhosis[a]

Type of infection	Community-acquired infections	Nosocomial infections[b]
SBP, spontaneous bacterial empyema (SBE), and spontaneous bacteraemia	Cefotaxime *or* ceftriaxone *or* amoxicillin/clavulanic acid	Piperacillin/tazobactam[c] or meropenem[d] ± glycopeptide[e]
UTI	*Uncomplicated:* Ciprofloxacin or cotrimoxazole *If sepsis:* Cefotaxime *or* ceftriaxone *or* amoxicillin/clavulanic acid	*Uncomplicated:* Nitrofurantoin or fosfomycin *If sepsis:* Piperacillin/tazobactam *or* meropenem glycopeptide
Pneumonia[f]	Amoxicillin/ clavulanic acid *or* ceftriaxone + macrolide *or* levofloxacin *or* moxifloxacin	Piperacillin/tazobactam[c] *or* meropenem/ ceftazidime + ciprofloxacin ± glycopeptide[e] should be added in patients with risk factors for MRSA[h]
Cellulitis	Amoxicillin/ clavulanic acid or ceftriaxone + oxacillin	Meropenem/ceftazidime[g] + oxacillin *or* glycopeptide[e]

"Modified from J Hepatol. 2014;60(6), Jalan R, Fernandez J, Wiest R, Schnabl B, Moreau R, Angeli P, et al., Bacterial infections in cirrhosis: a position statement based on the EASL Special Conference 2013, Pages 1310–24, Copyright (2014), with permission from European Association for the Study of the Liver"

[a] Abbreviations: *SBP* spontaneous bacterial peritonitis; *SBE* spontaneous bacterial empyema; *MRSA* methicillin-resistant *Staphylococcus aureus*

[b] Recommended empirical treatment also for healthcare-associated (HCA) urinary infections and pneumonia. Empirical antibiotic treatment of HCA spontaneous infections and cellulitis is decided on the basis of the severity of infection (patients with severe sepsis should receive the regimen proposed for nosocomial infections) and on the local epidemiology of MDR bacteria

[c] In areas with a low prevalence of multiresistant bacteria

[d] To cover extended-spectrum b-lactamase (ESBL)-producing Enterobacteriaceae

[e] IV vancomycin or teicoplanin in areas with a high prevalence MRSA and vancomycin-susceptible enterococci (VSE). Glycopeptides must be replaced by IV linezolid in areas with a high prevalence of vancomycin-resistant enterococci (VRE)

[f] Liver disease is considered as severe comorbidity for community-acquired pneumonia in guidelines

[g] active against *Pseudomonas aeruginosa*

[h] Ventilator-associated pneumonia, previous antibiotic therapy, nasal MRSA carriage

should be continued for 5 days if the source of infection has been removed, but for 7 days for other infections [46]. Possibility of MDR and fungal infection must be considered in non-responders or poor responders to appropriate antibiotic therapy and hence, a good antifungal agent must be added to the higher antibiotic regimen.

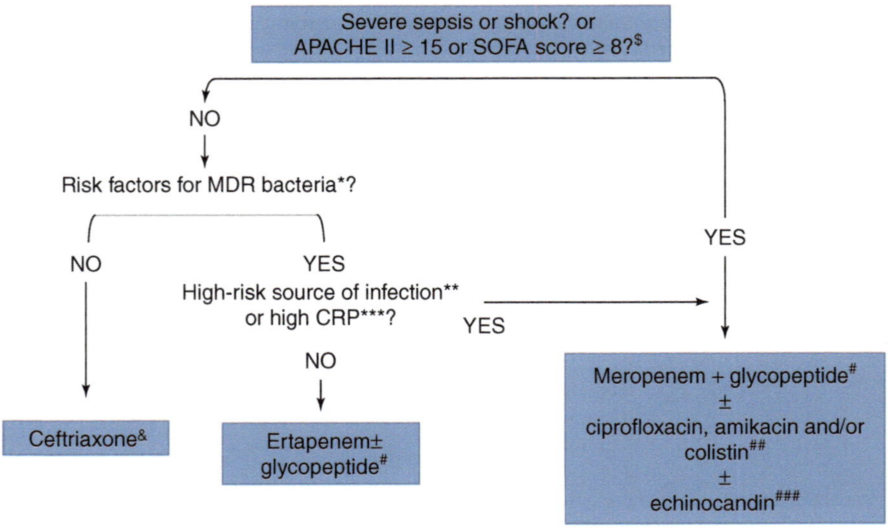

Fig. 4.1 Empirical antibiotic schedules suggested in critical care in the setting of a Spanish stewardship programme aimed at preventing the development of MDR bacteria. Empirical treatment is decided according to the severity of infection, the presence of risk factors for MDR bacteria, and the local epidemiology. Broader-spectrum antibiotics are used in the most severe infections, covering all possible pathogens.
$score values associated with a predicted hospital mortality ≥20%; *previous colonization, antibiotic treatment ≥5 days in the last 3 months, hospitalization ≥5 days in the last 3 months and nursing home/long-term care facility. In these patients, nasal and rectal swabs should be performed to look for MDR colonization; **high-risk infection: pneumonia, secondary peritonitis (high bacterial load) or high risk of severe complications (meningitis). Urinary tract infection, cellulitis, catheter infection and suspected infection are considered infections of moderate or low risk; ***C-reactive protein levels correlate with bacterial load and liver function: ≥25 mg/dL, 15 mg/dL and 10 mg/dL in Child–Pugh A, B, and C patients, respectively
&plus azithromycin in community-acquired pneumonia
#change glycopeptides to daptomycin in infections with high risk of bacteraemia (catheter, endocarditis) or to linezolid in pneumonia, cellulitis or meningitis; ##consider adding one or more of these antibiotics depending on the local epidemiology, recent antibiotic treatments (6 weeks) and source of infection; ###consider adding an echinocandin if two or more of the following criteria are present: multifocal colonization by Candida sp. (e.g., candiduria, rectal swab), antibiotic treatment or steroids, parenteral nutrition, gastroduodenal surgery or necrohaemorrhagic pancreatitis, renal replacement therapy
Abbreviations: *APACHE* Acute Physiology and Chronic Health Evaluation; *CRP* C-reactive protein; SOFA, Sequential Organ Failure Assessment. "Reprinted from Hepatology. 2016 Jun;63(6), Fernández J, Tandon P, Mensa J, Garcia-Tsao G, Antibiotic prophylaxis in cirrhosis: Good and bad, Pages 2019-31, Copyright (2015), with permission from American Association for the Study of Liver Diseases"

After the diagnosis of severe infections or sepsis, dosing strategies aimed at optimizing the antibiotics' pharmacokinetics/pharmacodynamics should also be applied within the first 48–72 h in order to improve clinical efficacy and minimize the selection of MDR strains. These strategies consist of the use of high antibiotic doses and of continuous or extended infusions in time-dependent antibiotics, like beta-lactams (Table 4.3) [47].

Table 4.3 Empiric antibiotic strategies and de-escalation rules implemented in intensive care units across Spain in critically ill patients as an example of antibiotic stewardship to prevent the selection of MDR bacteria

Antibiotic	Initial dose[g]	First 48 h[a]	At 72 h[a]
Cefotaxime	2 g	6–8 g/day in continuous infusion	1–2 g/8 h[b]
Ceftriaxone	2 g	1 g/12 h	1 g/12–24 h
Ceftazidime Meropenem	2 g	6 g/day in continuous infusion	1–2 g/8 h[b]
Piperacillin-tazobactam	4 (0.5) g	16 g/day in continuous infusion	4 (0.5) g/6–8 h[b]
Levofloxacin	1000 mg	500 mg/12 h	500 mg/24 h
Ciprofloxacin	600 mg	400 mg/8 h	400 mg/8–12 h
Fosfomycin[c]	4 g	200–300 mg/kg/day in continuous infusion	2 g/6 h
Tigecycline	200 mg[d]	100 mg/12h[d]	50–100 mg/12 h[d]
Metronidazole	1000–1500 mg	500 mg/6 h	500 mg/6–8 h
Linezolid	600 mg	600 mg/8 h	600 mg/12 h
Daptomycin	10 mg/kg	8–10 mg/kg/day	6–8 mg/kg/day
Vancomycin	20 mg/kg	15–20 mg/kg/8–12 h	Doses adjusted to C_{min} of 15 mg/L
Teicoplanin	12–15 mg/kg	8–12 mg/kg/day	8 mg/kg/day
Clindamycin	900 mg	600 mg/6 h	600 mg/8 h
Amikacin[e]	25 mg/kg	20 mg/kg/day[f]	Consider stopping or adjust the serum concentration
Gentamicin[e] Tobramycin[e]	7–9 mg/kg	7 mg/kg/day[f]	–
Colistin	6–9 MU	4.5 MU/12 h	4.5 MU/12 h

High doses of antibiotics are administered in the first 48 h to achieve high concentrations in plasma, thus ensuring a rapid decrease in bacterial load and preventing the selection of MDR bacteria

Abbreviations: C_{min} minimum or trough concentration; *MU* million units

"Reprinted from Hepatology. 2016 Jun;63(6), Fernández J, Tandon P, Mensa J, Garcia-Tsao G, Antibiotic prophylaxis in cirrhosis: Good and bad, Pages 2019–31, Copyright (2015), with permission from American Association for the Study of Liver Diseases"

[a] Recommended dose in patients with glomerular filtration rate > 60 mL/min

[b] In extended infusion (4 h)

[c] 13.5 mEq of Na^1 per gram of fosfomycin

[d] Recommended dose in Child–Pugh A patients (Child–Pugh B/C: initial dose of 100 mg followed by 50 mg/12 h)

[e] Aminoglycosides should be avoided in patients with cirrhosis due to the high risk of acute kidney injury. Their use is only indicated in patients with infection by XDR bacteria. Doses must be adjusted to plasma concentration obtained at second dose

[f] Adjusted body weight

[g] The initial dose is independent on renal function

4.5 Antibiotic-Associated Toxicities in Cirrhosis

Prescription of antibiotics in cirrhosis often presents a unique challenge to the physician. The metabolism of various antibiotics, including antitubercular drugs, is governed by the class of drug, its mechanism of action and by pharmacokinetic and pharmacodynamic principles. Patients with cirrhosis are at higher risk of developing hepatoxicity, nephrotoxicity and neurotoxicity due to alterations in metabolic pathways and concurrent renal dysfunction. Since an overwhelming majority of drugs are primarily metabolized and excreted by the hepatobiliary system, hepatocellular failure leads to impairment in drug handling while portosystemic shunting in cirrhosis causes alterations in drug action.

4.5.1 Hepatotoxicity

In addition to the altered metabolic pathways consequent to hepatocellular failure, factors like lifestyle and nutritional status may determine susceptibility to liver injury in patients with cirrhosis [48]. Malnutrition and fasting have been found to be associated with increased risk of Drug Induced Liver Injury (DILI). Conversely, overnutrition and obesity are risk factors for Nonalcoholic Fatty Liver Disease (NAFLD) which can be a risk factor for DILI [49–51]. Further, chronic alcohol consumption is associated with a state of chronic inflammation which can lead to mitochondrial damage, oxidative stress and predispose individuals to liver injury [51]. Chronic inflammation can also impair the detoxification and elimination mechanisms of the liver thereby aggravating cellular injury. However, although it has been claimed that underlying liver disease does not increase the risk of idiosyncratic DILI [52], once DILI occurs, it may lead to worse outcomes. Chronic hepatitis B and C, though, have been reported to be risk factors for antitubercular therapy (ATT) induced liver injury [53, 54]. It is worth mentioning here that Zimmerman, the father of DILI, had suggested that despite the lack of data suggesting that most hepatotoxic drugs were harmful in the setting of CLD, in the event of an occurrence of DILI, patients with impaired hepatic function could have worse outcomes [33].

Antimicrobials constitute one of the major causes of severe DILI and have been reported to be the single largest class of agents causing acute liver failure (ALF) [55]. Antibiotic-induced hepatotoxicity is mostly idiosyncratic. However, intrinsic properties of drugs do play a role in idiosyncratic reactions. Antibiotic-induced hepatotoxicity can present as hepatocellular, cholestatic, or mixed patterns of injury or even as granulomatous injury and steatohepatitis [56].

In the background of cirrhosis, diagnosing antibiotic-induced hepatotoxicity is difficult since it is usually a diagnosis of exclusion and requires a high degree of clinical suspicion. Other common causes of liver injury, like viral hepatitis, alcoholic hepatitis, and biliary tract disease, need to be ruled out prior to making a diagnosis of antibiotic-induced hepatotoxicity. Certain clinical indicators suggesting DILI include the appearance of rash, fever or eosinophilia, a 1–5-week duration of exposure to the drug and rapid reappearance of similar features upon rechallenge.

Although considered to be the gold standard, rechallenge is impractical and also unethical in current medical practice. Therefore, instruments have been devised to objectively assess DILI, the Roussel-Uclaf Causality Assessment Method (RUCAM) being one of the most frequently used.

The interval between antibiotic administration and the development of hepatotoxicity is variable. It may occur immediately or may take months to appear. It is important, therefore, to monitor patients even after they have been discharged from the hospital or have completed their treatment. Treatment consists of prompt withdrawal of the drug and management of hepatotoxicity as per existing guidelines.

4.5.2 Nephrotoxicity

Renal dysfunction occurs commonly in patients with cirrhosis and is attributable to a number of factors. These include AKI from complications of liver disease and infections, functional renal failure in cirrhosis—HRS, chronic kidney disease (IgA nephropathy), and systemic conditions, like polycystic kidney and liver disease. Patients with cirrhosis are thus at a significant risk of developing drug induced nephrotoxicity. Additionally, factors like reduced muscle mass and impaired metabolism of creatine to creatinine in cirrhosis render estimations of creatinine clearance based on serum creatinine measurements (e.g., Cockcroft–Gault equation) inaccurate [57]. A glomerular filtration rate (GFR) of less than 85% has been shown to be associated with a higher risk of nephrotoxicity in non-cirrhotic patients. Patients with cirrhosis and portal hypertension often have a GFR less than 85% of the normal [58]. Renal dysfunction in cirrhosis is a crucial determinant of prognosis and an important component of the MELD score.

Aminoglycosides and vancomycin are known to be nephrotoxic and should be used with caution in liver cirrhosis. They are indicated mainly in cases of severe infection with sepsis in which a combination of beta-lactam antibiotics with aminoglycoside is preferred for synergistic action. It has been suggested that a short course and a once-daily schedule of administration can minimize the risk of aminoglycoside-induced nephrotoxicity [52]. Vancomycin has been shown to be associated with higher mortality (HR = 1.640, CI = 1.119 to 2.405, $p = 0.011$) in acutely decompensated cirrhosis patients [59]. It is not clear whether this is due to resultant nephrotoxicity or the presence of drug-resistant bacteria.

Fluoroquinolones are frequently administered to patients with cirrhosis, especially in the setting of SBP. Significant changes in plasma levels or half-life have not been observed with ciprofloxacin administration, and therefore, no dosing adjustments are necessary in cirrhosis [60]. Reduced renal elimination of ofloxacin has been reported in cirrhosis and dose adjustment is required [61]. Fluroquinolones have also been reported to cause QTc interval prolongation in patients who have undergone transjugular intrahepatic portosystemic shunt, and this should be kept in mind [62].

Monitoring of renal function is important in cirrhosis and assumes more importance during antibiotic therapy. Owing to the multifactorial aetiology of renal impairment in cirrhosis, it is essential to rule out other causes of renal dysfunction before attributing it to antibiotics. Once renal dysfunction or renal failure occurs, it is equally important to modify medications, including antibiotics, as per existing guidelines.

4.5.3 Neurotoxicity

A number of antimicrobials are known to cause neurotoxicity. The antimicrobial classes predominantly causing neurotoxicity are fluoroquinolones, macrolides, sulphonamides, nitrofurans, and β-lactams. Age is an important risk factor for development of neurotoxicity. The mechanism of neurotoxicity varies depending upon the antimicrobial class involved. Presence of risk factors, like age, renal dysfunction, or the occurrence of drug interactions, increases the likelihood of neurotoxicity [63]. Therefore, drug dosing, use of concurrent medications, and the presence of comorbidities need to be taken into account in order to minimize the occurrence of neurotoxicity.

Antibiotics are an often underrecognized class of medications associated with delirium. Awareness of antibiotic-associated encephalopathy (AAE) is required in clinical decision making while evaluating patients with cirrhosis and hepatic encephalopathy. Phenotypically, AAE can be divided into three classes: seizures or myoclonus arising within days after antibiotic administration (cephalosporins and penicillin), psychosis arising within days after antibiotic administration (quinolones, macrolide and procaine penicillin) and cerebellar signs and MRI abnormalities weeks after initiation of antibiotics (metronidazole) [64].

Although approved for use in hepatic encephalopathy, neomycin is known to cause both nephrotoxicity and neurotoxicity including ototoxicity. Systemic absorption of neomycin is increased in hepatic and renal failure [65]. The rate of elimination of metronidazole is prolonged in patients with hepatic encephalopathy with consequent irreversible peripheral neurotoxicity and therefore, metronidazole is not recommended for the management of hepatic encephalopathy [66].

4.5.4 Other Toxicities

Cytopenias in cirrhosis are thought to be caused by hypersplenism and alcohol induced bone marrow suppression. However, it is quite possible that multiple other factors may be responsible for causing cytopenias in cirrhosis. It has been suggested that broad-spectrum antibiotics commonly used in cirrhosis can cause gut dysbiosis, leading to impaired haematopoiesis and increasing the susceptibility to infections [67].

Beta-lactam antibiotics should be used cautiously because of the propensity to induce leukopenia when administered in usually recommended dosages in patients with hepatic dysfunction [68]. Piperacillin/tazobactam has been reported to cause agranulocytosis, thrombocytopenia, and severe hepatic dysfunction [69]. Impaired hepatic metabolism leading to high antibiotic concentrations results in bone marrow suppression, and the risk increases with the severity of hepatic dysfunction. Therefore, it has been suggested that dosages of beta-lactam antibiotics should be reduced in the setting of hepatic dysfunction [68]. Quinolones and beta-lactam antibiotics have also been found to have a statistically significant association with thrombocytopenia [70].

Antimicrobials, like sulphonamides, dapsone, cotrimoxazole, sulphasalazine amoxicillin, ampicillin, minocycline, and antitubercular agents, have been implicated in drug induced skin injury along with DILI [71]. Concomitant occurrence of DILI and drug induced skin injury is not common and is associated with features of hypersensitivity like fever, rash, eosinophilia, lymphadenopathy, and mucositis. Although alterations in liver function tests are common in Stevens–Johnson Syndrome/Toxic Epidermal Necrolysis, severe hepatic injury is rare. Human Leukocyte Antigen (HLA) genotype is strongly associated with drug induced skin injury and hypersensitivity features as well as with Stevens–Johnson Syndrome/ Toxic Epidermal Necrolysis [71].

4.6 Antitubercular Therapy in Cirrhosis

ATT in cirrhosis deserves special mention. Patients with cirrhosis are at a greater risk for tuberculosis compared to non-cirrhotic patients, especially those with chronic alcohol intake and hepatitis C infection [72]. Antitubercular drugs are known to cause hepatotoxicity, and treatment of tuberculosis in patients with cirrhosis often gets complicated by the development of liver injury. Rifampicin is extensively metabolized in the liver and is eliminated in the bile. Hepatotoxicity is probably due to toxic idiosyncratic metabolic products or induction of an immunologic reaction [73]. Rifampicin can worsen liver function in cirrhosis, and the risk increases with concomitant use of isoniazid [74]. Isoniazid is known to cause DILI, especially in slow acetylators, elderly patients, patients with cirrhosis and those with underlying chronic hepatitis B and C [75–77]. Concomitant chronic alcohol use has also been reported to increase the risk of hepatotoxicity [78]. Although it has been used safely with liver enzyme monitoring in cirrhotic patients awaiting liver transplant [79] and has also been used to treat post-transplant tuberculosis [80, 81], a great degree of caution is required while prescribing isoniazid in cirrhosis, especially in combination with other antitubercular drugs. The half-life of pyrazinamide is increased in hepatic impairment [82] and therefore, therapy needs close monitoring in cirrhosis. Therefore, in patients with cirrhosis, it has been suggested that pyrazinamide should be substituted with a fluoroquinolone or an aminoglycoside as per the physician's discretion [83]. Ofloxacin can also be safely substituted for rifampicin and may be less hepatotoxic when combined with pyrazinamide compared to a combination of rifampicin with pyrazinamide [84]. Recommended ATT in Child class A cirrhosis is similar to that for non-cirrhosis population with close monitoring. Pyrazinamide is avoided in Child class B patients while isoniazid should not be concomitantly used with rifampicin. Isoniazid or rifampicin with ethambutol and fluoroquinolones are administered for 12 to 18 months. However, in Child class C patients, use of hepatotoxic ATT drugs is contraindicated; Ethambutol, fluoroquinolones and a second-line agent are administered for a duration of 12 to 18 months [34, 83].

4.7 Drug Resistance and MDR Infections

MDR bacterial infections negatively impact the prognosis in patients with decompensated liver disease and ACLF. The prevalence of MDR infections is gradually increasing. The prevalence of MDR bacterial infections in a cohort of culture-positive infections was found to be 29.2% [85]. In another study, MDR bacteria were isolated in 51% of cases with predominance of extended-spectrum b-lactamase producing Enterobacteriaceae, *Enterococcus faecium*, *Enterococcus faecalis*, *Pseudomonas aeruginosa,* and Methicillin-resistant *Staphylococcus aureus*. Extensively drug-resistant (XDR) bacteria were isolated in 6.2% cases, while one case of pan-drug-resistant (PDR) bacteria was reported. Therefore, strategies to combat the spread of antibiotic resistance in cirrhosis need to be considered urgently.

Factors independently associated with MDR bacterial infections include history of hospitalization in an intensive/intermediate care unit in the previous month and antibiotic therapy in the previous 3 months, while prophylaxis for SBP has also been found to be an independent risk factor for MDR infection [86–88]. Alcohol-associated liver disease and alcohol consumption have also been associated with greater rates of infection and antibiotic resistance [89].

4.8 Antibiotic Selection and Antibiotic Stewardship Programme

While prescribing antibiotics, it is important that multiple factors, such as the source of infection—community or nosocomial, history of recent antibiotic use or history of MDR infections, be considered [25]. Beta-Lactams are often preferred in treating community-acquired infections [90, 91]. However, while dealing with nosocomial infections, the pattern of local antibiotic resistance should be carefully looked at. Diagnosis of a bacterial infection warrants the initiation of empirical antibiotics [8]. Delay in initiation of antibiotic treatment has been shown to increase the risk of mortality in patients with cirrhosis and septic shock [92]. Broad-spectrum antibiotics should be considered in high-risk patients [91]. Therapy should, however, be tailored to the most appropriate single antibiotic after identifying the source of infection and the specific pathogen. Empiric antifungal therapy may be started in patients not responding to broad-spectrum antibiotics after 48–72 h. Initiation of empirical antibiotic treatment depends upon the following factors: type of infection, presence of risk factors for MDR bacterial infection, severity of infection and local resistance patterns. Particular emphasis should be put on the occurrence of likely adverse effects and the necessity to spare antibiotics active against MDR bacteria [25].

European Association for the Study of Liver (EASL) guidelines recommend the use of third-generation cephalosporins as the first-line antibiotic treatment for community-acquired SBP in regions with low rates of bacterial resistance while in regions with high rates of resistance, piperacillin/tazobactam or carbapenem should be considered [93]. In healthcare-associated and nosocomial SBP, piperacillin/tazobactam in areas with low prevalence of MDR and carbapenem in areas with high prevalence of ESBL producing Enterobacteriaceae are the recommended antimicrobial agents. Additionally, in areas with high prevalence of Gram-positive MDR bacteria, it is recommended that carbapenem should be combined with glycopeptides or daptomycin or linezolid.

Use of antibiotics, like vancomycin and aminoglycosides, may be required in case of severe infections in cirrhosis. Considering the known nephrotoxicity of these antibiotics, it is recommended that plasma levels of these antibiotics should be monitored [93].

Antibiotic stewardship programmes should be implemented in hospitals with emphasis on the prevention of antibiotic overuse and well-defined early de-escalation policies [94]. Early de-escalation policies and keeping the duration of antibiotic treatments to the minimum are key aspects to prevent antibiotic resistance. De-escalation should be based on bacterial susceptibility according to culture reports. Practices, like hand hygiene, barrier precaution, avoidance of unnecessary instrumentation, and control of ventilator-associated pneumonia, are equally important [95].

4.9 Conclusion

Cirrhosis is a multisystem disorder and presents a unique situation where multiple factors combine to render the patient susceptible to a wide variety of infections. Timely initiation of antibiotics can significantly reduce morbidity and mortality. However, antibiotic prescription in cirrhosis has to be rational and judicious, keeping in mind the growing problem of drug resistance and the altered pharmacodynamics and pharmacokinetics. Awareness of antibiotic-associated toxicities in cirrhosis, early recognition of adverse effects, and strict implementation of antibiotic stewardship programmes are extremely crucial while prescribing antibiotics in the setting of chronic liver disease and cirrhosis.

References

1. Moreau R, Jalan R, Gines P, et al. Acute-on-chronic liver failure is a distinct syndrome that develops in patients with acute decompensation of cirrhosis. Gastroenterology. 2013;144:1426–37, 1437.e1–9.
2. Fernández J, Acevedo J, Castro M, et al. Prevalence and risk factors of infections by multiresistant bacteria in cirrhosis: a prospective study. Hepatology. 2012;55:1551–61.
3. Gustot T, Durand F, Lebrec D, Vincent J-L, Moreau R. Severe sepsis in cirrhosis. Hepatology. 2009;50:2022–33.

4. Piano S, Tonon M, Vettore E, et al. Incidence, predictors and outcomes of acute-on-chronic liver failure in outpatients with cirrhosis. J Hepatol. 2017;67:1177–84.
5. Fernández J, Acevedo J, Wiest R, et al. Bacterial and fungal infections in acute-on-chronic liver failure: prevalence, characteristics and impact on prognosis. Gut. 2018;67:1870–80.
6. Arvaniti V, D'Amico G, Fede G, et al. Infections in patients with cirrhosis increase mortality four-fold and should be used in determining prognosis. Gastroenterology. 2010;139:1246–56, 1256.e1–5.
7. Foreman MG, Mannino DM, Moss M. Cirrhosis as a risk factor for sepsis and death: analysis of the National Hospital Discharge Survey. Chest. 2003;124:1016–20.
8. Jalan R, Fernandez J, Wiest R, et al. Bacterial infections in cirrhosis: a position statement based on the EASL special conference 2013. J Hepatol. 2014;60:1310–24.
9. Appenrodt B, Grünhage F, Gentemann MG, Thyssen L, Sauerbruch T, Lammert F. Nucleotide-binding oligomerization domain containing 2 (NOD2) variants are genetic risk factors for death and spontaneous bacterial peritonitis in liver cirrhosis. Hepatology. 2010;51:1327–33.
10. Nischalke HD, Berger C, Aldenhoff K, et al. Toll-like receptor (TLR) 2 promoter and intron 2 polymorphisms are associated with increased risk for spontaneous bacterial peritonitis in liver cirrhosis. J Hepatol. 2011;55:1010–6.
11. Soriano G, Sánchez E, Nieto JC, et al. Cytokine production in patients with cirrhosis and D299g and/or T399i toll-like receptor 4 polymorphisms. J Hepatol. 2013;58:S247–8.
12. Bauer TM, Steinbrückner B, Brinkmann FE, et al. Small intestinal bacterial overgrowth in patients with cirrhosis: prevalence and relation with spontaneous bacterial peritonitis. Am J Gastroenterol. 2001;96:2962–7.
13. Morencos FC, de las Heras Castaño G, Martín Ramos L, López Arias MJ, Ledesma F, Pons Romero F. Small bowel bacterial overgrowth in patients with alcoholic cirrhosis. Dig Dis Sci. 1995;40:1252–6.
14. Pande C, Kumar A, Sarin SK. Small-intestinal bacterial overgrowth in cirrhosis is related to the severity of liver disease. Aliment Pharmacol Ther. 2009;29:1273–81.
15. Chang CS, Chen GH, Lien HC, Yeh HZ. Small intestine dysmotility and bacterial overgrowth in cirrhotic patients with spontaneous bacterial peritonitis. Hepatology. 1998;28:1187–90.
16. Saitoh O, Sugi K, Lojima K, et al. Increased prevalence of intestinal inflammation in patients with liver cirrhosis. World J Gastroenterol. 1999;5:391–6.
17. Lorenzo-Zúñiga V, Bartolí R, Planas R, et al. Oral bile acids reduce bacterial overgrowth, bacterial translocation, and endotoxemia in cirrhotic rats. Hepatology. 2003;37:551–7.
18. Teltschik Z, Wiest R, Beisner J, et al. Intestinal bacterial translocation in rats with cirrhosis is related to compromised Paneth cell antimicrobial host defense. Hepatology. 2012;55:1154–63.
19. Assimakopoulos SF, Tsamandas AC, Tsiaoussis GI, et al. Altered intestinal tight junctions' expression in patients with liver cirrhosis: a pathogenetic mechanism of intestinal hyperpermeability. Eur J Clin Investig. 2012;42:439–46.
20. Assimakopoulos SF, Charonis AS. Uncovering the molecular events associated with increased intestinal permeability in liver cirrhosis: the pivotal role of enterocyte tight junctions and future perspectives. J Hepatol. 2013;59:1144–6.
21. Tritto G, Bechlis Z, Stadlbauer V, et al. Evidence of neutrophil functional defect despite inflammation in stable cirrhosis. J Hepatol. 2011;55:574–81.
22. Wasmuth HE, Kunz D, Yagmur E, et al. Patients with acute on chronic liver failure display "sepsis-like" immune paralysis. J Hepatol. 2005;42:195–201.
23. Malik R, Mookerjee RP, Jalan R. Infection and inflammation in liver failure: two sides of the same coin. J Hepatol. 2009;51:426–9.
24. Fasolato S, Angeli P, Dallagnese L, et al. Renal failure and bacterial infections in patients with cirrhosis: epidemiology and clinical features. Hepatology. 2007;45:223–9.
25. Fernández J, Gustot T. Management of bacterial infections in cirrhosis. J Hepatol. 2012;56:S1–12.
26. O'Leary JG, Reddy KR, Wong F, et al. Long-term use of antibiotics and proton pump inhibitors predict development of infections in patients with cirrhosis. Clin Gastroenterol Hepatol. 2015;13:753–9.e1-2.

27. Bajaj JS, O'Leary JG, Reddy KR, et al. Second infections independently increase mortality in hospitalized patients with cirrhosis: the north American consortium for the study of end-stage liver disease (NACSELD) experience. Hepatology. 2012;56:2328–35.
28. Merli M, Lucidi C, Giannelli V, et al. Cirrhotic patients are at risk for health care-associated bacterial infections. Clin Gastroenterol Hepatol. 2010;8:979–85.
29. Jalan R, Gines P, Olson JC, et al. Acute-on chronic liver failure. J Hepatol. 2012;57:1336–48.
30. Rodighiero V. Effects of liver disease on pharmacokinetics. An update. Clin Pharmacokinet. 1999;37:399–431.
31. Delcò F, Tchambaz L, Schlienger R, Drewe J, Krähenbühl S. Dose adjustment in patients with liver disease. Drug Saf. 2005;28:529–45.
32. Lewis JH. The rational use of potentially hepatotoxic medications in patients with underlying liver disease. Expert Opin Drug Saf. 2002;1:159–72.
33. Zimmerman HJ. Hepatotoxicity: the adverse effects of drugs and other chemicals on the liver. Lippincott Williams & Wilkins; 1999.
34. Amarapurkar DN. Prescribing medications in patients with decompensated liver cirrhosis. Int J Hepatol. 2011;2011:519526.
35. Bajaj JS, Liu EJ, Kheradman R, et al. Fungal dysbiosis in cirrhosis Gut. 2018;67:1146–54.
36. Brown GD, Denning DW, Gow NAR, Levitz SM, Netea MG, White TC. Hidden killers: human fungal infections. Sci Transl Med. 2012;4:165rv13.
37. Pappas PG, Kauffman CA, Andes DR, et al. Clinical practice guideline for the Management of Candidiasis: 2016 update by the Infectious Diseases Society of America. Clin Infect Dis. 2016;62:e1–50.
38. Wisplinghoff H, Bischoff T, Tallent SM, Seifert H, Wenzel RP, Edmond MB. Nosocomial bloodstream infections in US hospitals: analysis of 24,179 cases from a prospective nationwide surveillance study. Clin Infect Dis. 2004;39:309–17.
39. Kuti EL, Kuti JL. Pharmacokinetics, antifungal activity and clinical efficacy of anidulafungin in the treatment of fungal infections. Expert Opin Drug Metab Toxicol. 2010;6:1287–300.
40. Vekeman F, Weiss L, Aram J, et al. Retrospective cohort study comparing the risk of severe hepatotoxicity in hospitalized patients treated with echinocandins for invasive candidiasis in the presence of confounding by indication. BMC Infect Dis. 2018;18:438.
41. Glöckner A. Treatment and prophylaxis of invasive candidiasis with anidulafungin, caspofungin and micafungin: review of the literature. Eur J Med Res. 2011;16:167–79.
42. Bajaj JS, Heuman DM, Sanyal AJ, et al. Modulation of the metabiome by rifaximin in patients with cirrhosis and minimal hepatic encephalopathy. PLoS One. 2013;8:e60042.
43. Bass NM, Mullen KD, Sanyal A, et al. Rifaximin treatment in hepatic encephalopathy. N Engl J Med. 2010;362:1071–81.
44. Hanouneh MA, Hanouneh IA, Hashash JG, et al. The role of rifaximin in the primary prophylaxis of spontaneous bacterial peritonitis in patients with liver cirrhosis. J Clin Gastroenterol. 2012;46:709–15.
45. Vlachogiannakos J, Viazis N, Vasianopoulou P, Vafiadis I, Karamanolis DG, Ladas SD. Long-term administration of rifaximin improves the prognosis of patients with decompensated alcoholic cirrhosis. J Gastroenterol Hepatol. 2013;28:450–5.
46. Fernández J, Tandon P, Mensa J, Garcia-Tsao G. Antibiotic prophylaxis in cirrhosis: good and bad. Hepatology. 2016;63:2019–31.
47. Udy AA, Roberts JA, Lipman J. Clinical implications of antibiotic pharmacokinetic principles in the critically ill. Intensive Care Med. 2013;39:2070–82.
48. Ali N, Gupta N, Saravu K. Malnutrition as an important risk factor for drug-induced liver injury in patients on anti-tubercular therapy: an experience from a tertiary care center in South India. Drug Discov Ther. 2020;14:135–8.
49. Whitcomb DC, Block GD. Association of acetaminophen hepatotoxicity with fasting and ethanol use. JAMA. 1994;272:1845–50.
50. Li X, Gao P, Niu J. Metabolic comorbidities and risk of development and severity of drug-induced liver injury. Biomed Res Int. 2019;2019:8764093.

51. Cross FS, Long MW, Banner AS, Snider DE. Rifampin-isoniazid therapy of alcoholic and nonalcoholic tuberculous patients in a U.S. Public Health Service cooperative therapy trial. Am Rev Respir Dis. 1980;122:349–53.
52. Russo MW, Watkins PB. Are patients with elevated liver tests at increased risk of drug-induced liver injury? Gastroenterology. 2004;126:1477–80.
53. Wong WM, Wu PC, Yuen MF, et al. Antituberculosis drug-related liver dysfunction in chronic hepatitis B infection. Hepatology. 2000;31:201–6.
54. Patel PA, Voigt MD. Prevalence and interaction of hepatitis B and latent tuberculosis in Vietnamese immigrants to the United States. Am J Gastroenterol. 2002;97:1198–203.
55. Reuben A, Koch DG, Lee WM. Acute liver failure study group. Drug-induced acute liver failure: results of a U.S. multicenter, prospective study. Hepatology. 2010;52:2065–76.
56. Devarbhavi H, Andrade RJ. Drug-induced liver injury due to antimicrobials, central nervous system agents, and nonsteroidal anti-inflammatory drugs. Semin Liver Dis. 2014;34:145–61.
57. Orlando R, Mussap M, Plebani M, et al. Diagnostic value of plasma cystatin C as a glomerular filtration marker in decompensated liver cirrhosis. Clin Chem. 2002;48:850–8.
58. Lodise TP, Lomaestro B, Graves J, Drusano GL. Larger vancomycin doses (at least four grams per day) are associated with an increased incidence of nephrotoxicity. Antimicrob Agents Chemother. 2008;52:1330–6.
59. Habib S, Patel N, Yarlagadda S, et al. Safety and efficacy of antibiotics among acutely decompensated cirrhosis patients. J Gastroenterol Hepatol. 2018;33:1882–8.
60. Dixit RK, Satapathy SK, Kumar R, et al. Pharmacokinetics of ciprofloxacin in patients with liver cirrhosis. Indian J Gastroenterol. 2002;21:62–3.
61. Montay G, Gaillot J. Pharmacokinetics of fluoroquinolones in hepatic failure. J Antimicrob Chemother. 1990;26:61–7.
62. Vuppalanchi R, Juluri R, Ghabril M, et al. Drug-induced QT prolongation in cirrhotic patients with transjugular intrahepatic portosystemic shunt. J Clin Gastroenterol. 2011;45:638–42.
63. Mattappalil A, Mergenhagen KA. Neurotoxicity with antimicrobials in the elderly: a review. Clin Ther. 2014;36:1489–511.e4.
64. Bhattacharyya S, Darby RR, Raibagkar P, Castro LNG, Berkowitz AL. Antibiotic-associated encephalopathy. Neurology. 2016;86:963–71.
65. Veirup N, Kyriakopoulos C. Neomycin [Internet]. In: StatPearls. Treasure Island (FL): StatPearls Publishing; 2021 [cited 2021 Oct 1]. Available from: http://www.ncbi.nlm.nih.gov/books/NBK560603/
66. Loft S, Sonne J, Døssing M, Andreasen PB. Metronidazole pharmacokinetics in patients with hepatic encephalopathy. Scand J Gastroenterol. 1987;22:117–23.
67. Ianiro G, Tilg H, Gasbarrini A. Antibiotics as deep modulators of gut microbiota: between good and evil. Gut. 2016;65:1906–15.
68. Singh N, Yu VL, Mieles LA, Wagener MM. Beta-lactam antibiotic-induced leukopenia in severe hepatic dysfunction: risk factors and implications for dosing in patients with liver disease. Am J Med. 1993;94:251–6.
69. He Z-F, Wu X-A, Wang Y-P. Severe bone marrow suppression and hepatic dysfunction caused by piperacillin/tazobactam. Scand J Infect Dis. 2013;45:885–7.
70. Patil A, Khillan V, Thakur M, Kale P, Bihari C. Antimicrobial-induced Cytopenia and bone marrow Hypocellularity in patients with cirrhosis. Bone Marrow Res. 2018;2018:e4029648.
71. Devarbhavi H, Raj S. Drug-induced liver injury with skin reactions: drugs and host risk factors, clinical phenotypes and prognosis. Liver Int. 2019;39:802–11.
72. Lin Y-T, Wu P-H, Lin C-Y, et al. Cirrhosis as a risk factor for tuberculosis infection–a Nationwide longitudinal study in Taiwan. Am J Epidemiol. 2014;180:103–10.
73. Rifampin [Internet]. In: LiverTox: Clinical and Research Information on Drug-Induced Liver Injury. Bethesda (MD): National Institute of Diabetes and Digestive and Kidney Diseases; 2012 [cited 2021 Oct 1]. Available from: http://www.ncbi.nlm.nih.gov/books/NBK548314/
74. Gupta NK, Lewis JH. Review article: the use of potentially hepatotoxic drugs in patients with liver disease. Aliment Pharmacol Ther. 2008;28:1021–41.
75. Saito A, Nagayama N, Yagi O, et al. Tuberculosis complicated with liver cirrhosis. Kekkaku. 2006;81:457–65.

76. Hawkins MT, Lewis JH. Latest advances in predicting DILI in human subjects: focus on biomarkers. Expert Opin Drug Metab Toxicol. 2012;8:1521–30.
77. Isoniazid [Internet]. In: LiverTox: Clinical and Research Information on Drug-Induced Liver Injury. Bethesda (MD): National Institute of Diabetes and Digestive and Kidney Diseases; 2012 [cited 2021 Oct 1]. Available from: http://www.ncbi.nlm.nih.gov/books/NBK548754/
78. Kaneko Y, Nagayama N, Kawabe Y, et al. Drug-induced hepatotoxicity caused by anti-tuberculosis drugs in tuberculosis patients complicated with chronic hepatitis. Kekkaku. 2008;83:13–9.
79. Jahng AW, Tran T, Bui L, Joyner JL. Safety of treatment of latent tuberculosis infection in compensated cirrhotic patients during transplant candidacy period. Transplantation. 2007;83:1557–62.
80. Holty J-EC, Gould MK, Meinke L, Keeffe EB, Ruoss SJ. Tuberculosis in liver transplant recipients: a systematic review and meta-analysis of individual patient data. Liver Transplant. 2009;15:894–906.
81. Jafri S-M, Singal AG, Kaul D, Fontana RJ. Detection and management of latent tuberculosis in liver transplant patients. Liver Transplant. 2011;17:306–14.
82. Lacroix C, Tranvouez JL, Phan Hoang T, Duwoos H, Lafont O. Pharmacokinetics of pyrazinamide and its metabolites in patients with hepatic cirrhotic insufficiency. Arzneimittelforschung. 1990;40:76–9.
83. Kumar N, Kedarisetty CK, Kumar S, Khillan V, Sarin SK. Antitubercular therapy in patients with cirrhosis: challenges and options. World J Gastroenterol. 2014;20:5760–72.
84. Saigal S, Agarwal SR, Nandeesh HP, Sarin SK. Safety of an ofloxacin-based antitubercular regimen for the treatment of tuberculosis in patients with underlying chronic liver disease: a preliminary report. J Gastroenterol Hepatol. 2001;16:1028–32.
85. Fernández J, Prado V, Trebicka J, et al. Multidrug-resistant bacterial infections in patients with decompensated cirrhosis and with acute-on-chronic liver failure in Europe. J Hepatol. 2019;70:398–411.
86. Merli M, Lucidi C, Di Gregorio V, et al. The spread of multi drug resistant infections is leading to an increase in the empirical antibiotic treatment failure in cirrhosis: a prospective survey. PLoS One. 2015;10:e0127448.
87. Ariza X, Castellote J, Lora-Tamayo J, et al. Risk factors for resistance to ceftriaxone and its impact on mortality in community, healthcare and nosocomial spontaneous bacterial peritonitis. J Hepatol. 2012;56:825–32.
88. Tandon P, Delisle A, Topal JE, Garcia-Tsao G. High prevalence of antibiotic-resistant bacterial infections among patients with cirrhosis at a US liver center. Clin Gastroenterol Hepatol. 2012;10:1291–8.
89. Chan C, Levitsky J. Infection and alcoholic liver disease. Clin Liver Dis. 2016;20:595–606.
90. Bunchorntavakul C, Chavalitdhamrong D. Bacterial infections other than spontaneous bacterial peritonitis in cirrhosis. World J Hepatol. 2012;4:158–68.
91. Fernandez J, Arroyo V. Bacterial infections in cirrhosis: a growing problem with significant implications. Clin Liver Dis. 2013;2:102–5.
92. Arabi YM, Dara SI, Memish Z, et al. Antimicrobial therapeutic determinants of outcomes from septic shock among patients with cirrhosis. Hepatology. 2012;56:2305–15.
93. European Association for the Study of the Liver. EASL clinical practice guidelines for the management of patients with decompensated cirrhosis. J Hepatol. 2018;69:406–60.
94. Viale P, Giannella M, Bartoletti M, Tedeschi S, Lewis R. Considerations about antimicrobial stewardship in settings with epidemic extended-Spectrum β-lactamase-producing or Carbapenem-resistant Enterobacteriaceae. Infect Dis Ther. 2015;4:65–83.
95. Fernández J, Bert F, Nicolas-Chanoine M-H. The challenges of multi-drug-resistance in hepatology. J Hepatol. 2016;65:1043–54.

Ursodeoxycholic Acid in Liver Cirrhosis: An Evidence-Based Review

5

Kanokwan Pinyopornpanish

Abstract

Ursodeoxycholic acid (UDCA) is a drug with multiple hepatoprotectant and anticholestatic properties. It is used extensively for the dissolution of gallstones and for the treatment of various cholestatic liver diseases. UDCA modifies the constituents of the bile acid pool, stimulates hepatobiliary secretion, exerts cytoprotective effects, inhibits bile acid absorption by cholangiocytes, and exerts immunomodulatory action. These cytoprotective effects alleviate hepatic inflammation and provide potential anti-fibrotic property of this compound. The mechanism involved in the direct inhibitory fibrogenetic effects is unclear, and the data concerning it is extremely limited. In clinical studies, UDCA has been shown to delay the progression of fibrosis, stabilize portal pressure, and delay development of varices and clinical decompensation in patients with primary biliary cholangitis. The effects of UDCA on liver fibrosis and cirrhosis in other chronic cholestatic disorders show heterogeneous results. In non-cholestatic disorders, UDCA demonstrated limited clinical benefits, and currently, there is insufficient evidence to support its use in these conditions. It should be emphasized that there is a possibility that the treatment duration in the studies may not be of sufficient length for the drug to show the effects, as the fibrosis may progress slowly. Future studies are required to elucidate long-term clinical benefits in conditions, such as cirrhosis, and also to investigate any potential cirrhosis-related complications.

Keywords

Liver Fibrosis · Liver Cirrhosis, Biliary · Deoxycholic Acid · Polycyclic Compound · Cholestasis, Intrahepatic

K. Pinyopornpanish (✉)
Department of Internal Medicine, Faculty of Medicine, Chiang Mai University, Chiang Mai, Thailand

X. Qi, Y. Yang (eds.), *Pharmacotherapy for Liver Cirrhosis and Its Complications*, https://doi.org/10.1007/978-981-19-2615-0_5

5.1 Introduction

Ursodeoxycholic acid (UDCA; 3α,7β-dihydroxy-5β-cholanic acid), also known as ursodiol, is a secondary bile acid occurring in human bile. It is a hydrophilic bile acid accounting for a small proportion (1–3%) of the human bile acid pool [1]. It is the predominant bile acid of the bile of black bears. UDCA was first utilized for the dissolution of gallstones in the 1970s. This utilization was followed up by a lot of studies into various liver diseases, especially cholestatic liver diseases. There is abundant data supporting its use in patients with primary biliary cholangitis (PBC), and it is currently approved for first-line treatment of this condition. However, there are limited data regarding the effect of UDCA treatment on liver fibrosis, liver cirrhosis outcomes, and cirrhosis-related portal hypertension. This chapter will summarize current evidence pertinent to the mechanism of the action and effects of UDCA on liver fibrosis and portal hemodynamics, clinical evidence of UDCA use on hepatic fibrosis and potential cirrhosis-related complications in patients with chronic liver diseases, and clinical outcomes in patients with cirrhosis.

5.2 UDCA Mechanism of Action and its Effects on Liver Fibrosis

Many mechanisms have been proposed as being responsible for the hepatoprotective effects of UDCA. It is unclear, however, about which mechanism provides the major beneficial effects and the predominant mechanism may vary depending on the nature and severity of the liver disease. The mechanisms mainly considered to be responsible are summarized below [1–3].

5.2.1 Alteration of the Bile Acid Pool and Protection of Injured Cholangiocytes from Toxic Bile Acids

The magnitude of hydrophobicity of human bile acids in order should be lithocholic acid > deoxycholic acid > chenodeoxycholic acid > cholic acid > ursodeoxycholic acid [4]. The accumulation of hydrophobic bile acids is known to cause damage to cell membranes and also extracellular cytotoxicity especially when in excess. Therefore, in patients with cholestasis, bile retention promotes cholangiolar injury and inflammation. UDCA is a hydrophilic bile acid, and continuous therapeutic use can cause it to become the major bile acid in the bile pool (40–50% of total bile acid by continuous use of UDCA at a standard dose of 13–15 mg/kg per day). Hence, replacing hydrophobic bile acids with more hydrophilic UDCA lessens the toxicity of bile that may aggravate the activity of primary bile duct disease. This mechanism is thought to be the main mechanism of action of UDCA in patients with early cholestatic disorders when the bile excretory function is still reserved.

5.2.2 Stimulation of Impaired Hepatobiliary Secretion

UDCA causes biliary secretion of bile acids and other organic compounds in experimental models. This effect is also demonstrated in patients with PBC and primary sclerosing cholangitis (PSC) resulting in a decrease in endogenous, hydrophobic bile acid, chenodeoxycholic acid, and bilirubin. UDCA stimulates the elimination of toxic compounds from hepatocytes by stimulating the expression of transporter proteins that are needed for biliary secretion. It also stimulates HCO_3^- secretion by cholangiocytes and increases cytosolic free Ca^{2+} in cholangiocytes, resulting in increasing activity of Cl^- channels and promoting bicarbonate movement into the bile ducts. The stimulation of cholangiocellular calcium-dependent chloride/bicarbonate anion secretion is considered to be the mechanism responsible for the anticholestatic effect of UDCA in the diseases in which HCO_3^- secretion is impaired.

5.2.3 Hepatocytes and Cholangiocyte Cytoprotection

A variety of pathways involving the stabilization of plasma membranes and mitochondria and induction of subcellular anti-apoptotic pathways by UDCA offer cytoprotective effects against bile acid-induced apoptosis.

5.2.4 Inhibition of Absorption of Toxic, Hydrophobic, Endogenous Bile Salts

Under cholestatic conditions, UDCA use is associated with impaired apical uptake of hydrophobic bile acid by cholangiocytes, thus reducing the toxic bile acids within the cell.

5.2.5 Potential Immunomodulatory Effects

Modulation of cell-mediated immunity by UDCA has been observed. Human leukocyte antigen (HLA) class I and class II molecules are overexpressed by hepatocytes and cholangiocytes under chronic cholestasis conditions. This aberrant expression of HLA class I may induce recognition and subsequent destruction by cytotoxic T lymphocytes. UDCA reversal of aberrant HLA class I molecules has been demonstrated; however, this effect might be secondary to the anticholestatic properties of UDCA.

5.2.6 Mechanisms Involved in the Anti-Fibrosis Effects of UDCA

Protection of hepatic tissues against hepatic fibrogenesis by UDCA in a cholestatic-induced hepatic fibrosis rat model has been demonstrated [5]. Aforementioned

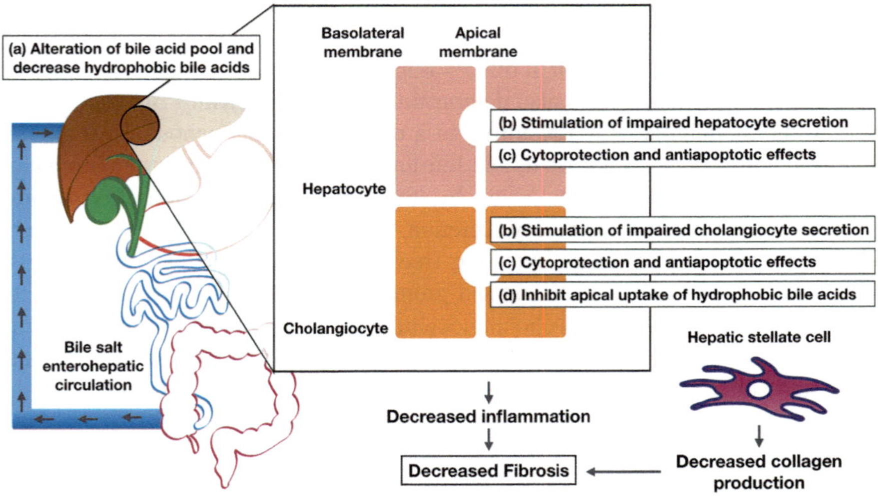

Fig. 5.1 Potential mechanisms of the action and anti-fibrosis effects of UDCA. (**a**) Alteration of the bile acid pool by replacing toxic, hydrophobic bile acids with non-toxic, more hydrophilic UDCA; (**b**) Stimulation of impaired hepatocyte and cholangiocyte secretion; (**c**) Cytoprotection and anti-apoptotic effects; (**d**) Inhibition of cholangiocyte apical uptake of hydrophobic bile acids. The mechanisms listed as A-D illustrate the anticholestatic effect of UDCA resulting in the decrease in hepatic inflammation and decrease in hepatic fibrosis in cholestatic liver disease. UDCA may also cause a decrease in the production of collagen by hepatic stellate cells, therefore, providing primary anti-fibrosis activity

multiple mechanisms involving the inhibitory pathogenic process of cholestatic liver disease and alleviation of cholangiocellular injury and inflammation by UDCA are considered to be responsible for its anti-fibrotic activity in cholestatic liver diseases. Data from an experimental study also shows that UDCA displays anti-fibrotic activity by decreasing collagen production by hepatic stellate cell (HSC) and cell survival [6]. Less severe liver fibrosis and lower hepatic expression of type I and type III collagens proteins were observed in a UDCA-treated rat model of liver fibrosis [7]. The mechanism underlying its direct anti-fibrotic activity is currently unclear, and data are scarce. The autophagy process was found to facilitate HSC activation, and inhibition of autophagy by UDCA has been proposed as demonstrated in a preclinical study [6]. This primary anti-fibrotic property of UDCA still needs to be confirmed, and further investigation is necessary. The potential mechanisms involved in the action of UDCA and the effects on liver fibrosis are summarized in Fig. 5.1.

5.3 The Effect of UDCA on Portal System Hemodynamics

UDCA affects systemic hemodynamics by decreasing diastolic blood pressure without significant alteration of splanchnic hemodynamics in healthy subjects [8]. A study using the nitric oxide (NO)-releasing derivatives of UDCA (NX-1000; 2

(acetyloxy) benzoic acid-3 (nitroxymethyl) phenyl ester) in patients with cirrhosis and portal hypertension also demonstrated changes in systolic blood pressure and hepatic blood flow without any reduction in portal pressure [9]. Therefore, based on current evidence, UDCA has no direct effect on portal hemodynamics.

5.4 The Effects of UDCA on Liver Fibrosis, Cirrhosis-Related Complications, and Cirrhosis Outcomes in Patients with Chronic Liver Diseases (Table 5.1)

5.4.1 Cholestatic Liver Diseases

5.4.1.1 Primary Biliary Cholangitis (PBC)

The use of UDCA showed remarkable beneficial effects on disease progression in patients with PBC. A dose-finding study showed that UDCA in a dosage of 13–15 mg/kg/day is the effective and preferred dose in patients with PBC [10]. UDCA therapy was found to significantly delay the progression of liver fibrosis and is associated with five-fold lower yearly fibrosis progression rate from early stage of the disease to extensive fibrosis or cirrhosis [11]. In earlier analysis, the effects on the development of portal hypertension complications were not demonstrated [12]. The likely explanation of this result might be because the disease progression is slow in PBC patients and the 2-year UDCA treatment used in clinical trials is probably not long enough to detect the difference from placebo. Reports of UDCA treatment with adequate duration of drug exposure showed that its use prevents the progression of portal hypertension in most patients receiving treatment [13]. Lower risk of the development of varices was observed in patients treated with UDCA for 4 years compared to placebo [14]. This is likely due to the improvement in liver architecture resulting in a decrease in portal venous outflow resistance in patients receiving UDCA. UDCA use is also associated with a reduction in the rate of liver transplantation or death in patients with PBC. The number needed to treat to prevent one liver transplantation or death within 5 years in patients with and without cirrhosis was 4 and 20, respectively [15].

It is estimated that 30–50% of patients receiving UDCA do not have a satisfactory response to the treatment. Multiple prognostic models have been proposed to evaluate the response [16, 17]. The Toronto criteria proposed by Kumagi et al. in 2010 demonstrated that histologic progression of fibrosis was associated with the lack of biochemical response after 2 years of treatment [18]. An alkaline phosphatase (ALP) of >1.67 × ULN (upper limit of normal) was associated with an increase in 1 stage of fibrosis progression at 2 years, and ALP of >1.76 × ULN was associated with an increase in 2 stage of fibrosis progression at 2 years [18]. The UDCA non-responders defined by other biochemical response criteria were related to significant development of liver cirrhosis and higher mortality than those who responded to treatment [19]. A recent study showed that UDCA use in PBC patients with compensated cirrhosis reduced clinical decompensation in patients who

Table 5.1 Summary of clinical evidences regarding the effects of UDCA use in liver fibrosis, cirrhosis-related complications, and cirrhosis outcomes in patients with chronic liver diseases

Liver diseases	UDCA doses	Effects	Results
Primary biliary cholangitis (UDCA responder)	13–15 mg/kg/day	Fibrosis/cirrhosis progression	Delayed
		Portal hypertension	Stabilized
		Development of varices	Reduced risk
		Liver transplantation and death	Reduced risk
Primary biliary cholangitis and compensated cirrhosis (UDCA responder)	13–14 mg/kg/day	Clinical decompensation	Reduced risk
Primary sclerosing cholangitis	13–15 mg/kg/day	Disease progression	No improvement
	17–23 mg/kg/day	Liver transplantation	No improvement
	28–30 mg/kg/day	Development of varices	Increased risk
Cystic fibrosis	10–20 mg/kg/day	Fibrosis improvement	Potential improvement in patients without cirrhosis
	20–25 mg/kg/day	Development of portal hypertension	No risk reduction
Cystic fibrosis and cirrhosis	10–20 mg/kg/day	Overall survival	No improvement
Progressive familial intrahepatic cholestasis (complete responder)	20–30 mg/kg/day	Fibrosis/cirrhosis improvement	Improved
Non-alcoholic steatohepatitis	13–15 mg/kg/day	Fibrosis improvement (histology)	No improvement
	23–28 mg/kg/day	Fibrosis improvement (histology)	No improvement
	28–35 mg/kg/day	Fibrosis improvement (serum fibrosis markers)	Improved
Autoimmune hepatitis	13–15 mg/kg/day	Fibrosis improvement	No improvement
Alcoholic cirrhosis (advanced disease with jaundice)	13–15 mg/kg/day	6-month survival	No improvement
Hepatitis C infection	600 mg/day	Fibrosis improvement	No improvement

responded to the treatment compared to those who showed partial response [20]. Therefore, in patients with PBC, UDCA exerts stabilization or delayed progression of fibrosis and reduction of cirrhosis-related complications in those who responded to treatment. The drug has therefore been described as safe and is recommended as the first-line therapy in patients with PBC. Patients treated with UDCA should be evaluated for biochemical response at 12 months after the initiation of treatment to identify those who are non-responders and who might not benefit from UDCA, and the introduction of second-line therapy is necessary.

5.4.1.2 Primary Sclerosing Cholangitis (PSC)

Standard dose UDCA treatment in patients with PSC is associated with improvement of liver biochemistries without demonstrating any delay in disease progression [21]. Treatment with UDCA at 17–23 mg/kg/day provided no significant benefit with regard to death or transplantation [22]. Despite considered as being an extremely safe therapy, a higher dosage of 28–30 mg/kg/day of UDCA use in patients with PSC was related to higher rates of adverse events, including the development of varices, death, or becoming eligible for liver transplantation in a treated group in comparison to placebo [23]. This study was terminated after 6 years due to the futility of the outcomes. The possible explanation of this result might be due to the toxic bile acids being produced from unabsorbed UDCA. It has been shown in animal models that UDCA aggravates bile infarcts and hepatocyte necrosis in the case of biliary obstruction, which is found in patients with PSC [23]. To date, there is no recommended pharmacological treatment for patients with PSC and the clinical benefits of taking UDCA are limited. High dose UDCA use in this condition increases adverse effects and should not be used.

5.4.1.3 Cystic Fibrosis (CF)

Cholestasis in the case of this genetic disease is caused by defective secretion of cholangiocellular bicarbonate. Thick biliary secretions in CF patients lead to biliary obstruction. Two-year treatment with UDCA is associated with a trend toward less fibrosis compared to baseline prior to treatment initiation in patients with CF [24]. Improvement of liver stiffness in patients treated with UDCA is demonstrated only in patients initiated onto UDCA based on Colombo criteria without liver cirrhosis [25]. A longitudinal population-based cohort study including over 3000 CF patients showed that UDCA improved overall survival only in patients without cirrhosis, but not in those with cirrhosis [26]. However, another large cohort demonstrated conflicting result showing that earlier use of UDCA did not change the incidence of severe liver disease defined as cirrhosis or portal hypertension development [27]. Furthermore, a recent study demonstrated that CF patients followed up in UDCA prescribing centers (41% of patients receiving UDCA) did not show a lower incidence of portal hypertension as compared to those followed in centers not prescribing UDCA (2.5% of patients receiving UDCA) [28]. The role of UDCA in CF patients has been controversial as the outcomes from the studies are inconsistent. The effect of UDCA in reducing the risk of severe liver disease with portal hypertension was not established, and the potential prevention of the progression of fibrosis when administered early before apparent liver damage is controversial. The data from several studies implies that this drug might have limited effects on liver fibrosis, and survival outcomes in patients with CF and liver cirrhosis.

5.4.1.4 Progressive Familial Intrahepatic Cholestasis (PFIC)

Pediatric patients with PFIC treated with UDCA at a dose of 20–30 mg/kg/day had a 42–46% chance of complete response to treatment with normalization of transaminases, gamma glutamyl transferase (GGT), and direct bilirubin [29]. In patients who had a complete response, decreased liver fibrosis was observed in all 4 patients with baseline fibrosis or cirrhosis who underwent a paired liver biopsy [29]. After 4.5 years of UDCA administration, a patient with PFIC type 3, an inherited disease characterized by a multidrug resistance protein 3 (MDR3) deficiency, exhibited the reversal of advanced fibrosis from METAVIR fibrosis stage 4 to stage 1 [30]. The use of UDCA in patients with PFIC results in fibrosis regression in patients who respond to treatment.

5.4.2 Other Liver Diseases

5.4.2.1 Non-alcoholic Steatohepatitis (NASH)

One of the proposed mechanisms involved in the development of NASH involves inflammatory processes and the administration of non-toxic UDCA might provide cytoprotective effects. UDCA use in an animal model of NASH showed anti-apoptotic and mitochondrial protective effects and reduction of pro-inflammatory cytokines [31]. The effects of UDCA use in NASH patients were evaluated in several clinical trials. The use of 13–15 mg/kg/day of UDCA for 2 years was not associated with any improvement of liver fibrosis in patients with biopsy-proven NASH [32]. The use of a higher dosage of 23–28 mg/kg/day of UDCA for 18 months also demonstrated negative improvement of liver fibrosis evaluated by liver histology compared to placebo [33]. Meanwhile, another study evaluated the effect of 28–35 mg/kg/day of UDCA for 12 months on liver fibrosis. The outcome was assessed by the changes in the serum marker associated with fibrosis (Fibrotest®), and improvement was shown in the surrogate marker of fibrosis with an excellent safety profile [34]. Therefore, current evidence shows no significant benefit of the use of UDCA up to 28 mg/kg/day dosage on liver fibrosis in patients with NASH. It is important to note that NASH has a slow progression disease and inadequate duration of treatment in these studies might cause negative results. A higher dosage of UDCA may result in the improvement of fibrosis, but to date this outcome has not been confirmed by histology, the reference standard for the evaluation of fibrosis in patients with NASH. Further study is needed to confirm this finding.

5.4.2.2 Autoimmune Hepatitis (AIH)

A small case series in 1998 demonstrated improvement of liver biochemistries, reduction of immunoglobulin G and anti-nuclear antibodies titer in 8 patients with AIH type 1 after 2 years of treatment with UDCA [35]. In 4 patients with baseline bridging fibrosis who had follow-up liver biopsy, histological improvement was seen in all cases without any changes in liver fibrosis. A study in patients with a suboptimal response to prednisolone or a combination treatment of prednisolone and azathioprine revealed unchanged liver fibrosis in patients treated with UDCA compared to placebo [36].

5.4.2.3 Cirrhosis Due to Alcohol-Related Liver Disease (ALD Cirrhosis)

UDCA use in patients with ALD cirrhosis and jaundice was evaluated in a randomized controlled trial, and no beneficial effect of UDCA on 6-month survival was observed [37]. Most of the participants in this study had advanced liver cirrhosis with a mean Child–Pugh score of 10, and approximately half of the patients in this study resumed their alcoholism, which might contribute to the poorer prognosis of patients in the study. Therefore, UDCA does not appear to provide any survival benefit in advanced alcoholic cirrhosis; however, the effects in patients with early cirrhosis and those abstaining from alcohol remained to be elucidated.

5.4.2.4 Viral Hepatitis C

UDCA use in combination with interferon therapy in patients with hepatitis C did not change the degree of portal fibrosis at the end of treatment compared to interferon monotherapy [38]. A study in hepatitis C cirrhosis patients showed a decrease in hepatic transaminases and GGT [39]. However, no data regarding the progression of liver fibrosis or long-term outcomes are available. These studies were all conducted prior to the era of direct acting antiviral agents treatment, which significantly improve liver-related outcomes. Therefore, the role of UDCA at present, especially in patients with fibrosis or cirrhosis after sustained virological response (SVR), should be further evaluated.

5.5 Conclusion

UDCA has multiple beneficial mechanisms for the treatment of cholestatic liver diseases. Reduction of hepatic inflammation may in turn decrease hepatic fibrogenesis. Few experimental studies suggest direct anti-fibrotic effects of UDCA, and further studies are required to expand current knowledge. UDCA has significant benefits in PBC patients who respond to treatment by delaying the progression of fibrosis, stabilizing portal pressure, decreasing the risk of the development of varices and liver decompensation. Induction of fibrosis regression was seen in patients with PFIC. In CF patients, data from observational studies suggested that UDCA does not prevent the development of portal hypertension. Based on current evidence, UDCA has no benefit in those with PSC, AIH, alcoholic cirrhosis, and hepatitis C infection. The result of using high dose UDCA in patients with NASH indicates the potential improvement of fibrosis, which needs to be confirmed in future studies. It is worth noting that the progression of fibrogenesis and cirrhosis is a slow process; therefore, adequate duration of UDCA treatment is important to evaluate the outcomes. The data regarding long-term effects of UDCA use in various liver diseases are lacking and more studies are warranted.

References

1. Beuers U. Drug insight: mechanisms and sites of action of ursodeoxycholic acid in cholestasis. Nat Clin Pract Gastroenterol Hepatol. 2006;3:318–28.
2. Paumgartner G, Beuers U. Mechanisms of action and therapeutic efficacy of ursodeoxycholic acid in cholestatic liver disease. Clin Liver Dis. 2004;8:67–81, vi.
3. Angulo P. Use of ursodeoxycholic acid in patients with liver disease. Curr Gastroenterol Rep. 2002;4:37–44.
4. Perez MJ, Briz O. Bile-acid-induced cell injury and protection. World J Gastroenterol. 2009;15:1677–89.
5. Tang N, Zhang Y, Liang Q, Liu Z, Shi Y. The role of ursodeoxycholic acid on cholestatic hepatic fibrosis in infant rats. Mol Med Rep. 2018;17:3837–44.
6. Ye HL, Zhang JW, Chen XZ, Wu PB, Chen L, Zhang G. Ursodeoxycholic acid alleviates experimental liver fibrosis involving inhibition of autophagy. Life Sci. 2020;242:117175.
7. Zhang LX, Liang TJ, Tan YR, Ren WH, Han GQ, Zhang J, et al. Protective effects of ursodeoxycholic acid against immune-mediated liver fibrosis in rats. Hepato-Gastroenterology. 2010;57:1196–202.
8. Schiedermaier P, Hansen S, Asdonk D, Brensing K, Sauerbruch T. Effects of ursodeoxycholic acid on splanchnic and systemic hemodynamics. A double-blind, cross-over, placebo-controlled study in healthy volunteers. Digestion. 2000;61:107–12.
9. Berzigotti A, Bellot P, De Gottardi A, Garcia-Pagan JC, Gagnon C, Spenard J, et al. NCX-1000, a nitric oxide-releasing derivative of UDCA, does not decrease portal pressure in patients with cirrhosis: results of a randomized, double-blind, dose-escalating study. Am J Gastroenterol. 2010;105:1094–101.
10. Angulo P, Dickson ER, Therneau TM, Jorgensen RA, Smith C, DeSotel CK, et al. Comparison of three doses of ursodeoxycholic acid in the treatment of primary biliary cirrhosis: a randomized trial. J Hepatol. 1999;30:830–5.
11. Corpechot C, Carrat F, Bonnand AM, Poupon RE, Poupon R. The effect of ursodeoxycholic acid therapy on liver fibrosis progression in primary biliary cirrhosis. Hepatology. 2000;32:1196–9.
12. Mayo MJ. Portal hypertension in primary biliary cirrhosis: a potentially reversible harbinger of demise. Gastroenterology. 2008;135:1450–1.
13. Huet PM, Vincent C, Deslaurier J, Cote J, Matsutami S, Boileau R, et al. Portal hypertension and primary biliary cirrhosis: effect of long-term ursodeoxycholic acid treatment. Gastroenterology. 2008;135:1552–60.
14. Lindor KD, Jorgensen RA, Therneau TM, Malinchoc M, Dickson ER. Ursodeoxycholic acid delays the onset of esophageal varices in primary biliary cirrhosis. Mayo Clin Proc. 1997;72:1137–40.
15. Harms MH, de Veer RC, Lammers WJ, Corpechot C, Thorburn D, Janssen HLA, et al. Number needed to treat with ursodeoxycholic acid therapy to prevent liver transplantation or death in primary biliary cholangitis. Gut. 2020;69:1502–9.
16. Pinyopornpanish K, Chadalavada P, Talal Sarmini M, Khoudari G, Alomari M, Padbidri V, et al. Simplified 6-month prediction scores for primary biliary cholangitis patients treated with ursodeoxycholic acid. Eur J Gastroenterol Hepatol. 2022;34:411–6.
17. Chen S, Duan W, You H, Jia J. A brief review on prognostic models of primary biliary cholangitis. Hepatol Int. 2017;11:412–8.
18. Kumagi T, Guindi M, Fischer SE, Arenovich T, Abdalian R, Coltescu C, et al. Baseline ductopenia and treatment response predict long-term histological progression in primary biliary cirrhosis. Am J Gastroenterol. 2010;105:2186–94.

19. Ornolfsson KT, Lund SH, Olafsson S, Bergmann OM, Bjornsson ES. Biochemical response to ursodeoxycholic acid among PBC patients: a nationwide population-based study. Scand J Gastroenterol. 2019;54:609–16.
20. John BV, Khakoo NS, Schwartz KB, Aitchenson G, Levy C, Dahman B, et al. Ursodeoxycholic acid response is associated with reduced mortality in primary biliary cholangitis with compensated cirrhosis. Am J Gastroenterol. 2021;116:1913–23.
21. Lindor KD. Ursodiol for primary sclerosing cholangitis. Mayo primary Sclerosing cholangitis-Ursodeoxycholic acid study group. N Engl J Med. 1997;336:691–5.
22. Olsson R, Boberg KM, de Muckadell OS, Lindgren S, Hultcrantz R, Folvik G, et al. High-dose ursodeoxycholic acid in primary sclerosing cholangitis: a 5-year multicenter, randomized, controlled study. Gastroenterology. 2005;129:1464–72.
23. Lindor KD, Kowdley KV, Luketic VA, Harrison ME, McCashland T, Befeler AS, et al. High-dose ursodeoxycholic acid for the treatment of primary sclerosing cholangitis. Hepatology. 2009;50:808–14.
24. Lindblad A, Glaumann H, Strandvik B. A two-year prospective study of the effect of ursodeoxycholic acid on urinary bile acid excretion and liver morphology in cystic fibrosis-associated liver disease. Hepatology. 1998;27:166–74.
25. van der Feen C, van der Doef HP, van der Ent CK, Houwen RH. Ursodeoxycholic acid treatment is associated with improvement of liver stiffness in cystic fibrosis patients. J Cyst Fibros. 2016;15:834–8.
26. Toledano MB, Mukherjee SK, Howell J, Westaby D, Khan SA, Bilton D, et al. The emerging burden of liver disease in cystic fibrosis patients: a UK nationwide study. PLoS One. 2019;14:e0212779.
27. Boelle PY, Debray D, Guillot L, Clement A, Corvol H, French CFMGSI. Cystic fibrosis liver disease: outcomes and risk factors in a large cohort of French patients. Hepatology. 2019;69:1648–56.
28. Colombo C, Alicandro G, Oliver M, Lewindon PJ, Ramm GA, Ooi CY, et al. Ursodeoxycholic acid and liver disease associated with cystic fibrosis: a multicenter cohort study. J Cyst Fibros. 2022;21:220–6.
29. Jacquemin E, Hermans D, Myara A, Habes D, Debray D, Hadchouel M, et al. Ursodeoxycholic acid therapy in pediatric patients with progressive familial intrahepatic cholestasis. Hepatology. 1997;25:519–23.
30. Frider B, Castillo A, Gordo-Gilart R, Bruno A, Amante M, Alvarez L, et al. Reversal of advanced fibrosis after long-term ursodeoxycholic acid therapy in a patient with residual expression of MDR3. Ann Hepatol. 2015;14:745–51.
31. Pathil A, Mueller J, Warth A, Chamulitrat W, Stremmel W. Ursodeoxycholyl lysophosphatidylethanolamide improves steatosis and inflammation in murine models of nonalcoholic fatty liver disease. Hepatology. 2012;55:1369–78.
32. Lindor KD, Kowdley KV, Heathcote EJ, Harrison ME, Jorgensen R, Angulo P, et al. Ursodeoxycholic acid for treatment of nonalcoholic steatohepatitis: results of a randomized trial. Hepatology. 2004;39:770–8.
33. Leuschner UF, Lindenthal B, Herrmann G, Arnold JC, Rossle M, Cordes HJ, et al. High-dose ursodeoxycholic acid therapy for nonalcoholic steatohepatitis: a double-blind, randomized, placebo-controlled trial. Hepatology. 2010;52:472–9.
34. Ratziu V, de Ledinghen V, Oberti F, Mathurin P, Wartelle-Bladou C, Renou C, et al. A randomized controlled trial of high-dose ursodesoxycholic acid for nonalcoholic steatohepatitis. J Hepatol. 2011;54:1011–9.
35. Nakamura K, Yoneda M, Yokohama S, Tamori K, Sato Y, Aso K, et al. Efficacy of ursodeoxycholic acid in Japanese patients with type 1 autoimmune hepatitis. J Gastroenterol Hepatol. 1998;13:490–5.

36. Czaja AJ, Carpenter HA, Lindor KD. Ursodeoxycholic acid as adjunctive therapy for problematic type 1 autoimmune hepatitis: a randomized placebo-controlled treatment trial. Hepatology. 1999;30:1381–6.
37. Pelletier G, Roulot D, Davion T, Masliah C, Causse X, Oberti F, et al. A randomized controlled trial of ursodeoxycholic acid in patients with alcohol-induced cirrhosis and jaundice. Hepatology. 2003;37:887–92.
38. Fabbri C, Marchetto S, Pezzoli A, Accogli E, Fusaroli P, Azzaroli F, et al. Efficacy of ursodeoxycholic acid in association with alpha-interferon for chronic hepatitis C in alpha-interferon non-responder patients. Eur J Gastroenterol Hepatol. 2000;12:511–5.
39. Lirussi F, Beccarello A, Bortolato L, Morselli-Labate AM, Crovatto M, Ceselli S, et al. Long-term treatment of chronic hepatitis C with ursodeoxycholic acid: influence of HCV genotypes and severity of liver disease. Liver. 1999;19:381–8.

Ursodeoxycholic Acid in Liver Cirrhosis: A Chinese Perspective

6

Wenkang Gao, Zhonglin Li, Huikuan Chu, Hang Yuan, Lilin Hu, Lin Yao, Li Zhang, Weijun Wang, Rong Lin, and Ling Yang

Abstract

Bile acids (BAs) not only play critical roles in liver-gut immune homeostasis but also participate in regulating lipid, glucose, and energy metabolism. BAs transporter defect or signaling pathways abnormal activation are linked to cholestasis, inflammation, fibrosis, carcinogenesis, and metabolic disorders. BAs and related signaling pathways have become attractive therapeutic targets for inflammation, fibrosis, and metabolic diseases, including type 2 diabetes mellitus and non-alcoholic fatty liver disease (NAFLD). Hydrophilic BAs, including ursodeoxycholic acid (UDCA), tauroursodeoxycholic (TUDCA), and 24-norursodeoxycholic (nor-UDCA), have hepatoprotective properties and are widely used in cholestatic liver diseases. Here, we provide an overview of the mechanism and recent clinical application of UDCA in hepatobiliary diseases, as well as BAs cross-talk with the gut microbiota in health and diseases. Targeting bile-acid signaling for liver cirrhosis is a promising and effective strategy. Evidences from clinical trials suggest that UDCA treatment has beneficial effects on cirrhosis.

Keywords

Bile acids · Cirrhosis · Cholestasis · Bile acid transport · Ursodeoxycholic acid

---

W. Gao · Z. Li · H. Chu · H. Yuan · L. Hu · L. Yao · L. Zhang · W. Wang · R. Lin · L. Yang (✉)
Division of Gastroenterology, Union Hospital, Tongji Medical College, Huazhong University of Science and Technology, Wuhan, China
e-mail: yanglinguh@hust.edu.cn

X. Qi, Y. Yang (eds.), *Pharmacotherapy for Liver Cirrhosis and Its Complications*, https://doi.org/10.1007/978-981-19-2615-0_6

6.1 Bile Acids and History of Ursodeoxycholic Acid

Bile is an important secretion necessary for the digestion and absorption of lipids in the gut. About 500 mg of cholesterol is converted into bile acids (BAs) in the adult liver each day. Newly synthesized BAs are transported into the lumen of the small intestine via the biliary duct, where they act as emulsifiers to help the digestion and absorption of dietary lipids, cholesterol, and fat-soluble nutrients [1]. The solubilized substances are incorporated into lipoproteins, which are delivered to the liver and metabolized. The enterohepatic circulation is a complex pathway in order to maintain the homeostasis of BAs. Generally, BAs move from the hepatocyte into canalicular bile, flow through the biliary tract and into the duodenum. Most BAs are actively recycled in the distal ileum, with a small fraction passively absorbed in the large intestine. Then, they are transported to the liver through portal vein, and efficiently taken up by the hepatocyte [2]. The majority of BAs (>95%) are effectively reabsorbed in the gut via the enterohepatic circulation, and the remaining 5% are newly synthesized in the liver [1].

Ursodeoxycholic acid (UDCA; 3α,7β-dihydroxy5β-cholanoic acid) is a primary component of human bile, physiologically. It is a type of hydrophilic BAs produced by intestinal bacteria and accounts for 1–3% of human BAs [3]. The earliest use of UDCA to cure diseases can be traced back more than 1000 years ago, when traditional Chinese medicine practitioners in the Tang Dynasty discovered the efficacy of bear bile in treating chronic liver diseases [4]. Until 1902, Hammarsten first found the presence of an unknown BA in the bile of the polar bear that he called "ursocholeinic acid." In 1927, the chemical form of UDCA was identified by Shoda firstly. In 1936, the characterization of the chemical structure of UDCA was done by Iwasaki, which promoted its sufficient synthesis for use in clinical practice [5]. Then, in the 1950s, it was proposed that the therapeutic effects of the bear bile were likely related to high concentrations of the taurine-conjugated form of UDCA and tauroursodeoxycholic (TUDCA) [6]. Subsequently, the therapeutical effect of UDCA in hepatobiliary diseases, such as gallbladder stones [7, 8] and primary biliary cirrhosis (PBC) [9], had been reported in succession.

Nowadays, UDCA has a defined role in preventing and treating patients with cholestatic liver diseases. Of note, UDCA also showed beneficial effects in some other diseases, including treating chronic heart failure [10], shrinking tumors [11], and improving vision [12]. This chapter will provide an overview of the mechanism and clinical application of hydrophilic BAs in hepatobiliary diseases, as well as BAs cross-talk with the gut microbiota in health and disease.

6.2 The Mechanisms of Bile Acids in Hepatobiliary Diseases

6.2.1 Bile Acid Transport, Bile Acid-Induced Toxicity, and Hepatocellular Adaptive Responses in Cholestasis

6.2.1.1 Bile Acid Transport

The transport of BAs is critical for maintaining the enterohepatic BAs circulation, and the regulation of BAs transporters is required for the maintenance of BAs homeostasis [13]. The transporters of BAs include a variety of transport proteins and enzymes located in hepatocytes, as follows: the sinusoidal transporter sodium taurocholate co-transporting polypeptide (NTCP/SLC10A1), members of the anion transporting polypeptide (OATPs/SLCO) family, conjugation enzymes, and the ATP-dependent efflux pump bile salt export pump (BSEP, also known as ABCB) [11, 13, 14]. These transporters are important for a rapid transition of BAs from blood to bile and maintain a low intracellular BA concentration [15, 16]. In the gut, apart from a few passive uptakes of BAs in the proximal small intestine and colon, they are actively absorbed mainly in the terminal ileum via an apical sodium-dependent BA transporter (ASBT) [17]. Then, BAs are bound to the ileal bile acid-binding protein (IBABP, also known as ileal lipid-binding protein ILBP and fatty acid-binding protein 6, FABP6) and exported into the portal blood via organic solute transporter alpha/beta (OSTα/OSTβ) [17]. Furthermore, the BAs in the enterocytes can induce the production of the intestinal peptide hormone fibroblast growth factor 15 (FGF15) in mice (a homolog of human FGF 19), which inhibits the BAs synthesis in hepatocytes in an endocrine manner [18], facilitates gallbladder refilling [19], and downregulates the expression of ASBT expression in a paracrine manner [20], altogether causing a reduction of circulating BAs.

6.2.1.2 Bile Acid-Induced Toxicity

The hydrophobicity of BAs depends on the number, position, and orientation of the hydroxyl groups, which are key factors in determining their degree of toxicity. Regarding the order of hydrophobicity of BAs, it is generally considered that UDCA < cholic acid (CA) < chenodeoxycholic acid (CDCA) < deoxycholic acid (DCA) < lithocholic acid (LCA) [21]. The accumulation of hydrophobic BAs in hepatocytes, like CDCA and DCA, has been considered as the main cause of liver injury in cholestatic liver disease. Hydrophobic BAs are known to directly injure isolated hepatocytes [22], cultured hepatocytes [23], and whole liver [24], but the mechanisms of their toxicity need to be further studied. Here are several hypotheses that may account for the cytotoxicity associated with the most hydrophobic BAs [25]. BAs can cause cell damage by their detergent effects on lipid components [26]. Moreover, it can also enhance the reactive oxygen species (ROS) generation that, in turn, oxidatively modify lipids, proteins, and nucleic acids, and eventually resulting in an increase in hepatocyte apoptosis [27]. Additionally, they can activate Kupffer cells to generate ROS, further aggravating the hepatocyte injury [28].

There are two main pathways of cell death caused by the accumulation of BAs within the hepatocyte; lower concentrations of BAs induce hepatocellular apoptosis [29–32], whereas higher concentrations induce necrosis [23, 33]. However, the contribution of these two types of cell death in promoting cholestatic liver injury is still in dispute. A brief introduction of them is as follows. Apoptosis is characterized by the maintenance of cellular ATP content. Hydrophobic BAs can induce apoptosis through the extrinsic death receptor-mediated pathway or the intrinsic mitochondria-mediated pathway according to the early evidence [34, 35]. It is confirmed recently that the changes of calcium signaling caused by ER stress can induce apoptosis as well [34, 35]. In contrast to BA-induced cell apoptosis, cellular necrosis is often induced by a high concentration of BAs with the character of cell swelling and intracellular and plasma membranes disruption. The mechanisms for BA-induced hepatocellular necrosis include direct membrane damage due to the detergent-like properties of hydrophobic BAs [26], depletion of ATP, ion dysregulation, mitochondrial and cellular swelling, plasma membrane failure, and cell lysis, releasing intracellular contents [22].

Conversely, as a hydrophilic BA, UDCA can treat cholestatic liver diseases by modulating hydrophobic BAs induced injury in hepatocytes. The hepatoprotective effects of hydrophilic BA have been found in different animal models, such as cholestatic liver diseases and metabolic diseases [36, 37]. And their potential mechanisms [38] like protection against liver inflammation and fibrosis will be discussed in the following paragraphs.

6.2.1.3 Hepatocellular Adaptive Responses in Cholestasis

Cholestasis is a blockage in bile flow caused by mechanical obstruction of biliary ducts or by hepatic transporter defects. During cholestasis, hepatic BAs synthesis and transport will be disturbed, the levels of intrahepatic BAs and plasma BAs will increase, and only small quantities of BAs will reach the colon to participate in enterohepatic circulation, which leads to the BAs profiles, localization and signal transduction alteration [35].

In order to avoid the damage from cholestasis, compensatory changes in the expression of hepatic BAs transporters occur [39]. These changes mainly include downregulation of BAs uptake and synthesis, and upregulation of BAs excretion through increased BSEP or transporters that are able to facilitate the BAs excretion [40, 41]. Several nuclear receptors will be involved in the responses above, such as farnesoid X receptor (FXR), pregnane X receptor (PXR), Constitutive Androstane Receptor (CAR), and the small heterodimer partner (SHP), as well as FGF19 [13, 40]. FXR is a BA-activated nuclear receptor, which influences a myriad of pathways in hepatocytes and other hepatic nonparenchymal cells, including Kupffer cells, endothelial cells, and hepatic stellate cells [13]. FXR/SHP in hepatocytes represses BAs synthesis by mediating a downregulation of NTCP and cholesterol 7α-hydroxylase (CYP7A1) to repress. FXR can also promote BA excretion through directly upregulating BSEP [13]. In humans, hepatic production of FGF-19 may also induce the downregulation of CYP7A1 [42]. Furthermore, a variety of alternative excretory transporters are upregulated during cholestasis, such as the heteromeric transporter OSTα/β and the ABC transporters MRP3 and MRP4, which are often located on the basolateral membrane of hepatocytes, and their expression levels are low under normal physiological conditions [13]. Therefore, if BA secretion is impaired, adaptive responses reduce the accumulation of BAs in the liver and protect hepatocytes against damage to a certain extent. If these responses are insufficient, apoptosis or necrosis of liver cells may occur inevitably [16].

6.2.2 Bile Acids and Cholangiocytes in Cholestasis

Cholangiocytes are polarized epithelial cells lining the intra- and extrahepatic bile ducts, which play a key role in bile composition and flow by solute transport processes [43]. Despite comprising ~5% of the cells in the liver, cholangiocytes account for up to 30% of total bile flow in humans, with the other 70% originating from hepatocyte canalicular secretion [44]. Cholangiocytes contain a large number of transporters that can secret large amounts of bicarbonate, water, and chloride. Specifically, secretin stimulates the apical insertion of intracellular vesicles containing anion exchange protein 2 (AE2), cystic fibrosis transmembrane conductance regulator (CFTR), and aquaporin 1 (AQP1), resulting in chloride secretion through CFTR that is exchanged with bicarbonate via AE2. This bicarbonate generates osmotic force and facilitates the movement of water through AQP1. An alkaline barrier, also called "biliary bicarbonate umbrella", was formed by the biliary secretion of bicarbonate which can render the BAs polar, de-protonated, and membrane impermeable [45]. Moreover, biliary bicarbonate neutralizes gastric acid contained in food and facilitates the absorption of nutrients [46].

Cholangiocytes also express BAs transporters (like ASBT) that contribute to the absorption of conjugated BAs. Also, passive absorption of protonated unconjugated BA can occur. Cholangiocytes reuptake BAs and then secret them into the peribiliary plexuses blood. This process is called as "cholehepatic shunt pathway," which is an alternative mechanism to the enterohepatic circulation of BAs, and leads to BAs return to hepatocytes for re-secretion into bile, enhancing its choleretic effect. Furthermore, several experiments indicated that the concentration and composition of BAs may activate different signaling pathways (i.e., calcium protein kinase C, phosphoinositide 3-kinase, mitogen-activated protein kinase, and extracellular signal-regulated protein kinase) to regulate the function of cholangiocytes.

Cholangiocyte damage is a major manifestation in certain cholestatic diseases, thus, the responses of cholangiocytes to injury are also important for understanding the pathophysiology and treatment of cholestatic diseases [43, 47]. Once cholangiocytes are injured, they transform into a neuroendocrine phenotype and cause bile duct hyperplasia, a common histological manifestation of cholestatic liver diseases [48]. Injury of biliary cells can either be immune mediated or non-immune mediated, such as drug-induced liver injury, mechanical biliary obstruction, and so on. Whatever the cause, the accumulation of toxic BAs in the bile ducts will damage cholangiocytes through cholangiocyte membrane disruption, induction of autophagy, and mediation of the secretion of pro-inflammatory and pro-fibrotic factors [48]. In addition, "bicarbonate umbrella" is formed by secreted bicarbonate and cholangiocyte glycocalyx, which can protect the apical membrane of cholangiocytes against BAs induced damage [45, 49].

6.2.3 Hepatoprotective Properties of Hydrophilic Bile Acids (UDCA, TUDCA, nor-UDCA)

Hydrophilic BAs are usually used as therapeutic approaches for cholestasis, including UDCA, TUDCA, and nor-UDCA. TUDCA is the taurine conjugate of UDCA. In cholestasis, UDCA and TUDCA can counteract many of the cellular changes induced by hydrophobic BAs. Their hepatoprotective properties [4] are summarized as follows. (1) Hydrophilic BAs, such as UDCA, can stabilize cell membrane structure and prevent hydrophobic BAs from damaging the cell membrane. (2) Hydrophilic BAs can also inhibit cell apoptosis mainly through blocking mitochondrial damage. (3) Treatment with hydrophilic BAs can promote bicarbonate secretion by several mechanisms including an increase in the anion exchanger 2 expressions. The detergent effects of hydrophobic BAs will be antagonized by bicarbonate. (4) Hydrophilic BAs also have various functions, such as preventing oxidative stress, regulating immunity, and alleviating the damage caused by cholestasis together with the above mechanisms.

24-norursodeoxycholic (nor-UDCA) is a non-amidated, side chain-shortened C23 derivative of UDCA. Instead of undergoing a full enterohepatic circulation, like other conjugated BAs, nor-UDCA undergoes cholehepatic shunting. Since a nor-UDCA anion is secreted into canalicular bile in the unconjugated form, it is protonated by a hydrogen ion derived from carbonic acid that was generated by the hydration of luminal CO_2, a process catalyzed by cholangiocellular carbonic anhydrase [50, 51]. The protonated BA is absorbed, thus generating a bicarbonate anion. Nor-UDCA passes through the cholangiocyte, returns to the sinusoids via the periductular capillary plexus, and is re-secreted into bile. This process is termed "cholehepatic shunting", which generates bicarbonate anion, reinforcing the "biliary bicarbonate umbrella". Cholehepatic shunting also enables "ductular targeting" to injured bile ducts, which plays a critical role of direct anti-inflammatory, anti-fibrosis, and anti-proliferation [52, 53].

Recently, hydrophilic tetrahydroxylated bile acids (THBA) have attracted the attention of researchers. THBA is more hydrophilic and less cytotoxic than the di- or tri-hydroxylated BAs, which can suppress BA-induced liver damage in mice [54]. Scientists found that feeding THBA to $Mdr2^{-/-}$ mice led to lower levels of toxic secondary BA, LCA, compared with the mice fed the base diet, while feeding of UDCA at equivalent doses led to an average increase in LCA of more than one thousand-fold in the feces and 300-fold in plasma. While the significance of such an increase in LCA was not explored [3], it does find possible adverse consequences of raising LCA during UDCA treatment. For example, treatment with UDCA has been reported to increase the incidence of colon cancer in primary sclerosing cholangitis (PSC) patients with inflammatory bowel disease, where most colon carcinomas develop in the early years after UDCA treatment. Thus, the finding that THBA feeding leads to lower or unchanged LCA production in comparison to UDCA and other BA derivatives may have special implications in terms of the therapeutic potential of THBA for reducing the toxicity of the BA pool.

6.2.3.1 Hydrophilic Bile Acids and Liver Inflammation

The BAs-induced inflammation plays an important role in the process of liver injury [55]. Thus, the modulation of the inflammatory responses via hydrophilic BAs is a potential target in treating cholestasis. UDCA was approved in 1997 for treatment in PBC at a dose of 13–15 mg/kg/day. Many clinical studies showed that UDCA improved liver biochemical indexes, delayed the progress of diseases, and increased survival free of liver transplantation [56–58]. A study evaluated the efficacy of TUDCA by analyzing 199 Chinese PBC patients who received TUDCA or UDCA for 24 weeks. A similar proportion of patients in both groups achieved a 25% or 40% reduction in ALP compared to baseline values. In addition, a phase II study of 159 patients with PSC treated with placebo vs. 500, 1000, or 1500 mg of nor-UDCA showed that nor-UDCA reduced ALP levels in a dose-dependent manner. Of note, the anti-inflammatory effect of nor-UDCA is more obvious when compared to UDCA in *S. mansoni* induced liver injury, and nor-UDCA can directly repress antigen presentation of antigen-presenting cells and subsequent T-cell activation in vitro [59].

Except for PBC and PSC, hydrophilic BAs have also achieved a good result in other chronic liver diseases. In a mouse model of hepatic ischemia reperfusion (HIR), TUDCA attenuated HIR injury by improving liver function in vivo and decreasing hepatocyte apoptosis in vitro. Moreover, TUDCA diminishes the expression and secretion of pro-inflammatory cytokines IL-1β, IL-6, and TNF-α by suppressing ER stress in Kupffer cells via the IRE1α/TRAF2/NF-κB pathway [60]. Likewise, in a non-alcoholic fatty liver disease (NAFLD) model, TUDCA alleviates gut inflammatory responses via downregulation of pro-inflammatory cytokines, such as IL-1β, CCL2, CCL4, and Icam1, and improves intestinal barrier function by increasing levels of tight junction molecules and the solid chemical barrier [61].

6.2.3.2 Hydrophilic Bile Acids and Liver Fibrosis

Chronic liver inflammation will cause liver fibrosis, cirrhosis and, even hepatocellular carcinoma. Hepatic fibrosis is a pathological process that results from the excessive accumulation of extracellular matrix (ECM) proteins, which replace the damaged normal liver tissue. There are two main causes of chronic liver injuries: hepatoxic injury (caused by hepatitis B or hepatitis C virus) and cholesterol injury (like PBC and PSC). Upon removal of the etiological source of the chronic injury, liver fibrosis can be reversed [62]. The transcription of proteins, such as BSEP and CYP7A1, participating in numerous signaling pathways, such as BAs synthesis, detoxification, and fibrogenesis, play a key role in the pathogenesis of cholestatic liver fibrosis [41, 63, 64]. A recent study found that NTCP expression is linearly associated with the severity of liver fibrosis, and antagonizing BAs uptake may be a therapeutic target for preventing disease progression [65].

Many experiments confirmed that hydrophilic BAs could inhibit liver fibrosis in different disease models [66–70], but its detailed mechanism remains to be investigated. The latest study revealed that UDCA displayed antifibrotic role by protecting HSC against the production of collagen and inhibiting cellular viability involving autophagy inhibition [71]. Notably, in the Mdr2$^{-/-}$ mice, a model of sclerosing cholangitis, nor-UDCA strongly reversed biliary fibrosis and injury, which was superior to UDCA treatment [72]. Similarly, in a rat model of thioacetamide-induced liver fibrosis, although nor-UDCA and UDCA exhibited therapeutic effects on fibrosis, nor-UDCA was more effective than UDCA, especially in the experiment with liver fibrosis regression. A similar role has also been reported for TUDCA. A study confirmed that TUDCA could inhibit carbon tetrachloride-induced liver fibrosis in rats [73], and its beneficial effects may be attributed to decreased hepatic unfolded protein response signaling and apoptotic cell death [74].

6.2.3.3 Hydrophilic Bile Acids and Liver Lipid Metabolism

FXR, a dedicated BA receptor, plays a critical role in lipid homeostasis. Prior studies revealed that FXR agonists can reduce circulating triglycerides (TGs) [75] and hepatic steatosis [76]. This beneficial remodeling of lipid metabolism is regulated by the FXR-SHP axis, which represses sterol regulatory element-binding protein 1c (SREBP1c), a master regulator of hepatic de novo lipogenesis [77], and by FXR-dependent interference of ChREBP binding to the liver pyruvate kinase (LPK) promoter [78]. Similarly, whole-body FXR$^{-/-}$ mice display an increase in serum TGs and cholesterol levels, together with an accumulation of hepatic lipid deposits and enhanced levels of lipogenic genes in the liver [79–81].

However, whether hydrophilic BAs, like UDCA, can lower the lipid levels is now uncertain and needs to be further studied. In basic research, UDCA is usually recognized as an agent with lipid-lowering activity. For instance, UDCA-treated mice showed higher expression levels of ABCG8, ABCB11, and CYP27A1, and lower expression levels of LXR and PPAR-α, which suggested that UDCA can improve lipid metabolism [82]. UDCA significantly inhibited lipid accumulation in a NAFLD cell model, which may repress the activation of AKT/mTOR/SREBP-1 signaling pathway [83]. But in clinical trials, it remains difficult to draw a firm conclusion. Some studies observed a significant decrease in total cholesterol levels after UDCA treatment [84–87]; however, other studies found no beneficial effect on lipid metabolism [88–91]. A meta-analysis [92] pooled the data from 15 randomized placebo-controlled trials and summarized the impact of UDCA on circulating lipid concentrations. Total cholesterol was reduced after UDCA treatment, while LDL-C, HDL-C, and TG were not significantly altered by UDCA administration. Moreover, UDCA reduced the levels of total cholesterol and LDL-C without affecting TG and HDL-C in PBC patients.

6.2.3.4 Hydrophilic Bile Acids and Gut Microbiome

There is a close and bidirectional interplay between BAs and the gut microbiota: the gut microbiome shapes the BAs pool, and cholestasis may alter intestinal microbial communities. Few studies have focused on the gut microbiota in cholestatic liver diseases [93, 94]. Notably, a recent study found that the diversity of gut microbiota reduced significantly in PBC patients, which is partially relieved by UDCA administration [95]. Similarly, reduced intraindividual bacterial diversity has been found in stool samples from PSC patients [96], but it remains unknown if they are primary or secondary to the bile secretory failure present in cholestatic disorders. Moreover, loss of gut microbiota in mdr2$^{-/-}$ mice, a mouse model of PSC deficient of canalicular transporter of phospholipid that can induce biliary injury, can also lead to increased liver damage [97]. Furthermore, the germ-free mdr2$^{-/-}$ mice exhibited significantly more severe liver chemistry and histological injuries compared to the control group [36]. These findings suggested the importance of commensal microbiota and its metabolites in protecting against injuries to bile duct.

Recent studies explored the effects of UDCA on gut microbiota composition in human and mice models [98–100]. Interestingly, UDCA influenced bacterial populations inducing a marked decrease in abundance of *Bifidobacterium*, *Lactobacillus*, and *Lactobacillaceae* [98]. UDCA could also improve colitogenic dysbiosis. A recent study indicated that UDCA, TUDCA, or glycoursodeoxycholic (GUDCA) equally lowered the severity of dextran sodium sulfate-induced colitis in mice and ameliorated colitis-associated fecal dysbiosis at the phylum level [101]. In a human study, the UDCA treatment can increase the abundances of *F. prausnitzii*, but reduce *Ruminococcus gnavus*, and this finding was associated with the lower risk of colorectal adenoma in men than in women [99]. In general, hydrophilic BAs seem to be a protective substance in both health and disease, but it remains to be determined if these effects are relevant to the therapeutic action of hydrophilic BAs.

6.3 Clinical Applications of Hydrophilic Bile Acids (UDCA, TUDCA, nor-UDCA) in Cirrhosis

6.3.1 Primary Biliary Cirrhosis

6.3.1.1 UDCA

PBC is characterized by progressive immune-mediated destruction of the small-to-medium-sized bile ducts, resulting in chronic cholestasis, portal inflammation, and fibrosis that can develop to cirrhosis, and even liver failure [102]. The diagnosis is based on anti-mitochondrial antibody (AMA) or anti-nuclear antibody (ANA) positive in the presence of a cholestatic biochemical profile, histologic confirmation being mandatory only in seronegative cases [103]. These patients usually have fatigue and pruritus, both of which occur independently of disease severity. It is prevalent among women, white patients, and patients 60–70 years old [104].

UDCA is the only drug approved by the US Food and Drug Administration and the European Association for the Study of the Liver for the treatment of PBC [105]. UDCA is the 7-β-epimer of the primary bile acid chenodeoxycholic acid, a naturally-occurring hydrophilic BA. The inflammation state created by BA accumulation in hepatocytes resulted in cell necrosis and apoptosis. UDCA increases the elimination of toxic substances from hepatocytes by inhibiting intestinal absorption of BAs and increasing biliary BAs secretion. The secretion stimulation depends on a dual MAPK- and integrin-dependent mechanism and activating hepatocytes and cholangiocytes vesicular exocytosis as well as carrier insertion into their apical membranes [106, 107] Meanwhile, it stimulates the secretion of a bicarbonate-rich fluid from cholangiocytes, which decreases cholestasis. Finally, UDCA augments micelle formation to prevent the toxic effect of BAs to cell membranes [108]. It is also reported that the gut microbial profile in PBC patients is altered and partially restored after UDCA therapy [95].

UDCA has been shown to improve serum hepatic biochemistries and prevent histological progression [109, 110], but it could not relieve the symptoms of fatigue and pruritus [111]. A retrospective review including 550 patients with PBC who accepted UDCA treatment or placebo control revealed that UDCA improved the survival free of liver transplantation [58]. The survival rate of patients with stage 1 or 2 disease was similar to that of a healthy control population when given long-term UDCA [112]. A meta-analysis of 4845 patients enrolled in long-term cohort studies revealed that UDCA treatment improved the transplant-free survival of 90% at 5 years, 78% at 10 years, and 66% at 15 years, compared with 79% at 5 years, 59% at 10 years, and 32% at 15 years in untreated group [56]. The latest research in 2021 showed that in a cohort of predominantly male patients with cirrhosis, UDCA response contributes to a reduction in decompensation, all-cause, and liver-related death or transplantation, with the highest benefit in patients with portal hypertension [113]. African American and Asian American/American Indian/Pacific Island (ASINPI) patients who did not receive UDCA had significantly higher mortality than white patients [114].

The recommended dose of UDCA is 13–15 mg/kg per day for all patients with PBC, usually for life, unless intolerance occurs. Loose stool, headache, and mild weight gain are the most frequently reported adverse effects of UDCA [115]. High doses of UDCA (28–30 mg/kg/day) is not recommended especially for patients with varices or liver transplantation, because UDCA has slight side effects which may be ineffective and harmful [115]. UDCA should be given to all PBC patients lifelong, including during pregnancy and breastfeeding [105]. What is more, preventive UDCA after liver transplantation for PBC reduces the risk of disease recurrence, graft loss, and death [116].

About 40% of patients will not have an adequate biochemical response to UDCA, who have relative risk of 5.51 (95% CI 1.70–15.99) of death or liver transplantation compared with those with a response [117]. Women presenting at younger than age 50 has the lowest response rates and highest levels of symptoms [118]. Besides, serum vitamin D level is also associated with disease severity and response to UDCA in PBC [119].

Stratification to recognize those high-risk patients with shorter survival using serum liver tests has been evaluated extensively across different cohorts worldwide, which is suggested for all patients following 1 year of UDCA therapy. This stratification is fundamental to recognizing those patients that should be considered for new disease-modifying therapy.

There are several classifications to define incomplete response to UDCA [120] (Table 6.1).

However, large-scale follow-up data have recently shown that even an incomplete response to UDCA in PBC is associated with better survival [127], which strongly suggests that UDCA therapy in PBC must be continued for life, regardless of biochemical response.

Table 6.1 Classifications to define incomplete response to UDCA

Definition of Incomplete -response	Duration of response	Classification	Reference
ALP ≥3x ULN or AST ≥2x ULN or Bilirubin >1 mg/dl	1 year	Paris-1	[121]
ALP ≥1.5x ULN or AST ≥1.5x ULN or Bilirubin >1 mg/dl	1 year	Paris-2	[122]
Bilirubin ≥1x ULN and/or Albumin <1x ULN	1 year	Rotterdam	[123]
ALP >1.67x ULN	2 years	Toronto	[124]
ALP ≥2 x ULN	1 year	Rochester-II	[125]
Decrease in ALP ≤ 40% and ALP ≥ 1x ULN	1 year	Barcelona	[117]
Decrease in GGT ≤ 70% and GGT ≥ 1 ULN	6 months	Ehime	[126]

ALP Alkaline phosphatase; *AST* Aspartate Aminotransferase; *GGT* Gamma-glutamyl transferase; *ULN* Upper limit of normal

Table 6.2 Continuous Prognostic Scores for UDCA-treated patients with PBC

Scoring parameters	Time	Classification	Reference
Bilirubin, ALP, and AST (or ALT); baseline: Albumin and platelets	1 year	UK-PBC	[129]
Bilirubin, ALP, albumin, and platelet count; baseline: Age	1 year	GLOBE	[130]

PBC patient outcomes can be predicted by biochemical indexes. The GLOBE and UK-PBC risk scoring systems were proven to be good predictors for future cirrhosis-related complications [120, 128] (Table 6.2).

6.3.1.2 Combined with Obeticholic Acid, Fibrates, Corticosteroids, and Other Drugs

No unified treatment was recommended to PBC patients who have an incomplete response to UDCA. UDCA combination with obeticholic acid (OCA), fibrates, and budesonide may be effective, but long-term efficacy is still a needed step to study.

6.3.1.3 Combined with Obeticholic Acid

For those adult PBC patients who are incompletely responsive to UDCA for at least 1 year or cannot tolerate UDCA as monotherapy, OCA was firstly recommended by EMA and FDA as a combined drug of UDCA [120, 131]. OCA can regulate BA synthesis, absorption, transport, secretion, and metabolism as an FXR agonist [132, 133]. A randomized control study assessed the effect of OCA on BA hepatobiliary excretion in PBC patients with an inadequate response to UDCA [134]. This study showed that, compared to placebo, OCA increased the transport of the conjugated BA tracer ^{11}C-CSar and accelerated the transportation of endogenous conjugated BAs from hepatocytes into biliary canaliculi, which revealed that OCA can reduce the time hepatocytes are exposed to potentially cytotoxic BAs. A research revealed that OCA demonstrated choleretic and antifibrotic effects by regulating FXR as well as immune response and inflammation [135]. Several other researches suggested that OCA reduced ALP levels compared with placebo along with or without UDCA [136–138]. OCA 5 mg once daily is recommended for adult PBC patients who are in inadequate biochemical response to the UDCA treatment with adequate doses for at least 1 year or who are intolerant to UDCA. If ALP or total bilirubin level has not gained any adequate reduction after 6 month-treatment at this dose, the OCA dosage can be increased to the maximum recommended dose of 10 mg/day once daily. The side effects of OCA are itch and dyslipidemia. As the benefit is not well determined in decompensated PBC patients, OCA is not recommended for these patients [131].

6.3.1.4 Combined with Fibrates

As agonists of peroxisome proliferator-activated receptors (PPARs), fibrates have anti-inflammatory, anticholestatic, and antifibrotic functions [139, 140]. Several placebo-controlled trials showed that patients treated with bezafibrate in combination with UDCA had a higher biochemical response and lower predicted mortality or need for liver transplantation than those treated with placebo plus UDCA [116, 141, 142]. Another study revealed that bezafibrate combined with UDCA significantly decreased the predicted risk of mortality [143]. Besides, bezafibrate also has a function of improving pruritus, fibrosis, and inflammatory histological scores [141, 144]. Overall, bezafibrate is the only drug currently available to improve symptoms, serological indicators, and prognosis in PBC patients. In spite of this, there are still several PBC patients who had a low response to bezafibrate combined with UDCA. Similarly, fenofibrate combined with UDCA for those PBC patients who have an inadequate response to UDCA can also improve serological indicators [145, 146] as well as fibrosis and ductular injury [147], and enhance transplant-free and decompensation-free survival [148]. But there were also some side effects of using fibrates, including myalgias, elevation in serum bilirubin levels/creatinine levels/aminotransaminase levels. At the same time, fibrates are also not recommended to treat PBC patients with decompensated liver cirrhosis.

6.3.1.5 Combined with Corticosteroids

The role of glucocorticoids in treating PBC inflammation is controversial [140], especially when UDCA is combined use of budesonide. Budesonide, as an agonist of PXR/glucocorticoid receptor (GR), is also involved in the synthesis, transport, and metabolism of BA, with high receptor affinity and high primary metabolism [149]. Several studies illustrated that budesonide improved the level of ALP and liver histology compared to placebo when combined with UDCA [150, 151] In addition, budesonide has severe osteoporosis complications and minor action of improving biochemical parameters as well as liver histology [152]. Besides, a recent placebo-controlled randomized trial disclosed that the addition of budesonide improved liver-related serological parameters, but had little effect on liver histology [153]. The effect of budesonide is closely related to the disease stage of PBC. Steroid-related side effects are the main adverse effects of budesonide, and also include portal vein thrombosis as well as osteoporosis [154]. Therefore, budesonide is not suitable for the treatment of advanced stage of PBC.

6.3.1.6 Combined with Other Drugs

PBC is a type of disease associated with an autoimmune state, and the role of several immunosuppressants and immunomodulators has been evaluated over the past few decades, such as methotrexate [155, 156], colchicine [157], azathioprine [158] and so on. However, the effects of these drugs were largely unsatisfactory, with patients showing no significant improvement in serological indicators, liver pathology, and overall survival, and/or reporting unacceptable risk of adverse events [159–162]. These demonstrated that autoimmune characteristics only partly reflected the nature of PBC.

6.3.2 Primary Sclerosing Cholangitis (PSC)

PSC is a rare disease with unknown etiology. It is mainly manifested as chronic progressive cholestasis, which eventually leads to end-stage liver disease. Multifocal intrahepatic or extrahepatic bile duct inflammation and fibrotic stenosis are the main characteristics [163]. Inflammatory bowel disease (IBD), which occurs most frequently in men aged 30–40, may be an important risk factor for 60%–80% of patients [164]. In addition, the risk of developing hepatobiliary or colorectal cancer is very high. About 40% of PSC patients die of cancer, with a mortality rate four times that of the general population [165]. Currently, the treatment of PSC has not been determined.

A number of studies since 1992 found that low-dose (13-15 mg/kg) and medium-dose (17–23 mg/L) UDCA had significant effects on improving liver biochemical indexes of PSC patients [166, 167]. However, there was no statistically significant improvement in mortality, liver transplantation, and cholangiocarcinoma [168–170]. In addition, high doses (28-32 mg/kg) of UDCA can lead to PSC progression to cirrhosis, esophageal varices, cholangiocellular carcinoma (CCA), colorectal dysplasia, liver transplantation, or death [115]. There are currently conflicting treatment guidelines for PSC. In 2019, the British Gastroenterological Association recommended that UDCA should not be routinely treated in newly diagnosed PSC patients [171]. As recommended by the British Gastroenterology Association, the American Association for the Study of Liver Diseases (AASLD) clinical practice guidelines do not recommend UDCA for patients with PSC [172]. However, the European Association for the Study of the Liver (EASL) has no specific recommendation on whether UDCA can be used for PSC [173]. For patients already using UDCA, discontinuation of UDCA leads to deterioration of liver symptoms, biochemical indices, and Mayo risk scores [174]. Therefore, patients already treated with UDCA need to decide whether to continue UDCA treatment after 6 months of use based on biochemical reactions and itching relief [175]. At present, the optimal dose of UDCA is 17–23 mg/kg, which has the most significant improvement on liver biochemical indexes [176], and the usual dosage for most doctors is 20 mg/kg.

TUDCA is a hydrophilic BA that is a taurine conjugate of UDCA. The role of UDCA in the liver is mostly generated by the non-conjugated form and its taurine conjugated TUDCA, and there is little difference between the two [4]. Eight patients with pancreatic cancer-induced biliary tract obstruction, but no liver or intestinal disease, were randomly treated with TUDCA and UDCA, and their absorption and BA secretion were similar [177]. Toxicity of BAs is inversely proportional to hydrophilicity, and coupling with taurine makes UDCA more polar, which indicates that TUDCA has a higher therapeutic effect [178–180]. In patients with cholestatic liver disease treated with UDCA or TUDCA, 85% of the PBC cholestase decreased, but not in the PSC group [181]. At present, the efficacy of TUDCA on PSC is still lacking more evidence, and further exploration is needed.

Nor-UDCA and UDCA have similar physiological structure, with one methylene less side chain than UDCA, relatively resistant to amidation, hepatobiliary shunting and the ability to directly stimulate bile duct cells to secrete bicarbonate. It has a strong ability to resist biliary tract injury caused by BAs [45] and has a bright prospect for the treatment of cholestatic liver and bile duct diseases. In typical PSC models of multidrug resistance gene 2 knockout mice ($Mdr2^{-/-}$), nor-UDCA significantly improved sclerosing cholangitis in mice [72]. Nor-UDCA also reduced liver damage in selective bile duct ligation (SBDL) mice, while UDCA was significantly more toxic to common bile duct ligation (CBDL) mice [182]. A multicenter randomized controlled trial of 161 patients with PSC found significant reductions in ALP levels after 12 weeks of nor-UDCA500 mg/day, 1000 mg/day, and 1500 mg/day, showing a good safety profile similar to placebo. There was no difference between itch reports and comfort groups [183]. Nor-UDCA is currently being evaluated in a phase III clinical study in patients with PSC (ClinicalTrials.gov, NCT01755507).

6.3.3 NAFLD-Related Cirrhosis

NAFLD has become one of the most common chronic liver diseases in the world, which is associated with obesity, hyperlipidemia, hyperlipidemia, type 2 diabetes, and metabolic syndrome [184, 185]. Non-alcoholic steatohepatitis (NASH), a subtype of NAFLD, has hepatocellular necrosis, inflammation, and fibrosis, and can lead to cirrhosis and even liver cancer in some patients [185]. Currently, there are no FDA-approved therapeutic drugs for this disease, and lifestyle changes, such as diet modification and exercise, are effective treatment methods [185]. BAs not only promote intestinal fat digestion and absorption but also act as ligands to bind BA receptors and regulate lipid metabolism and glucose metabolism through various signaling pathways [186–188]. Meanwhile, there is evidence that BA homeostasis is imbalanced in NASH patients [189], so BA analogs and their compounds affecting BA signaling pathways are expected to be effective drugs for the treatment of NAFLD/NASH.

UDCA, a hydrophilic BA with several hepatoprotective properties, has also been tested in NAFLD/NASH, but the results appear to be less than satisfactory. Treatment studies of UDCA in NAFLD reported a decade ago showed improvement in NAFLD transaminases with both low [190] and high dose [191] therapies, but this was not confirmed in large cohort studies that also used lower [192] and higher [193] dose treatments for more than 1 year. Therefore, there has been controversy about the efficacy of UDCA in NAFLD, and enthusiasm for its research in the disease has waned. The results of two recently conducted trials were again opposite, with one conventional dose (20 mg/kg/day), short-term (3 weeks) therapy demonstrating increased liver steatosis, disease activity and fibrosis in patients treated with UDCA [91, 194], while the other 6-month UDCA treatment at a dose of 15 mg/kg/day produced significant normalization of liver enzymes and improvement in lipids and liver steatosis [69]. Overall, the question of whether UDCA plays a role in NAFLD that is more beneficial or more detrimental has not been confirmed at this experimental stage, so it is not recommended in the current guidelines as a treatment for NAFLD [195]. However, some trials have shown beneficial effects of UDCA in combination with other drugs (e.g., vitamin E, curcumin) [190, 196, 197], and this may be considered in the future. The UDCA derivative nor-UDCA has been shown to improve steatohepatitis in a mouse model of NASH [198], and a recent phase II trial in patients with the disease also significantly reduced transaminase levels [199], indicating a potential therapeutic role for nor-UDCA in NAFLD disease.

OCA is a semi-synthetic analog of CDCA, a highly selective receptor agonist for FXR [200]. FXR expression in the terminal ileum and liver plays a role in the treatment of NAFLD [201]. When intestinal BA levels are elevated, the reabsorbed BAs enter the enterocytes to activate FXR and release human FGF19, which reaches the liver and binds to FGF receptor 4 (FGFR4), inhibiting BA synthesis by directly inhibiting the expression of CYP7A1 [202]. Hepatic FXR activation also inhibits CYP7A1, which manifests to promote bile excretion. In addition, in animal models of liver disease, FXR activation inhibits adipogenesis to reduce steatosis and exerts anti-inflammatory and antifibrotic effects [203, 204]. Thus, the results of the OCA Phase II and Phase III clinical trials in NASH showed considerable beneficial effects of OCA - improvement of fibrosis [204, 205]. However, OCA treatment also decreased HDL and increased LDL cholesterol [204], increasing cardiovascular risk, while its side effect of pruritus was surprising and disappointing, so the development of an alternative to OCA without pruritic side effects is an urgent priority.

6.3.4 Drug-Induced Cholestasis

Drug-induced cholestasis is common and accounts for approximately 17% of all hepatic adverse drug reactions (ADRs) [206]. Some drugs only cause simple cholestasis, such as estrogens, anabolic steroids. Some drugs can induce cholestatic hepatitis, drug-induced sclerosing cholangitis, and the vanishing bile duct syndrome (VBDS), some cases even progress to cholestatic cirrhosis. Chlorpromazine, ketoconazole, and amoxycillin-clavulanate are typical drugs. There is no pretreatment for drug-induced cholestasis, but early recognition and prompt drug withdrawal are the more important [206]. According to the published individual case reports and open cohort studies, UDCA is effective to relieve jaundice, pruritus, fatigue, and liver biochemical abnormalities in approximately two-thirds of treated cases [206–210]. Considering the important methodological limitations, it is difficult to preclude a generalization of the results on some retrospective and prospective cohort studies [211–213]. High-quality controlled studies are required to explore the effect of UDCA in drug-induced cholestasis. However, it is difficult to conduct these experiments, given that a wide variety of drugs have been involved and the nature of these cases has been isolated [214].

6.3.5 Intrahepatic Cholestasis of Pregnancy

Intrahepatic cholestasis of pregnancy (ICP) is one of the most common pregnancy-specific liver diseases, which often occurs in the second and third trimester of pregnancy. Clinical syndromes of ICP include generalized pruritus and elevated BAs, with normal or abnormal liver function. ICP is associated with multiple adverse pregnancy outcomes, including preterm birth (iatrogenic and spontaneous), amniotic fluid staining, neonatal depression, respiratory distress syndrome, and increased risk of stillbirth [215]. In normal pregnancies, BAs are transported from the fetus to the mother, whereas in ICP pregnancies, placental transport occurs in the opposite direction. As a result, both maternal and fecal BA levels increased. Increased levels of total bile acid (TBA) are associated with the induction of oxidative stress and apoptosis, resulting in damage to liver cells and other tissues, and an increased risk of harmful effects on the fetus with increased levels of TBA in maternal blood [216].

UDCA is the therapeutic choice for ICP. The mechanism includes the replacement of hydrophobic BAs to ensure the protection of hepatocyte membranes and to stimulate the expulsion of BAs from the fetus through the placenta [216]. Since 1991, after the publication of the first article showing that UDCA can improve serum bile salt levels and pruritus symptoms, many articles further confirmed that UDCA is effective on pruritus and in decreasing liver transaminase and bilirubin in ICP patients [217, 218]. A meta-analysis found that UDCA also can effectively improve fetal prognosis [219]. The incidence of fetal distress/asphyxia was lower in the UDCA group than in the placebo group, but the difference was not statistically significant [219]. However, an RCT trial involving 605 women found that UDCA treatment, although harmless, did not reduce maternal BA concentrations, nor can it reduce the adverse perinatal outcomes in women with ICP [220]. Meanwhile, a large meta-analysis of 5557 ICP cases and 165,136 controls showed that BAs are important for fetal prognosis, however, UDCA treatment did not significantly affect the relationship between BA levels and fetal prognosis [221]. Therefore, the relevance of UDCA for the treatment of ICP should be reconsidered. UDCA is still the first-line treatment for ICP and is recommended in six national guidelines for the management of ICP.

Although the usefulness of UDCA is now in doubt, no studies have been published to date to report any adverse effects of UDCA on mothers or fetuses. But Chappell recommended that the lack of evidence of in vivo benefits should prevent further routine clinical use of UDCA, which does no harm but avoids unproven treatment for women [221]. In conclusion, the findings of the latest study undermine the role of UDCA as a first-line treatment for ICP, and more research is needed to further explore the implications of UDCA for pregnant women and fetuses.

6.3.6 Total Parenteral Nutrition-Associated Cholestasis

Long-term total parenteral nutrition treatment is a risk factor to cause transient or persistent liver damage, manifested as cholestasis with increased serum ALP and bilirubin levels [222]. Clinical studies indicated that orally administered UDCA in doses of 10–30 mg/kg body weight per day is effective to improve cholestatic abnormalities caused by parenteral nutrition-associated cholestasis in neonates [223–226]. Recently, a retrospective research in neonates demonstrated that UDCA therapy was associated with a faster decline of conjugated bilirubin and greater weight gain, but not associated with the duration of parenteral nutrition-associated liver disease [227]. UDCA is recommended to treat parenteral nutrition-associated cholestasis by the American Society for Parenteral and Enteral Nutrition Clinical Guidelines (2014). However, this suggestion is lacking of high-quality evidence, and more relevant studies are required to verify its effect [228]. Evidence of a benefit of the application of UDCA in adults with parenteral nutrition-associated liver disease is more limited, with a single study showing that treatment with an average of 11.2 mg oral UDCA/kg body weight per day is related to a decline in GGT and ALT levels, but not ALP, AST, or bilirubin levels [229].

6.3.7 Chronic Graft-Versus-Host Disease Involving the Liver

Graft-versus-host disease (GVHD) is a common complication following allogeneic bone marrow transplantation with cholestasis and veno-occlusive disease. Up to now, preliminary studies indicated that short-term treatment with UDCA improves the cholestasis in GVHD [230]. A prospective, single-center study showed that the long-term treatment of UDCA results in clinical and biochemical beneficial effects in individuals with limited GVHD of the liver. The data suggests that long-term therapy is safe and tolerable [231]. Another randomized, open-label multicenter research indicated that in addition to short-term benefits, UDCA prophylaxis improves long-term survival and reduces non-relapse mortality without causing any adverse effects [232].

6.3.8 Liver Disease in Cystic Fibrosis

Cystic fibrosis (CF) is an autosomal recessive disease that occurs more often in Caucasians. The odds of the disease are about 1/2000–3000 [233]. The mutations of the CFTR gene lead to dysfunction of chloride channels in the apical epithelial cells of the gut, pancreas, and bile duct systems, and cause dehydration of secretions and mucus hyperplasia, while affecting bile production, leading to multisystem disease [234–236].

While CF predominantly causes damage in the lung, now people are shedding more light on how to deal with the extrapulmonary manifestations of CF for advances in patient care have altered the course of CF and led to a significant increase in life expectancy. The clinical manifestations of CFLD may include elevated liver enzymes, cholangitis, and hepatic steatosis, as well as focal fibrosis and focal cirrhosis [236]. CF is now considered the third leading cause of death following respiratory and transplant complications.

UDCA is currently the primary treatment for primary liver disease and can improve the flow of BAs by inducing the flow of hydrogen carbonate bile [237], but its use as a CFID treatment remains controversial. A population-based longitudinal cohort study from the UK has found that the prevalence of CFID is slowly increasing. After stratifying patients for cirrhosis of the liver, the use of UDCA was found to be associated with longer survival, especially in patients without cirrhosis, but not in patients with cirrhosis [238]. Another study reported that UDCA can reduce cirrhosis in patients with mild liver disease, thereby preventing the development of cirrhosis, which is consistent with earlier observational studies in CF patients with mild liver disease [239]. We, therefore, suspect that UDCA might have a beneficial effect in patients with early or mild CF disease. However, most studies prove it of no obvious effect to use UDCA for the long-term survival of CFID. A review based on four RCTs concluded that UDCA treatment had no significant effect on CF patients, except for a slight effect on liver enzyme reduction, but given that these studies were short-term trials, there is no enough evidence to support the UDCA's role in improving survival [237]. A multicenter cohort study found that using UDCA did not reduce the incidence of portal hypertension [240].

In short, more evidences are needed to confirm the effect of UDCA in CTID. In the future, RCTs which involve a larger sample size and longer observation time are required. Due to the absence of additional useful medicine for CFID, it is still recommended to start UDCA treatment once diagnosed with CFID.

6.3.9 Progressive Familial Intrahepatic Cholestasis

Progressive familial intrahepatic cholestasis (PFIC) is an autosomal recessive disorder that results from defect in bile secretion and is characterized by intrahepatic cholestasis. PFIC is usually onsets in infancy and childhood and can lead to liver cirrhosis. According to the gene mutation location, PFIC is divided into three types. Type1 (PFIC1) is defective in ATP8B1 gene which encodes the FIC1 protein. Type2 (PFIC2) has mutations in ABCB11 gene encoding BSEP. Type 3 (PFIC3) is associated with mutations in ABCB4 gene encoding the canalicular translocator of phosphatidylcholine MDR3 [241–243]. The severity of liver disease and the response to pharmacological therapy vary among PFIC children. Cholestatic jaundice and pruritus are the main clinical presentations. PFIC1/2 usually manifests with normal serum gamma-glutamyl transpeptidase (GGT) while that is raised in patients with PFIC3. Although the optimal strategy for the treatment of PFIC has not been fully defined, liver transplantation has been considered to be a definitive therapy, with a survival rate of approximately 92% at 5 years at present [244]. The combination of UDCA and standard nutritional support, including adequate calories, supplementation of fat-soluble vitamins, and medium-chain triglycerides, is the essential treatment for PFIC. UDCA 20–30 mg/kg/day for 2–4 years is safe and decreases the ALT and GGT levels and improves the nutritional condition, hepatosplenomegaly, and pruritus [245, 246]. Currently, UDCA is the first-line therapy for patients with ABCB4 deficiency (PFIC III). Its efficacy is associated with the type of ABCB4 variant and the changes in MDR3 expression/function which result from the former factors. For patients with normal or reduced MDR3 activity, UDCA can be used as an effective treatment method, and it improves the liver function, even restores it to be normal. However, patients with nearly complete or complete loss of MDR3 function are ineffective with the treatment of UDCA [247, 248]. In addition, studies have shown that UDCA can induce the insertion of Bsep into the microtubule membrane of hepatocytes, thereby increasing the microtubule expression of Bsep, which can be used for the treatment of patients with ABCB11 deficiency (PFIC II) [249, 250]. In patients with ATP8B1 deficiency (PFIC I), the efficacy of UDCA is not ideal. For these patients, partial biliary diversion surgery is an option worth considering [251].

6.3.10 Other Pediatric Cholestatic Disorders

Pediatric cholestatic disorders include biliary atresia, Alagille syndrome, BA synthesis defects, ductal plate abnormalities, including Caroli syndrome and congenital hepatic fibrosis, and certain metabolic diseases [252]. In addition to liver transplantation in childhood, UDCA is an adjunctive therapy for pediatric cholestatic diseases, especially for biliary atresia [253, 254]. Despite the compelling evidence lacking to verify its exact effect, given the low side effect risk profile of standard-dose UDCA (10–20 mg/kg/day), it is often used in those children who suffer from pediatric chronic cholestasis [252].

References

1. Russell DW. The enzymes, regulation, and genetics of bile acid synthesis. Annu Rev Biochem. 2003;72:137–74.
2. Hofmann AF. The enterohepatic circulation of bile acids in mammals: form and functions. Frontiers in bioscience (Landmark edition). 2009;14:2584–98.
3. Hofmann AF. Pharmacology of ursodeoxycholic acid, an enterohepatic drug. Scand J Gastroenterol Suppl. 1994;204:1–15.
4. Cabrera D, Arab JP, Arrese M. UDCA, NorUDCA, and TUDCA in liver diseases: a review of their mechanisms of action and clinical applications. Handb Exp Pharmacol. 2019;256:237–64.
5. Lazaridis KN, Gores GJ, Lindor KD. Ursodeoxycholic acid 'mechanisms of action and clinical use in hepatobiliary disorders'. J Hepatol. 2001;35:134–46.
6. Li S, Tan HY, Wang N, et al. Substitutes for bear bile for the treatment of liver diseases: research Progress and future perspective. Evid Based Complement Alternat Med. 2016;2016:4305074.
7. Leuschner U, Leuschner M, Sieratzki J, et al. Gallstone dissolution with ursodeoxycholic acid in patients with chronic active hepatitis and two years follow-up. A pilot study. Dig Dis Sci. 1985;30:642–9.
8. Nakagawa S, Makino I, Ishizaki T, et al. Dissolution of cholesterol gallstones by ursodeoxycholic acid. Lancet. 1977;2:367–9.
9. Poupon R, Chrétien Y, Poupon RE, et al. Is ursodeoxycholic acid an effective treatment for primary biliary cirrhosis? Lancet. 1987;1:834–6.
10. von Haehling S, Schefold JC, Jankowska EA, et al. Ursodeoxycholic acid in patients with chronic heart failure: a double-blind, randomized, placebo-controlled, crossover trial. J Am Coll Cardiol. 2012;59:585–92.
11. Goossens JF, Bailly C. Ursodeoxycholic acid and cancer: from chemoprevention to chemotherapy. Pharmacol Ther. 2019;203:107396.
12. Pardue MT, Allen RS. Neuroprotective strategies for retinal disease. Prog Retin Eye Res. 2018;65:50–76.
13. Halilbasic E, Claudel T, Trauner M. Bile acid transporters and regulatory nuclear receptors in the liver and beyond. J Hepatol. 2013;58:155–68.
14. Trauner M, Boyer JL. Bile salt transporters: molecular characterization, function, and regulation. Physiol Rev. 2003;83:633–71.
15. Jansen PL, Ghallab A, Vartak N, et al. The ascending pathophysiology of cholestatic liver disease. Hepatology. 2017;65:722–38.
16. Woolbright BL, Jaeschke H. Therapeutic targets for cholestatic liver injury. Expert Opin Ther Targets. 2016;20:463–75.
17. Dawson PA, Lan T, Rao A. Bile acid transporters. J Lipid Res. 2009;50:2340–57.
18. Inagaki T, Choi M, Moschetta A, et al. Fibroblast growth factor 15 functions as an enterohepatic signal to regulate bile acid homeostasis. Cell Metab. 2005;2:217–25.
19. Choi M, Moschetta A, Bookout AL, et al. Identification of a hormonal basis for gallbladder filling. Nat Med. 2006;12:1253–5.
20. Sinha J, Chen F, Miloh T, et al. Beta-klotho and FGF-15/19 inhibit the apical sodium-dependent bile acid transporter in enterocytes and cholangiocytes. Am J Physiol Gastrointest Liver Physiol. 2008;295:G996–G1003.
21. Thomas C, Pellicciari R, Pruzanski M, et al. Targeting bile-acid signalling for metabolic diseases. Nat Rev Drug Discov. 2008;7:678–93.
22. Spivey JR, Bronk SF, Gores GJ. Glycochenodeoxycholate-induced lethal hepatocellular injury in rat hepatocytes. Role of ATP depletion and cytosolic free calcium. J Clin Invest. 1993;92:17–24.
23. Galle PR, Theilmann L, Raedsch R, et al. Ursodeoxycholate reduces hepatotoxicity of bile salts in primary human hepatocytes. Hepatology. 1990;12:486–91.

24. Sokol RJ, McKim JM Jr, Goff MC, et al. Vitamin E reduces oxidant injury to mitochondria and the hepatotoxicity of taurochenodeoxycholic acid in the rat. Gastroenterology. 1998;114:164–74.
25. Attili AF, Angelico M, Cantafora A, et al. Bile acid-induced liver toxicity: relation to the hydrophobic-hydrophilic balance of bile acids. Med Hypotheses. 1986;19:57–69.
26. Billington D, Evans CE, Godfrey PP, et al. Effects of bile salts on the plasma membranes of isolated rat hepatocytes. Biochem J. 1980;188:321–7.
27. Sokol RJ, Straka MS, Dahl R, et al. Role of oxidant stress in the permeability transition induced in rat hepatic mitochondria by hydrophobic bile acids. Pediatr Res. 2001;49:519–31.
28. Ljubuncic P, Fuhrman B, Oiknine J, et al. Effect of deoxycholic acid and ursodeoxycholic acid on lipid peroxidation in cultured macrophages. Gut. 1996;39:475–8.
29. Rodrigues CM, Fan G, Ma X, et al. A novel role for ursodeoxycholic acid in inhibiting apoptosis by modulating mitochondrial membrane perturbation. J Clin Invest. 1998;101:2790–9.
30. Rodrigues CM, Ma X, Linehan-Stieers C, et al. Ursodeoxycholic acid prevents cytochrome c release in apoptosis by inhibiting mitochondrial membrane depolarization and channel formation. Cell Death Differ. 1999;6:842–54.
31. Yerushalmi B, Dahl R, Devereaux MW, et al. Bile acid-induced rat hepatocyte apoptosis is inhibited by antioxidants and blockers of the mitochondrial permeability transition. Hepatology. 2001;33:616–26.
32. Patel T, Bronk SF, Gores GJ. Increases of intracellular magnesium promote glycodeoxycholate-induced apoptosis in rat hepatocytes. J Clin Invest. 1994;94:2183–92.
33. Sokol RJ, Winklhofer-Roob BM, Devereaux MW, et al. Generation of hydroperoxides in isolated rat hepatocytes and hepatic mitochondria exposed to hydrophobic bile acids. Gastroenterology. 1995;109:1249–56.
34. Faubion WA, Guicciardi ME, Miyoshi H, et al. Toxic bile salts induce rodent hepatocyte apoptosis via direct activation of Fas. J Clin Invest. 1999;103:137–45.
35. Higuchi H, Bronk SF, Takikawa Y, et al. The bile acid glycochenodeoxycholate induces trail-receptor 2/DR5 expression and apoptosis. J Biol Chem. 2001;276:38610–8.
36. Mariotti V, Cadamuro M, Spirli C, et al. Animal models of cholestasis: an update on inflammatory cholangiopathies. Biochim Biophys Acta Mol basis Dis. 2019;1865:954–64.
37. Mariotti V, Strazzabosco M, Fabris L, et al. Animal models of biliary injury and altered bile acid metabolism. Biochim Biophys Acta Mol basis Dis. 2018;1864:1254–61.
38. Perez MJ, Briz O. Bile-acid-induced cell injury and protection. World J Gastroenterol. 2009;15:1677–89.
39. Arrese M, Trauner M. Molecular aspects of bile formation and cholestasis. Trends Mol Med. 2003;9:558–64.
40. Arrese M, Karpen SJ. Nuclear receptors, inflammation, and liver disease: insights for cholestatic and fatty liver diseases. Clin Pharmacol Ther. 2010;87:473–8.
41. Wagner M, Zollner G, Trauner M. Nuclear receptor regulation of the adaptive response of bile acid transporters in cholestasis. Semin Liver Dis. 2010;30:160–77.
42. Jansen PL, Schaap FG, Beuers UH. Fibroblast growth factor 19, an anticholestatic drug produced by human liver. Gastroenterology. 2012;142:e29–30.
43. Banales JM, Huebert RC, Karlsen T, et al. Cholangiocyte pathobiology. Nat Rev Gastroenterol Hepatol. 2019;16:269–81.
44. Banales JM, Prieto J, Medina JF. Cholangiocyte anion exchange and biliary bicarbonate excretion. World J Gastroenterol. 2006;12:3496–511.
45. Hohenester S, Wenniger LM, Paulusma CC, et al. A biliary HCO3- umbrella constitutes a protective mechanism against bile acid-induced injury in human cholangiocytes. Hepatology. 2012;55:173–83.
46. Tabibian JH, Masyuk AI, Masyuk TV, et al. Physiology of cholangiocytes. Comprehensive. Physiology. 2013;3:541–65.
47. Sato K, Meng F, Giang T, et al. Mechanisms of cholangiocyte responses to injury. Biochim Biophys Acta Mol basis Dis. 2018;1864:1262–9.

48. Cheung AC, Lorenzo Pisarello MJ, LaRusso NF. Pathobiology of biliary epithelia. Biochim Biophys Acta Mol basis Dis. 2018;1864:1220–31.
49. Beuers U, Trauner M, Jansen P, et al. New paradigms in the treatment of hepatic cholestasis: from UDCA to FXR, PXR and beyond. J Hepatol. 2015;62:S25–37.
50. Hofmann AF, Zakko SF, Lira M, et al. Novel biotransformation and physiological properties of norursodeoxycholic acid in humans. Hepatology. 2005;42:1391–8.
51. Yoon YB, Hagey LR, Hofmann AF, et al. Effect of side-chain shortening on the physiologic properties of bile acids: hepatic transport and effect on biliary secretion of 23-nor-ursodeoxycholate in rodents. Gastroenterology. 1986;90:837–52.
52. Lazarević S, Đanić M, Goločorbin-Kon S, et al. Semisynthetic bile acids: a new therapeutic option for metabolic syndrome. Pharmacol Res. 2019;146:104333.
53. Trauner M, Halilbasic E, Claudel T, et al. Potential of nor-Ursodeoxycholic acid in Cholestatic and metabolic disorders. Digestive Diseases (Basel, Switzerland). 2015;33:433–9.
54. Sheps JA, Wang R, Wang J, et al. The protective role of hydrophilic tetrahydroxylated bile acids (THBA). Biochim Biophys Acta Mol Cell Biol Lipids. 2021;1866:158925.
55. Li M, Cai SY, Boyer JL. Mechanisms of bile acid mediated inflammation in the liver. Mol Asp Med. 2017;56:45–53.
56. Lammers WJ, van Buuren HR, Hirschfield GM, et al. Levels of alkaline phosphatase and bilirubin are surrogate end points of outcomes of patients with primary biliary cirrhosis: an international follow-up study. Gastroenterology. 2014;147:1338–49.e5. quiz e15
57. Poupon RE, Bonnand AM, Chrétien Y, et al. The UDCA-PBC Study Group. Ten-year survival in ursodeoxycholic acid-treated patients with primary biliary cirrhosis. Hepatology. 1999;29:1668–71.
58. Poupon RE, Lindor KD, Cauch-Dudek K, et al. Combined analysis of randomized controlled trials of ursodeoxycholic acid in primary biliary cirrhosis. Gastroenterology. 1997;113:884–90.
59. Sombetzki M, Fuchs CD, Fickert P, et al. 24-nor-ursodeoxycholic acid ameliorates inflammatory response and liver fibrosis in a murine model of hepatic schistosomiasis. J Hepatol. 2015;62:871–8.
60. Xu X, Wang M, Li JZ, et al. Tauroursodeoxycholic acid alleviates hepatic ischemia reperfusion injury by suppressing the function of Kupffer cells in mice. Biomedicine & Pharmacotherapy = Biomedecine & pharmacotherapie. 2018;106:1271–81.
61. Wang W, Zhao J, Gui W, et al. Tauroursodeoxycholic acid inhibits intestinal inflammation and barrier disruption in mice with non-alcoholic fatty liver disease. Br J Pharmacol. 2018;175:469–84.
62. Kisseleva T, Brenner D. Molecular and cellular mechanisms of liver fibrosis and its regression. Nat Rev Gastroenterol Hepatol. 2021;18:151–66.
63. Cai SY, Boyer JL. The role of bile acids in cholestatic liver injury. Anna Translational Med. 2021;9:737.
64. Fickert P, Fuchsbichler A, Moustafa T, et al. Farnesoid X receptor critically determines the fibrotic response in mice but is expressed to a low extent in human hepatic stellate cells and periductal myofibroblasts. Am J Pathol. 2009;175:2392–405.
65. Salhab A, Amer J, Lu Y, et al. Sodium(+)/taurocholate cotransporting polypeptide as target therapy for liver fibrosis. Gut. 2021; https://doi.org/10.1136/gutjnl-2020-323345. Online ahead of print.
66. Buko VU, Lukivskaya OY, Naruta EE, et al. Protective effects of Norursodeoxycholic acid versus Ursodeoxycholic acid on Thioacetamide-induced rat liver fibrosis. J Clin Exp Hepatol. 2014;4:293–301.
67. Corpechot C, Carrat F, Bonnand AM, et al. The effect of ursodeoxycholic acid therapy on liver fibrosis progression in primary biliary cirrhosis. Hepatology. 2000;32:1196–9.
68. Mas N, Tasci I, Comert B, et al. Ursodeoxycholic acid treatment improves hepatocyte ultrastructure in rat liver fibrosis. World J Gastroenterol. 2008;14:1108–11.

69. Nadinskaia M, Maevskaya M, Ivashkin V, et al. Ursodeoxycholic acid as a means of preventing atherosclerosis, steatosis and liver fibrosis in patients with nonalcoholic fatty liver disease. World J Gastroenterol. 2021;27:959–75.
70. Pan XL, Zhao L, Li L, et al. Efficacy and safety of tauroursodeoxycholic acid in the treatment of liver cirrhosis: a double-blind randomized controlled trial. Journal of Huazhong University of Science and Technology Medical sciences. 2013;33:189–94.
71. Ye HL, Zhang JW, Chen XZ, et al. Ursodeoxycholic acid alleviates experimental liver fibrosis involving inhibition of autophagy. Life Sci. 2020;242:117175.
72. Fickert P, Wagner M, Marschall HU, et al. 24-norUrsodeoxycholic acid is superior to ursodeoxycholic acid in the treatment of sclerosing cholangitis in Mdr2 (Abcb4) knockout mice. Gastroenterology. 2006;130:465–81.
73. Wang D, Yang L, Huang J-M, et al. Tauroursodeoxycholic acid inhibits carbon tetrachloride-induced liver fibrosis in rats. World Chinese J Digestol 2010:1979–84.
74. Paridaens A, Raevens S, Devisscher L, et al. Modulation of the unfolded protein response by tauroursodeoxycholic acid counteracts apoptotic cell death and fibrosis in a mouse model for secondary biliary liver fibrosis. Int J Mol Sci. 2017;18.
75. de Groot P, Scheithauer T, Bakker GJ, et al. Donor metabolic characteristics drive effects of faecal microbiota transplantation on recipient insulin sensitivity, energy expenditure and intestinal transit time. Gut. 2020;69:502–12.
76. Pathak P, Liu H, Boehme S, et al. Farnesoid X receptor induces Takeda G-protein receptor 5 cross-talk to regulate bile acid synthesis and hepatic metabolism. J Biol Chem. 2017;292:11055–69.
77. Watanabe M, Houten SM, Wang L, et al. Bile acids lower triglyceride levels via a pathway involving FXR, SHP, and SREBP-1c. J Clin Invest. 2004;113:1408–18.
78. Caron S, Huaman Samanez C, Dehondt H, et al. Farnesoid X receptor inhibits the transcriptional activity of carbohydrate response element binding protein in human hepatocytes. Mol Cell Biol. 2013;33:2202–11.
79. Duran-Sandoval D, Cariou B, Percevault F, et al. The farnesoid X receptor modulates hepatic carbohydrate metabolism during the fasting-refeeding transition. J Biol Chem. 2005;280:29971–9.
80. Kong B, Luyendyk JP, Tawfik O, et al. Farnesoid X receptor deficiency induces nonalcoholic steatohepatitis in low-density lipoprotein receptor-knockout mice fed a high-fat diet. J Pharmacol Exp Ther. 2009;328:116–22.
81. Sinal CJ, Tohkin M, Miyata M, et al. Targeted disruption of the nuclear receptor FXR/BAR impairs bile acid and lipid homeostasis. Cell. 2000;102:731–44.
82. Fan N, Meng K, Zhang Y, et al. The effect of ursodeoxycholic acid on the relative expression of the lipid metabolism genes in mouse cholesterol gallstone models. Lipids Health Dis. 2020;19:158.
83. Hu J, Hong W, Yao KN, et al. Ursodeoxycholic acid ameliorates hepatic lipid metabolism in LO2 cells by regulating the AKT/mTOR/SREBP-1 signaling pathway. World J Gastroenterol. 2019;25:1492–501.
84. Balan V, Dickson ER, Jorgensen RA, et al. Effect of ursodeoxycholic acid on serum lipids of patients with primary biliary cirrhosis. Mayo Clin Proc. 1994;69:923–9.
85. Méndez-Sánchez N, González V, Chávez-Tapia N, et al. Weight reduction and ursodeoxycholic acid in subjects with nonalcoholic fatty liver disease. A double-blind, placebo-controlled trial. Ann Hepatol. 2004;3:108–12.
86. Miettinen TA, Färkkilä M, Vuoristo M, et al. Serum cholestanol, cholesterol precursors, and plant sterols during placebo-controlled treatment of primary biliary cirrhosis with ursodeoxycholic acid or colchicine. Hepatology. 1995;21:1261–8.
87. Mouillot T, Beylot M, Drai J, et al. Effect of bile acid supplementation on endogenous lipid synthesis in patients with short bowel syndrome: a pilot study. Clinical Nutrition (Edinburgh, Scotland). 2020;39:928–34.

88. Battezzati PM, Podda M, Bianchi FB, et al. Italian multicenter group for the study of UDCA in PBC. Ursodeoxycholic acid for symptomatic primary biliary cirrhosis. Preliminary analysis of a double-blind multicenter trial. J Hepatol. 1993;17:332–8.
89. Braga MF, Grace MG, Lenis J, et al. Efficacy and safety of ursodeoxycholic acid in primary, type IIa or IIb hypercholesterolemia: a multicenter, randomized, double-blind clinical trial. Atherosclerosis. 2009;203:479–82.
90. Fromm H, Roat JW, Gonzalez V, et al. Comparative efficacy and side effects of ursodeoxycholic and chenodeoxycholic acids in dissolving gallstones. A double-blind controlled study. Gastroenterology. 1983;85:1257–64.
91. Mueller M, Thorell A, Claudel T, et al. Ursodeoxycholic acid exerts farnesoid X receptor-antagonistic effects on bile acid and lipid metabolism in morbid obesity. J Hepatol. 2015;62:1398–404.
92. Simental-Mendía LE, Simental-Mendía M, Sánchez-García A, et al. Impact of ursodeoxycholic acid on circulating lipid concentrations: a systematic review and meta-analysis of randomized placebo-controlled trials. Lipids Health Dis. 2019;18:88.
93. Li Y, Tang R, Leung PSC, et al. Bile acids and intestinal microbiota in autoimmune cholestatic liver diseases. Autoimmun Rev. 2017;16:885–96.
94. Quigley EM. Primary biliary cirrhosis and the microbiome. Semin Liver Dis. 2016;36:349–53.
95. Tang R, Wei Y, Li Y, et al. Gut microbial profile is altered in primary biliary cholangitis and partially restored after UDCA therapy. Gut. 2018;67:534–41.
96. Kummen M, Holm K, Anmarkrud JA, et al. The gut microbial profile in patients with primary sclerosing cholangitis is distinct from patients with ulcerative colitis without biliary disease and healthy controls. Gut. 2017;66:611–9.
97. Tabibian JH, O'Hara SP, Trussoni CE, et al. Absence of the intestinal microbiota exacerbates hepatobiliary disease in a murine model of primary sclerosing cholangitis. Hepatology. 2016;63:185–96.
98. Kim DJ, Yoon S, Ji SC, et al. Ursodeoxycholic acid improves liver function via phenylalanine/tyrosine pathway and microbiome remodelling in patients with liver dysfunction. Sci Rep. 2018;8:11874.
99. Pearson T, Caporaso JG, Yellowhair M, et al. Effects of ursodeoxycholic acid on the gut microbiome and colorectal adenoma development. Cancer Med. 2019;8:617–28.
100. Winston JA, Rivera A, Cai J, et al. Secondary bile acid ursodeoxycholic acid alters weight, the gut microbiota, and the bile acid pool in conventional mice. PLoS One. 2021;16:e0246161.
101. Van den Bossche L, Hindryckx P, Devisscher L, et al. Ursodeoxycholic acid and its taurine- or glycine-conjugated species reduce Colitogenic Dysbiosis and equally suppress experimental colitis in mice. Appl Environ Microbiol 2017; 83:e02766–16.
102. Selmi C, Bowlus CL, Gershwin ME, et al. Primary biliary cirrhosis. Lancet. 2011;377:1600–9.
103. Terziroli Beretta-Piccoli B, Mieli-Vergani G, Vergani D, et al. The challenges of primary biliary cholangitis: what is new and what needs to be done. J Autoimmun. 2019;105:102328.
104. Lu M, Li J, Haller IV, et al. Factors associated with prevalence and treatment of primary biliary cholangitis in United States health systems. Clin Gastroenterol Hepatol. 2018;16:e6.
105. Easl E. EASL clinical practice guidelines: the diagnosis and management of patients with primary biliary cholangitis. J Hepatol. 2017;67:145–72.
106. Haussinger D, Kurz AK, Wettstein M, et al. Involvement of integrins and Src in tauroursodeoxycholate-induced and swelling-induced choleresis. Gastroenterology. 2003;124:1476–87.
107. Kurz AK, Graf D, Schmitt M, et al. Tauroursodesoxycholate-induced choleresis involves p38(MAPK) activation and translocation of the bile salt export pump in rats. Gastroenterology. 2001;121:407–19.
108. Poupon R. Ursodeoxycholic acid and bile-acid mimetics as therapeutic agents for cholestatic liver diseases: an overview of their mechanisms of action. Clin Res Hepatol Gastroenterol. 2012;36:S3–12.
109. Angulo P, Batts KP, Therneau TM, et al. Long-term ursodeoxycholic acid delays histological progression in primary biliary cirrhosis. Hepatology. 1999;29:644–7.

110. Combes B, Carithers RL Jr, Maddrey WC, et al. A randomized, double-blind, placebo-controlled trial of ursodeoxycholic acid in primary biliary cirrhosis. Hepatology. 1995;22:759–66.
111. Carey EJ, Ali AH, Lindor KD. Primary biliary cirrhosis. Lancet (London, England). 2015;386:1565–75.
112. Corpechot C, Carrat F, Bahr A, et al. The effect of ursodeoxycholic acid therapy on the natural course of primary biliary cirrhosis. Gastroenterology. 2005;128:297–303.
113. John BV, Khakoo NS, Schwartz KB, et al. Ursodeoxycholic acid response is associated with reduced mortality in primary biliary cholangitis with compensated cirrhosis. Am J Gastroenterol. 2021;116:1913–23.
114. Gordon SC, Wu KH, Lindor K, et al. Ursodeoxycholic acid treatment preferentially improves overall survival among African Americans with primary biliary cholangitis. Am J Gastroenterol. 2020;115:262–70.
115. Lindor KD, Kowdley KV, Luketic VA, et al. High-dose ursodeoxycholic acid for the treatment of primary sclerosing cholangitis. Hepatology. 2009;50:808–14.
116. Corpechot C, Rousseau A, Chazouillères O. Switching vs. add-on strategy in PBC treatment: lessons from UDCA and bezafibrate experience. J Hepatol. 2020;72:1210–1.
117. Pares A, Caballeria L, Rodes J. Excellent long-term survival in patients with primary biliary cirrhosis and biochemical response to ursodeoxycholic acid. Gastroenterology. 2006;130:715–20.
118. Carbone M, Mells GF, Pells G, et al. Sex and age are determinants of the clinical phenotype of primary biliary cirrhosis and response to ursodeoxycholic acid. Gastroenterology. 2013;144:560–9 e7. quiz e13-4
119. Guo GY, Shi YQ, Wang L, et al. Serum vitamin D level is associated with disease severity and response to ursodeoxycholic acid in primary biliary cirrhosis. Aliment Pharmacol Ther. 2015;42:221–30.
120. Montano-Loza AJ, Corpechot C. Definition and Management of Patients with Primary Biliary Cholangitis and an incomplete response to therapy. Clin Gastroenterol Hepatol. 2021;19:2241–51.e1.
121. Corpechot C, Abenavoli L, Rabahi N, et al. Biochemical response to ursodeoxycholic acid and long-term prognosis in primary biliary cirrhosis. Hepatology. 2008;48:871–7.
122. Corpechot C, Chazouilleres O, Poupon R. Early primary biliary cirrhosis: biochemical response to treatment and prediction of long-term outcome. J Hepatol. 2011;55:1361–7.
123. Kuiper EM, Hansen BE, de Vries RA, et al. Improved prognosis of patients with primary biliary cirrhosis that have a biochemical response to ursodeoxycholic acid. Gastroenterology. 2009;136:1281–7.
124. Kumagi T, Guindi M, Fischer SE, et al. Baseline ductopenia and treatment response predict long-term histological progression in primary biliary cirrhosis. Am J Gastroenterol. 2010;105:2186–94.
125. Momah N, Silveira MG, Jorgensen R, et al. Optimizing biochemical markers as endpoints for clinical trials in primary biliary cirrhosis. Liver Int. 2012;32:790–5.
126. Azemoto N, Abe M, Murata Y, et al. Early biochemical response to ursodeoxycholic acid predicts symptom development in patients with asymptomatic primary biliary cirrhosis. J Gastroenterol. 2009;44:630–4.
127. Harms MH, van Buuren HR, Corpechot C, et al. Ursodeoxycholic acid therapy and liver transplant-free survival in patients with primary biliary cholangitis. J Hepatol. 2019;71:357–65.
128. Efe C, Tascilar K, Henriksson I, et al. Validation of risk scoring Systems in Ursodeoxycholic Acid-Treated Patients with Primary Biliary Cholangitis. Am J Gastroenterol. 2019;114:1101–8.
129. Carbone M, Sharp SJ, Flack S, et al. The UK-PBC risk scores: derivation and validation of a scoring system for long-term prediction of end-stage liver disease in primary biliary cholangitis. Hepatology. 2016;63:930–50.

130. Lammers WJ, Hirschfield GM, Corpechot C, et al. Development and validation of a scoring system to predict outcomes of patients with primary biliary cirrhosis receiving Ursodeoxycholic acid therapy. Gastroenterology. 2015;149:e4.
131. Lindor KD, Bowlus CL, Boyer J, et al. Primary biliary cholangitis: 2018 practice guidance from the American Association for the Study of Liver Diseases. Hepatology. 2019;69:394–419.
132. Chávez-Talavera O, Tailleux A, Lefebvre P, et al. Bile acid control of metabolism and inflammation in obesity, type 2 diabetes, dyslipidemia, and nonalcoholic fatty liver disease. Gastroenterology. 2017;152:1679–94.e3.
133. Jia W, Wei M, Rajani C, et al. Targeting the alternative bile acid synthetic pathway for metabolic diseases. Protein Cell. 2021;12:411–25.
134. Kjærgaard K, Frisch K, Sørensen M, et al. Obeticholic acid improves hepatic bile acid excretion in patients with primary biliary cholangitis. J Hepatol. 2021;74:58–65.
135. Gomez E, Garcia Buey L, Molina E, et al. Effectiveness and safety of obeticholic acid in a southern European multicentre cohort of patients with primary biliary cholangitis and suboptimal response to ursodeoxycholic acid. Aliment Pharmacol Ther. 2021;53:519–30.
136. Hirschfield GM, Mason A, Luketic V, et al. Efficacy of obeticholic acid in patients with primary biliary cirrhosis and inadequate response to ursodeoxycholic acid. Gastroenterology. 2015;148:751–61.e8.
137. Kowdley KV, Luketic V, Chapman R, et al. A randomized trial of obeticholic acid monotherapy in patients with primary biliary cholangitis. Hepatology. 2018;67:1890–902.
138. Nevens F, Andreone P, Mazzella G, et al. A placebo-controlled trial of Obeticholic acid in primary biliary cholangitis. N Engl J Med. 2016;375:631–43.
139. Bolier R, de Vries ES, Parés A, et al. Fibrates for the treatment of cholestatic itch (FITCH): study protocol for a randomized controlled trial. Trials. 2017;18:230.
140. Gulamhusein AF, Hirschfield GM. Primary biliary cholangitis: pathogenesis and therapeutic opportunities. Nat Rev Gastroenterol Hepatol. 2020;17:93–110.
141. Reig A, Sesé P, Parés A. Effects of Bezafibrate on outcome and pruritus in primary biliary cholangitis with suboptimal Ursodeoxycholic acid response. Am J Gastroenterol. 2018;113:49–55.
142. Tanaka A, Hirohara J, Nakano T, et al. Association of bezafibrate with transplant-free survival in patients with primary biliary cholangitis. J Hepatol. 2021;75:565–71.
143. Honda A, Tanaka A, Kaneko T, et al. Bezafibrate improves GLOBE and UK-PBC scores and long-term outcomes in patients with primary biliary cholangitis. Hepatology. 2019;70:2035–46.
144. Sorda JA, González Ballerga E, Barreyro FJ, et al. Bezafibrate therapy in primary biliary cholangitis refractory to ursodeoxycholic acid: a longitudinal study of paired liver biopsies at 5 years of follow up. Aliment Pharmacol Ther. 2021;54:1202–12.
145. Grigorian AY, Mardini HE, Corpechot C, et al. Fenofibrate is effective adjunctive therapy in the treatment of primary biliary cirrhosis: a meta-analysis. Clin Res Hepatol Gastroenterol. 2015;39:296–306.
146. Zhang Y, Li S, He L, et al. Combination therapy of fenofibrate and ursodeoxycholic acid in patients with primary biliary cirrhosis who respond incompletely to UDCA monotherapy: a meta-analysis. Drug Des Devel Ther. 2015;9:2757–66.
147. Wang L, Sun K, Tian A, et al. Fenofibrate improves GLOBE and UK-PBC scores and histological features in primary biliary cholangitis. Minerva Med 2021. https://doi.org/10.23736/S0026-4806.21.07316-X. Online ahead of print.
148. Cheung AC, Lapointe-Shaw L, Kowgier M, et al. Combined ursodeoxycholic acid (UDCA) and fenofibrate in primary biliary cholangitis patients with incomplete UDCA response may improve outcomes. Aliment Pharmacol Ther. 2016;43:283–93.
149. Jung D, Fantin AC, Scheurer U, et al. Human ileal bile acid transporter gene ASBT (SLC10A2) is transactivated by the glucocorticoid receptor. Gut. 2004;53:78–84.
150. Leuschner M, Maier KP, Schlichting J, et al. Oral budesonide and ursodeoxycholic acid for treatment of primary biliary cirrhosis: results of a prospective double-blind trial. Gastroenterology. 1999;117:918–25.

151. Rautiainen H, Kärkkäinen P, Karvonen AL, et al. Budesonide combined with UDCA to improve liver histology in primary biliary cirrhosis: a three-year randomized trial. Hepatology. 2005;41:747–52.
152. Angulo P, Jorgensen RA, Keach JC, et al. Oral budesonide in the treatment of patients with primary biliary cirrhosis with a suboptimal response to ursodeoxycholic acid. Hepatology. 2000;31:318–23.
153. Hirschfield GM. Beuers U, Kupcinskas L, et al. A placebo-controlled randomised trial of budesonide for PBC following an insufficient response to UDCA. J Hepatol. 2021;74:321–9.
154. Hempfling W, Grunhage F, Dilger K, et al. Pharmacokinetics and pharmacodynamic action of budesonide in early- and late-stage primary biliary cirrhosis. Hepatology. 2003;38:196–202.
155. Combes B, Emerson SS, Flye NL, et al. Methotrexate (MTX) plus ursodeoxycholic acid (UDCA) in the treatment of primary biliary cirrhosis. Hepatology. 2005;42:1184–93.
156. Hendrickse MT, Rigney E, Giaffer MH, et al. Low-dose methotrexate is ineffective in primary biliary cirrhosis: long-term results of a placebo-controlled trial. Gastroenterology. 1999;117:400–7.
157. Gong Y, Gluud C. Colchicine for primary biliary cirrhosis: a Cochrane Hepato-biliary group systematic review of randomized clinical trials. Am J Gastroenterol. 2005;100:1876–85.
158. Gong Y, Christensen E, Gluud C. Azathioprine for primary biliary cirrhosis. Cochrane Database Syst Rev 2007:Cd006000.
159. Giljaca V, Poropat G, Stimac D, et al. Methotrexate for primary biliary cirrhosis. Cochrane Database Syst Rev 2010:Cd004385.
160. Harms MH, van Buuren HR, van der Meer AJ. Improving prognosis in primary biliary cholangitis–therapeutic options and strategy. Best Pract Res Clin Gastroenterol. 2018;34-35:85–94.
161. Kaplan MM, Cheng S, Price LL, et al. A randomized controlled trial of colchicine plus ursodiol versus methotrexate plus ursodiol in primary biliary cirrhosis: ten-year results. Hepatology. 2004;39:915–23.
162. Saffioti F, Gurusamy KS, Eusebi LH, et al. Pharmacological interventions for primary biliary cholangitis: an attempted network meta-analysis. Cochrane Database Syst Rev 2017; 3:Cd011648.
163. Karlsen TH, Folseraas T, Thorburn D, et al. Primary sclerosing cholangitis - a comprehensive review. J Hepatol. 2017;67:1298–323.
164. Rawla P, Sunkara T, Raj JP. Role of biologics and biosimilars in inflammatory bowel disease: current trends and future perspectives. J Inflamm Res. 2018;11:215–26.
165. Boonstra K, Weersma RK, van Erpecum KJ, et al. Population-based epidemiology, malignancy risk, and outcome of primary sclerosing cholangitis. Hepatology. 2013;58:2045–55.
166. Beuers U, Spengler U, Kruis W, et al. Ursodeoxycholic acid for treatment of primary sclerosing cholangitis: a placebo-controlled trial. Hepatology. 1992;16:707–14.
167. Olsson R, Boberg KM, de Muckadell OS, et al. High-dose ursodeoxycholic acid in primary sclerosing cholangitis: a 5-year multicenter, randomized, controlled study. Gastroenterology. 2005;129:1464–72.
168. Shi J, Li Z, Zeng X, et al. Ursodeoxycholic acid in primary sclerosing cholangitis: meta-analysis of randomized controlled trials. Hepatol Res. 2009;39:865–73.
169. Poropat G, Giljaca V, Stimac D, et al. Bile acids for primary sclerosing cholangitis. Cochrane Database Syst Rev. 2011;2011:Cd003626.
170. Triantos CK, Koukias NM, Nikolopoulou VN, et al. Meta-analysis: ursodeoxycholic acid for primary sclerosing cholangitis. Aliment Pharmacol Ther. 2011;34:901–10.
171. Chapman MH, Thorburn D, Hirschfield GM, et al. British Society of Gastroenterology and UK-PSC guidelines for the diagnosis and management of primary sclerosing cholangitis. Gut. 2019;68:1356–78.
172. Chapman R, Fevery J, Kalloo A, et al. Diagnosis and management of primary sclerosing cholangitis. Hepatology. 2010;51:660–78.

173. EASL. EASL clinical practice guidelines: management of cholestatic liver diseases. J Hepatol, 2009:237–67.
174. Wunsch E, Trottier J, Milkiewicz M, et al. Prospective evaluation of ursodeoxycholic acid withdrawal in patients with primary sclerosing cholangitis. Hepatology. 2014;60:931–40.
175. Lazaridis KN, LaRusso NF. Primary Sclerosing cholangitis. N Engl J Med. 2016;375:1161–70.
176. Lindor KD, Kowdley KV, Harrison ME. ACG clinical guideline: primary Sclerosing cholangitis. Am J Gastroenterol. 2015;110:646–59. quiz 60
177. Rudolph G, Kloeters-Plachky P, Sauer P, et al. Intestinal absorption and biliary secretion of ursodeoxycholic acid and its taurine conjugate. Eur J Clin Investig. 2002;32:575–80.
178. Heuman DM, Bajaj R. Ursodeoxycholate conjugates protect against disruption of cholesterol-rich membranes by bile salts. Gastroenterology. 1994;106:1333–41.
179. Heuman DM, Mills AS, McCall J, et al. Conjugates of ursodeoxycholate protect against cholestasis and hepatocellular necrosis caused by more hydrophobic bile salts. In vivo studies in the rat. Gastroenterology. 1991;100:203–11.
180. Tsukahara K, Kanai S, Ohta M, et al. Taurine conjugate of ursodeoxycholate plays a major role in the hepatoprotective effect against cholestasis induced by taurochenodeoxycholate in rats. Liver. 1993;13:262–9.
181. Reggiani A, Dizioli P, Quattrocchi D, et al. Intrahepatic cholestasis: clinical and nosological classification. Critical survey of personal experience. Minerva Gastroenterol Dietol. 1997;43:71–81.
182. Fickert P, Pollheimer MJ, Silbert D, et al. Differential effects of norUDCA and UDCA in obstructive cholestasis in mice. J Hepatol. 2013;58:1201–8.
183. Fickert P, Hirschfield GM, Denk G, et al. norUrsodeoxycholic acid improves cholestasis in primary sclerosing cholangitis. J Hepatol. 2017;67:549–58.
184. Sanyal AJ. Past, present and future perspectives in nonalcoholic fatty liver disease. Nat Rev Gastroenterol Hepatol. 2019;16:377–86.
185. Sheka AC, Adeyi O, Thompson J, et al. Nonalcoholic Steatohepatitis: A Review. JAMA. 2020;323:1175–83.
186. Arab JP, Karpen SJ, Dawson PA, et al. Bile acids and nonalcoholic fatty liver disease: molecular insights and therapeutic perspectives. Hepatology. 2017;65:350–62.
187. Lefebvre P, Cariou B, Lien F, et al. Role of bile acids and bile acid receptors in metabolic regulation. Physiol Rev. 2009;89:147–91.
188. Li Y, Jadhav K, Zhang Y. Bile acid receptors in non-alcoholic fatty liver disease. Biochem Pharmacol. 2013;86:1517–24.
189. Segovia-Miranda F, Morales-Navarrete H, Kücken M, et al. Three-dimensional spatially resolved geometrical and functional models of human liver tissue reveal new aspects of NAFLD progression. Nat Med. 2019;25:1885–93.
190. Dufour JF, Oneta CM, Gonvers JJ, et al. Randomized placebo-controlled trial of ursodeoxycholic acid with vitamin e in nonalcoholic steatohepatitis. Clin Gastroenterol Hepatol. 2006;4:1537–43.
191. Ratziu V, de Ledinghen V, Oberti F, et al. A randomized controlled trial of high-dose ursodesoxycholic acid for nonalcoholic steatohepatitis. J Hepatol. 2011;54:1011–9.
192. Lindor KD, Kowdley KV, Heathcote EJ, et al. Ursodeoxycholic acid for treatment of nonalcoholic steatohepatitis: results of a randomized trial. Hepatology. 2004;39:770–8.
193. Leuschner UF, Lindenthal B, Herrmann G, et al. High-dose ursodeoxycholic acid therapy for nonalcoholic steatohepatitis: a double-blind, randomized, placebo-controlled trial. Hepatology. 2010;52:472–9.
194. Mueller M, Castro RE, Thorell A, et al. Ursodeoxycholic acid: effects on hepatic unfolded protein response, apoptosis and oxidative stress in morbidly obese patients. Liver Int. 2018;38:523–31.

195. Chalasani N, Younossi Z, Lavine JE, et al. The diagnosis and management of nonalcoholic fatty liver disease: practice guidance from the American Association for the Study of Liver Diseases. Hepatology. 2018;67:328–57.
196. Gheibi S, Gouvarchin Ghaleh HE, Motlagh BM, et al. Therapeutic effects of curcumin and ursodexycholic acid on non-alcoholic fatty liver disease. Biomedicine & Pharmacotherapy = Biomedecine & Pharmacotherapie. 2019;115:108938.
197. Pietu F, Guillaud O, Walter T, et al. Ursodeoxycholic acid with vitamin E in patients with nonalcoholic steatohepatitis: long-term results. Clin Res Hepatol Gastroenterol. 2012;36:146–55.
198. Beraza N, Ofner-Ziegenfuss L, Ehedego H, et al. Nor-ursodeoxycholic acid reverses hepatocyte-specific nemo-dependent steatohepatitis. Gut. 2011;60:387–96.
199. Traussnigg S, Schattenberg JM, Demir M, et al. Norursodeoxycholic acid versus placebo in the treatment of non-alcoholic fatty liver disease: a double-blind, randomised, placebo-controlled, phase 2 dose-finding trial. Lancet Gastroenterol Hepatol. 2019;4:781–93.
200. Mudaliar S, Henry RR, Sanyal AJ, et al. Efficacy and safety of the farnesoid X receptor agonist obeticholic acid in patients with type 2 diabetes and nonalcoholic fatty liver disease. Gastroenterology. 2013;145:574–82.e1.
201. Yuan L, Bambha K. Bile acid receptors and nonalcoholic fatty liver disease. World J Hepatol. 2015;7:2811–8.
202. Jahn D, Rau M, Hermanns HM, et al. Mechanisms of enterohepatic fibroblast growth factor 15/19 signaling in health and disease. Cytokine Growth Factor Rev. 2015;26:625–35.
203. Verbeke L, Mannaerts I, Schierwagen R, et al. FXR agonist obeticholic acid reduces hepatic inflammation and fibrosis in a rat model of toxic cirrhosis. Sci Rep. 2016;6:33453.
204. Younossi ZM, Ratziu V, Loomba R, et al. Obeticholic acid for the treatment of non-alcoholic steatohepatitis: interim analysis from a multicentre, randomised, placebo-controlled phase 3 trial. Lancet (London, England). 2019;394:2184–96.
205. Neuschwander-Tetri BA, Loomba R, Sanyal AJ, et al. Farnesoid X nuclear receptor ligand obeticholic acid for non-cirrhotic, non-alcoholic steatohepatitis (FLINT): a multicentre, randomised, placebo-controlled trial. Lancet (London, England). 2015;385:956–65.
206. Velayudham LS, Farrell GC. Drug-induced cholestasis. Expert Opin Drug Saf. 2003;2:287–304.
207. Piotrowicz A, Polkey M, Wilkinson M. Ursodeoxycholic acid for the treatment of flucloxacillin-associated cholestasis. J Hepatol. 1995;22:119–20.
208. Agca E, Akcay A, Simsek H. Ursodeoxycholic acid for terbinafine-induced toxic hepatitis. Ann Pharmacother. 2004;38:1088–9.
209. Katsinelos P, Vasiliadis T, Xiarchos P, et al. Ursodeoxycholic acid (UDCA) for the treatment of amoxycillin-clavulanate potassium (Augmentin)-induced intra-hepatic cholestasis: report of two cases. Eur J Gastroenterol Hepatol. 2000;12:365–8.
210. Studniarz M, Czubkowski P, Cielecka-Kuszyk J, et al. Amoxicillin/clavulanic acid-induced cholestatic liver injury after pediatric liver transplantation. Ann Transplant. 2012;17:128–31.
211. Asgarshirazi M, Shariat M, Dalili H, et al. Ursodeoxycholic acid can improve liver transaminase quantities in children with anticonvulsant drugs hepatotoxicity: a pilot study. Acta Med Iran. 2015;53:351–5.
212. Lang SM, Ortmann J, Rostig S, et al. Ursodeoxycholic acid attenuates hepatotoxicity of multidrug treatment of mycobacterial infections: a prospective pilot study. International journal of mycobacteriology. 2019;8:89–92.
213. Wree A, Dechêne A, Herzer K, et al. Steroid and ursodesoxycholic acid combination therapy in severe drug-induced liver injury. Digestion. 2011;84:54–9.
214. Yu YC, Mao YM, Chen CW, et al. CSH guidelines for the diagnosis and treatment of drug-induced liver injury. Hepatol Int. 2017;11:221–41.
215. Wood AM, Livingston EG, Hughes BL, et al. Intrahepatic cholestasis of pregnancy: a review of diagnosis and management. Obstet Gynecol Surv. 2018;73:103–9.
216. Piechota J, Jelski W. Intrahepatic cholestasis in pregnancy: review of the literature. J Clin Med 2020; 9.

217. Grand'Maison S, Durand M, Mahone M. The effects of ursodeoxycholic acid treatment for intrahepatic cholestasis of pregnancy on maternal and fetal outcomes: a meta-analysis including non-randomized studies. J Obstet Gynaecol Can. 2014;36:632–41.
218. Joutsiniemi T, Timonen S, Leino R, et al. Ursodeoxycholic acid in the treatment of intrahepatic cholestasis of pregnancy: a randomized controlled trial. Arch Gynecol Obstet. 2014;289:541–7.
219. Bacq Y, Sentilhes L, Reyes HB, et al. Efficacy of ursodeoxycholic acid in treating intrahepatic cholestasis of pregnancy: a meta-analysis. Gastroenterology. 2012;143:1492–501.
220. Chappell LC, Bell JL, Smith A, et al. Ursodeoxycholic acid versus placebo in women with intrahepatic cholestasis of pregnancy (PITCHES): a randomised controlled trial. Lancet (London, England). 2019;394:849–60.
221. Kumar P, Kulkarni A. UDCA therapy in intrahepatic cholestasis of pregnancy? J Hepatol. 2020;72:586–7.
222. Calmus Y, Gane P, Rouger P, et al. Hepatic expression of class I and class II major histocompatibility complex molecules in primary biliary cirrhosis: effect of ursodeoxycholic acid. Hepatology. 1990;11:12–5.
223. Chen CY, Tsao PN, Chen HL, et al. Ursodeoxycholic acid (UDCA) therapy in very-low-birth-weight infants with parenteral nutrition-associated cholestasis. J Pediatr. 2004;145:317–21.
224. De Marco G, Sordino D, Bruzzese E, et al. Early treatment with ursodeoxycholic acid for cholestasis in children on parenteral nutrition because of primary intestinal failure. Aliment Pharmacol Ther. 2006;24:387–94.
225. Levine A, Maayan A, Shamir R, et al. Parenteral nutrition-associated cholestasis in preterm neonates: evaluation of ursodeoxycholic acid treatment. Journal of Pediatric Endocrinology & Metabolism: JPEM. 1999;12:549–53.
226. Spagnuolo MI, Iorio R, Vegnente A, et al. Ursodeoxycholic acid for treatment of cholestasis in children on long-term total parenteral nutrition: a pilot study. Gastroenterology. 1996;111:716–9.
227. Thibault M, McMahon J, Faubert G, et al. Parenteral nutrition-associated liver disease: a retrospective study of ursodeoxycholic acid use in neonates. The Journal of Pediatric Pharmacology and Therapeutics. 2014;19:42–8.
228. Wales PW, Allen N, Worthington P, et al. A.S.P.E.N. clinical guidelines: support of pediatric patients with intestinal failure at risk of parenteral nutrition-associated liver disease. JPEN J Parenter Enteral Nutr. 2014;38:538–57.
229. Beau P, Labat-Labourdette J, Ingrand P, et al. Is ursodeoxycholic acid an effective therapy for total parenteral nutrition-related liver disease? J Hepatol. 1994;20:240–4.
230. Fried RH, Murakami CS, Fisher LD, et al. Ursodeoxycholic acid treatment of refractory chronic graft-versus-host disease of the liver. Ann Intern Med. 1992;116:624–9.
231. Arat M, Idilman R, Soydan EA, et al. Ursodeoxycholic acid treatment in isolated chronic graft-vs.-host disease of the liver. Clin Transpl. 2005;19:798–803.
232. Ruutu T, Juvonen E, Remberger M, et al. Improved survival with ursodeoxycholic acid prophylaxis in allogeneic stem cell transplantation: long-term follow-up of a randomized study. Biol Blood Marrow Transplant. 2014;20:135–8.
233. Sakiani S, Kleiner DE, Heller T, et al. Hepatic manifestations of cystic fibrosis. Clin Liver Dis. 2019;23:263–77.
234. Al Sinani S, Al-Mulaabed S, Al Naamani K, et al. Cystic fibrosis liver disease: know more. Oman Med J. 2019;34:482–9.
235. Rafeeq MM, Murad HAS. Cystic fibrosis: current therapeutic targets and future approaches. J Transl Med. 2017;15:84.
236. Staufer K. Current treatment options for cystic fibrosis-related liver disease. Int J Mol Sci 2020;21:8586.
237. Cheng K, Ashby D, Smyth RL. Ursodeoxycholic acid for cystic fibrosis-related liver disease. Cochrane Database Syst Rev. 2017;9:Cd000222.
238. Toledano MB, Mukherjee SK, Howell J, et al. The emerging burden of liver disease in cystic fibrosis patients: a UK nationwide study. PLoS One. 2019;14:e0212779.

239. van der Feen C, van der Doef HP, van der Ent CK, et al. Ursodeoxycholic acid treatment is associated with improvement of liver stiffness in cystic fibrosis patients. J Cyst Fibros. 2016;15:834–8.
240. Colombo C, Alicandro G, Oliver M, et al. Ursodeoxycholic acid and liver disease associated with cystic fibrosis: a multicenter cohort study. J Cyst Fibros. 2022;21:220–6.
241. Davit-Spraul A, Fabre M, Branchereau S, et al. ATP8B1 and ABCB11 analysis in 62 children with normal gamma-glutamyl transferase progressive familial intrahepatic cholestasis (PFIC): phenotypic differences between PFIC1 and PFIC2 and natural history. Hepatology. 2010;51:1645–55.
242. Jacquemin E, De Vree JM, Cresteil D, et al. The wide spectrum of multidrug resistance 3 deficiency: from neonatal cholestasis to cirrhosis of adulthood. Gastroenterology. 2001;120:1448–58.
243. van Mil SW, Houwen RH, Klomp LW. Genetics of familial intrahepatic cholestasis syndromes. J Med Genet. 2005;42:449–63.
244. Wanty C, Joomye R, Van Hoorebeek N, et al. Fifteen years single center experience in the management of progressive familial intrahepatic cholestasis of infancy. Acta Gastro-Enterol Belg. 2004;67:313–9.
245. Jacquemin E, Hermans D, Myara A, et al. Ursodeoxycholic acid therapy in pediatric patients with progressive familial intrahepatic cholestasis. Hepatology. 1997;25:519–23.
246. Agarwal S, Lal BB, Rawat D, et al. Progressive familial intrahepatic cholestasis (PFIC) in Indian children: clinical Spectrum and outcome. J Clin Exp Hepatol. 2016;6:203–8.
247. Gordo-Gilart R, Andueza S, Hierro L, et al. Functional analysis of ABCB4 mutations relates clinical outcomes of progressive familial intrahepatic cholestasis type 3 to the degree of MDR3 floppase activity. Gut. 2015;64:147–55.
248. Khabou B, Mahjoub B, Barbu V, et al. Phenotypic variability in Tunisian PFIC3 patients harboring a complex genotype with a differential clinical outcome of UDCA treatment. Clinica Chimica acta. 2018;486:122–8.
249. Gonzales E, Grosse B, Schuller B, et al. Targeted pharmacotherapy in progressive familial intrahepatic cholestasis type 2: evidence for improvement of cholestasis with 4-phenylbutyrate. Hepatology. 2015;62:558–66.
250. Kagawa T, Orii R, Hirose S, et al. Ursodeoxycholic acid stabilizes the bile salt export pump in the apical membrane in MDCK II cells. J Gastroenterol. 2014;49:890–9.
251. van der Woerd WL, Houwen RH, van de Graaf SF. Current and future therapies for inherited cholestatic liver diseases. World J Gastroenterol. 2017;23:763–75.
252. Kriegermeier A, Green R. Pediatric Cholestatic liver disease: review of bile acid metabolism and discussion of current and emerging therapies. Front Med. 2020;7:149.
253. Verkade HJ, Bezerra JA, Davenport M, et al. Biliary atresia and other cholestatic childhood diseases: advances and future challenges. J Hepatol. 2016;65:631–42.
254. Burns J, Davenport M. Adjuvant treatments for biliary atresia. Translational Pediatrics. 2020;9:253–65.

7 Human Serum Albumin Infusion in Liver Cirrhosis

Zhaohui Bai, Meijuan Zou, Xiaoying Zhang,
and Gang Cheng

Abstract

Liver cirrhosis and its complications cause a substantial health burden in the world. Important progress over the past years has improved our understanding of the pathogenesis and treatment of the liver cirrhosis. But current management remains through targeted strategies aimed at preventing or treating specific complications. Human serum albumin (HSA) may be a multi-target disease-modifying treatment drug for the management of patients with decompensated cirrhosis. It could not only promote plasma volume expansion, but also adjust several other pathophysiological alterations of decompensated cirrhosis by binding damaging molecules, modulating inflammation and immune response, and exerting anti-oxidation. In the current chapter, we briefly reviewed the mechanisms and evidences of HSA infusion in liver cirrhosis and its complications.

Keywords

Liver cirrhosis · Complications · Albumin · Management

Z. Bai · M. Zou · G. Cheng (✉)
NMPA Key Laboratory for Research and Evaluation of Drug Regulatory Technology, Shenyang Pharmaceutical University, Shenyang, China

X. Zhang
Key Laboratory of Active Components of Chinese Medicine Screening and Evaluation, School of Traditional Chinese Materia Medica, Shenyang Pharmaceutical University, Shenyang, China

X. Qi, Y. Yang (eds.), *Pharmacotherapy for Liver Cirrhosis and Its Complications*, https://doi.org/10.1007/978-981-19-2615-0_7

7.1 Introduction

Liver cirrhosis is widely prevalent in the world, and it imposes a substantial health burden in many countries [1, 2]. There were 10.6 million cases of decompensated cirrhosis and 112 million cases of compensated cirrhosis globally in 2017 [3]. It is caused by long-term inflammation, which induces the replacement of the healthy liver parenchyma with fibrotic tissue and regenerative nodules [4]. With the progression of liver cirrhosis, the development of decompensated events, which mainly include variceal bleeding, ascites, hepatic encephalopathy (HE), hepatorenal syndrome (HRS), and bacterial infections, indicates that liver cirrhosis has entered the decompensation period [5]. Previous studies showed that portal hypertension, circulatory dysfunction, inflammation, and metabolism and mitochondrial dysfunction may be the pathophysiological mechanism of the development of decompensation events [6]. Current approach regarding the management of patients with decompensated cirrhosis is based on strategies targeted at preventing or treating each complication, and few studies have been designed to explore the influence of overall prognosis by certain drug in decompensated cirrhosis [7, 8]. Recently, the concept of disease-modifying agents has been proposed, which is defined that a certain intervention was prescribed to effectively improve the course of the disease independently from the treatment or prevention of a specific complication [9, 10]. Among the candidates of disease-modifying agents, human serum albumin (HSA) is the hot topic and the most promising drug [10]. Several previous randomized controlled trials (RCTs) explored the effect of HSA on the prognosis of patients with decompensated cirrhosis, which mainly included ANSWER [11], MACHT [12], and ATTIRE [13] studies. However, the conclusions among them were controversial. Notably, the populations, the intervention of control group, and the HSA infusion strategy may be important factors that cause the inconsistent results of these three RCTs [14]. In the current chapter, we attempt to comprehensively summarize the physical and chemical properties, pharmacological properties, and the application evidences of HSA in decompensated cirrhosis.

7.2 Physical and Chemical Properties of HSA

HSA is a 66.5 kDa negatively charged protein with high solubility and stability, encoded on chromosome 4 [15]. HSA is composed of 585 amino acids and is a monomeric multi-domain macromolecule, which includes an abundance of charged residues, such as lysine and aspartic acids [16, 17]. HSA includes 3 homologous domains (I-III), each containing two subdomains (A and B) composed of 4 and 6 α-helices, respectively. The subdomains move relative to one another by means of flexible loops provided by proline residues, which helps accommodate the binding of an array of substance [17] (Fig. 7.1). Additionally, HSA contains 35 cysteine residues, most of which form disulfide bridges (17 in all), contributing to overall tertiary structure. However, it also contains 1 free cysteine-derived, redox active, thiol

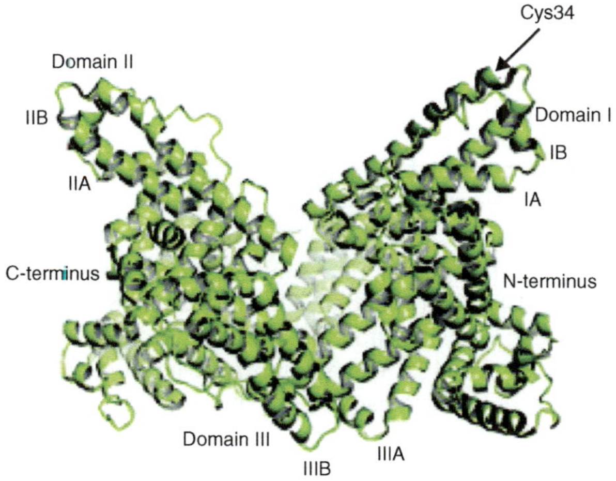

Fig. 7.1 HSA structure. HSA has a single polypeptide sequence formed by 585 amino acids. At position 34, the cysteine residue is free and available for reaction with other molecules. The protein has a heart-like shape, possessing three homologous domains I-III, each domain is divided into A and B subdomains. This figure refers to "*Carvalho JR, Verdelho Machado M. New Insights About Albumin and Liver Disease. Ann Hepatol 2018; 17:547–60*"

(-SH) group (Cys-34). Cys-34 is capable of thiolation (HSA-S-R) and nitrosylation (HSA-S-NO), thereby contributing to several physiological functions [17, 18] (Fig. 7.1).

7.3 Physiology of HSA and its Potential Effects on Liver Cirrhosis

In healthy body, the content of HSA ranges from 35 g/L to 50 g/L in blood and it is synthesized by liver hepatocytes and rapidly excreted into the bloodstream at the rate of about 10 g to 15 g per day [19]. Based on the physical and chemical properties, HSA has oncotic and non-oncotic functions [20]. For the oncotic function, HSA is responsible for approximately 75% of plasma colloid oncotic pressure, because the negative charges surrounding the protein molecules attract sodium, thus holding water [17]. For the non-oncotic function, HSA has functions of solubilization, antioxidant, immunomodulation, capillary permeability, hemostatic effects, and endothelial stabilization, which are based on the ligand-binding properties [17, 21, 22]. As known, the synthesis of HSA is significantly decreased in cirrhotic patients, due to the destruction of liver cell structure [15]. And the new concept of "effective albumin concentration" had also been proposed, which means that not only the concentration of HSA decreases in liver cirrhosis, but the quality of HSA also changes [21, 23]. Additionally, in liver cirrhosis, the systemic inflammation, oxidative stress, circulatory dysfunction, and immune dysfunction play important role among the development of complications and the worse outcomes [6, 24–26]. Therefore, the therapeutic potential of HSA in liver cirrhosis and its complications is very promising.

7.4 The Application of HSA in Liver Cirrhosis in the Real World

In 2015, a survey performed by the American Association for the Study of Liver Disease (AASLD) [27], which included 225 AASLD members, investigated the use of HSA in liver cirrhosis. The results showed that there was variation in the indications for HSA use among these participants as follows, 91% for HRS, 90% for spontaneous bacterial peritonitis (SBP), 24% for infections other than SBP, 57% for hypotension, 31% for refractory ascites, 23% for hyponatremia, 22% for hypoalbuminemia, 21% for edema, 9% for variceal bleeding, and 3% for HE. In 2018, another European survey [28], which involved 101 hepatologists from 86 hospitals, regarding the use of HSA in patients with cirrhosis showed that almost all participants agree that HSA is indicated for the prevention of post-paracentesis circulatory dysfunction (PPCD) (98%), renal failure after SBP (93%), and for the diagnosis and treatment of HRS (98%). Additionally, 52% of participants agree that HSA infusion should be performed into the long-term management of ascites, 56% in non-SBP infections, 56% in hypoalbuminemia, 37% in hyponatremia, 41% in HE, and 18% in severe muscle cramps. HRS, SBP, and PPCD were supported by the AASLD and European Association for the Study of the Liver (EASL) guidelines [7, 29]. The remaining indications were not supported by solid scientific evidence in clinical practice.

7.5 The Evidences of HSA in Liver Cirrhosis and its Complications

7.5.1 HSA and HRS

HRS is the result of a worsened circulatory dysfunction in liver cirrhosis. The splanchnic arterial vasodilatation and the development of cirrhotic cardiomyopathy in liver cirrhosis result in severe underfilling perfusion of the organs, including kidney, thereby leading to renal failure [30, 31]. Systematic inflammation is associated with the development of complications in liver cirrhosis [6], including HRS [32]. Additionally, systemic inflammation is also significantly associated the prognosis of liver cirrhosis [33]. HSA has been recommended as the first-line options of the management of HRS in current guidelines [7, 34, 35]. The mechanism may be that HSA could improve HRS by improving the circulatory dysfunction and the systematic inflammation. Furthermore, a large number of RCTs explored the effect of HSA plus vasoactive drugs on the management of HRS, and the results showed that HSA plus vasoactive drugs could significantly improve the renal function and increase the rate of HRS reversal than HSA alone, but not significant in the survival of type-1 HRS [36–38]. A meta-analysis, which included 25 RCTs and involved 1263 participants, suggested that HSA plus noradrenaline had fewer adverse events than HSA plus terlipressin, and HSA plus midodrine or plus octreotide or HSA alone had lower rate of HRS reversal than HSA plus terlipressin [39].

7.5.2 HSA and Bacterial Infections

Cirrhotic patients have an increased risk of developing bacterial infections [40, 41], and it presents at admission or develops during hospitalization in 25–35% of cirrhotic patients [42, 43]. Cirrhosis is associated with inherent and external factors, which can increase susceptibility to and progression of infections [44]. Inherent factors regarding infections in cirrhosis mainly include immune dysfunction, reduction in bile flow, and changes in gut microbial composition and function [44, 45]. External factors include the overuse of proton pump inhibitors, alcohol intake, frailty, multiple antibiotic courses, repeated hospital admissions, and invasive procedures [46]. Antibiotics are the cornerstone of bacterial infections treatment [47], and HSA infusion could also play an important role in the management of infections in liver cirrhosis, especially in the SBP. Notably, SBP was another indication of the use of HSA infusion in liver cirrhosis, which was recommended by current guidelines [7, 34]. SBP is defined as a bacterial infection of ascitic fluid without any intra-abdominal surgically treatable source of infection, which is the most common infection in cirrhosis-related infections [34, 48]. The prevalence of SBP in outpatients is 1.5–3.5% and approximately 10% in hospitalized patients [49], and the in-hospital mortality is approximately 25% [50]. Several previous RCTs confirmed the effect of HSA infusion on SBP. In 1999, an RCT [51], which included 126 cirrhotic patients with SBP, explored the effects of HSA on the prevention of renal impairment and death. Patients were assigned to cefotaxime group ($n = 63$) and cefotaxime plus HSA group ($n = 63$). Cefotaxime was given daily in doses that varied according to the serum creatinine level, and HSA was given at a dose of 1.5 g/kg of body weight at the time of diagnosis, followed by 1 g/kg on day 3. The results showed that cefotaxime plus HSA group had a significantly lower incidence of renal impairment (10% vs. 33%, $P = 0.002$) and in-hospital mortality (10% vs. 29%, $P = 0.01$) than cefotaxime group. Another RCT [52], which included 20 cirrhotic patients with SBP, compared the effects between HSA and hydroxyethyl starch on SBP. Patients were assigned to ceftriaxone plus HSA group ($n = 10$) and ceftriaxone plus hydroxyethyl starch group ($n = 10$). Both plasma expanders were given at the same dose (1.5 g/kg body weight after baseline measurements and 1 g/kg body weight on day 3). The results showed that HSA infusion was associated with a significant increase in arterial pressure and a suppression of plasma renin activity, indicating an improvement in circulatory function, but not in the hydroxyethyl starch group. Additionally, HSA could improve the endothelial function. However, for the non-SBP infections in liver cirrhosis, the role of HSA infusion remains unclear in current clinical practice [7, 41, 48]. Previous RCTs regarding the role of HSA infusion in the management of cirrhotic patients with non-SBP infections were controversial. In 2012, a RCT [53], which included 110 patients with liver cirrhosis and non-SBP infections, explored the effect of HSA infusion on the survival and renal function. Patients were assigned to antibiotics plus HSA group (n = 56) and antibiotics alone group (n = 54). The dosage of HSA was 1.5 g/kg body weight at diagnosis and 1 g/kg body weight at day 3. The results showed that HSA infusion plus antibiotics could improve the renal and circulatory function. However, HSA could not significantly improve the overall survival (antibiotics plus HSA: 14.3% vs. antibiotics alone: 18.5%), but HSA infusion was an independent predictor of survival after adjustment for other prognostic factors. In 2015, another RCT [54], which included 193 cirrhotic patients with a Child-Pugh score > 8 and sepsis unrelated to SBP, explored the effects of HSA on the renal failure rate and mortality. Patients were assigned to antibiotics plus HSA group (n = 96) and antibiotics alone group (n = 97). The results showed that HSA infusion could delay the onset of renal failure (mean time to onset, antibiotics plus HSA: 29.0 ± 21.8 vs. antibiotics alone: 11.7 ± 9.1 days, P = 0.018), but the 3-month renal failure rate (HSA: 14.3% vs. control: 13.5%; P = 0.88) and 3-month mortality (antibiotics plus HSA: 28.1% vs. antibiotics alone: 20.6%, P = 0.16) were similar between two groups. A recent RCT [55], which included 118 patients with cirrhosis and non-SBP infections, explored the effects of HSA infusion on the in-hospital mortality. Patients were assigned to antibiotics plus HSA group (n = 61) and antibiotics alone group (n = 57). The results showed that there was no significant difference in the in-hospital mortality between these two groups (antibiotics plus HSA: 13.1% vs. antibiotics alone: 10.5% in the control group, P = 0.66). Additionally, only in antibiotics plus HSA group, the circulatory and renal functions had an improvement.

7.5.3 HSA and Ascites

Ascites is the most common complication of liver cirrhosis, which is related to visceral vasodilation, activation of renin-angiotensin-aldosterone and sympathetic-adrenal systems, and increased secretion of antidiuretic hormone [34]. Additionally, it is also related to low plasma osmotic pressure, which is secondary to reduced hepatic capacity in synthesis of HSA [34]. Management of cirrhotic ascites mainly includes restriction of salt and water, diuretics, paracentesis, peritoneal dialysis, transjugular intrahepatic portosystemic shunt (TIPS), and liver transplantation [34]. HSA has been used for a long time in patients with liver cirrhosis and ascites [56]. For patients with liver cirrhosis and tense or refractory ascites and undergoing large-volume paracentesis (LVP) (>5 L), HSA is recommended as the first-line drug to prevent the PPCD, which is secondary to LVP [7, 34]. In contrast, for the cirrhotic patients with ascites and without LVP, the role of HSA infusion remains controversial. In 1999, an RCT [57], which included 126 patients with liver cirrhosis and ascites, suggested that the HSA could improve the response to diuretics. HSA group had higher cumulative rate of response to diuretic ($P < 0.05$) and shorter hospital stay ($P < 0.05$) than control group. However, the mortality was similar between these two groups. In 2018, the ANSWER study [11], which included 431 patients with cirrhosis and persistent uncomplicated ascites, explored the effects of long-term HSA infusion on the prevention of cirrhosis-related complications and outcomes. Patients were randomly assigned to standard medical treatment (SMT) ($n = 213$) and SMT plus HSA ($n = 218$). The dosage of HSA was 40 g twice weekly for 2 weeks, and then 40 g weekly. The results showed that SMT plus HSA group had a significantly higher 18-month survival rate than SMT group (77% vs. 66%; $P = 0.028$), and resulted in a 38% reduction in the mortality hazard ratio. Additionally, 71 patients had at least one paracentesis in the SMT plus HSA group and 116 in the SMT group. The probability of free of paracentesis throughout the study was almost twice in the SMT plus HA group (HR = 0.48; 62% vs. 34%; $P < 0.0001$). Besides the benefit on ascites management, long-term HSA infusion also could prevent the development of many other complications of liver cirrhosis. The incidence rate ratio of SBP, non-SBP bacterial infections, renal dysfunction, type-1 HRS, grade 3 or 4 HE, and potential diuretic-induced side effects was significantly reduced by 30% to 67.5% in patients receiving SMT plus HSA. MACHT study [12] explored the role of HSA in patients with ascites and awaiting liver transplantation. There were 196 patients included and assigned to receive midodrine plus HSA group ($n = 99$) and placebo group ($n = 97$). The dosage of HSA was 40 g/15 days. The results showed that there were no significant differences between both groups in the incidence for the development of complications of liver cirrhosis during follow-up (37% vs. 43%, $P = 0.402$) and 1-year mortality (7% vs. 5%, $P = 0.527$).

7.5.4 HSA and HE

HE is a common complication and one of the most debilitating manifestations of liver disease, severely affecting the life quality of patients. The incidence of overt and covert HE during the clinical course of liver cirrhosis is 30–40% and 20–80%, respectively [58]. Except for the well-known drugs, such as lactulose, rifaximin, and L-ornithine-L-aspartate [59–61], the role of HSA infusion for the management of HE has been widely and increasingly recognized, but remains controversial. Generally, hyperammonemia seems as the core pathogenesis of HE [62, 63], however, several studies showed that the systemic inflammation and oxidative stress also play potential role in the pathogenesis of HE [25, 64–66], which could be the therapeutic target of HSA. Practically, low serum albumin level could significantly increase the incidence and mortality of overt HE in patients with cirrhosis [67]. In 2013, an RCT [68], which included 56 patients with cirrhosis and overt HE, explored the effect of HSA on HE. Patients were assigned to HSA ($n = 26$) and saline ($n = 30$) groups. The dosage of HSA was 1.5 g/kg on day 1 and 1.0 g/kg on day 3. The results suggested that HSA could significantly improve the 90-day survival (69.2% vs. 40.0%; $P = 0.02$) than saline, but the percentage of patients without HE at day 4 had no difference between both groups (57.7% vs. 53.3%; $P > 0.05$). In 2017, another RCT [69], which included 120 patients with cirrhosis and overt HE, evaluated the effects of HSA plus lactulose vs. lactulose alone for the treatment of overt HE. Patients were assigned to HSA plus lactulose (n = 60) and lactulose ($n = 60$) groups. The dosage of HSA was 1.5 g/kg/day and continued till complete recovery of HE or a maximum of 10 days. The results showed that HSA plus lactulose group had a significantly higher complete reversal rate of HE (75% vs. 53.3%, $P = 0.03$) and a significantly lower mortality (18.3% vs. 31.6%, $P < 0.05$) than lactulose alone group. In the real world, our cohort study [70], which involved 708 cirrhotic patients and 182 cirrhotic overt HE patients, explored the effects of HSA on the prevention and treatment of overt HE. For the prevention of HE, HSA could significantly decrease the incidence of overt HE (4.20% vs. 12.70%, $P < 0.001$). For the treatment of HE, HSA could significantly improve overt HE (84.60% vs. 68.10%, $P = 0.009$) and decrease in-hospital mortality (7.70% vs. 19.80%, $P = 0.018$). Generally, a latest meta-analysis [71] also suggested that HSA infusions were associated with lower risks for development (OR = 0.53) and death (OR = 0.36) of overt HE in liver cirrhosis.

7.5.5 HSA and Hyponatremia

Hyponatremia is a confusing problem in the management of patients with liver cirrhosis [72]. As one of the important components of the MELD-Na score, patients with liver cirrhosis and hyponatremia generally have worse outcomes [73, 74]. Hyponatremia is defined as serum sodium level < 135 mmol/L [7, 34], and the prevalence is approximately 50% in liver cirrhosis [75]. Hypervolemic hyponatremia accounts for 90% of cases in liver cirrhosis [76]. Hyperdynamic circulation and splanchnic vasodilation, which are caused by portal hypertension and systematic inflammation in liver cirrhosis, play important role in the development of hyponatremia [24, 77]. They can activate the renin-angiotensin-aldosterone system and the abnormal secretion of antidiuretic hormone, thereby inducing the development of hypervolemic or dilutional hyponatremia [78]. Among the current guidelines, the management of hyponatremia in liver cirrhosis mainly included water restriction, vasopressin receptor-2 antagonists, correction of hypokalemia, and hypertonic saline [7, 34], but the effects remain unsatisfactory. HSA could be a potential drug for hyponatremia in liver cirrhosis, and the related evidences are lacking [7]. In 2007, a published abstract of an RCT explored the effect of HSA on cirrhosis with refractory ascites and hyponatremia. Twenty-four cirrhotic patients were included. HSA group patients were treated with HSA (40 g/day) plus fluid restriction and sodium restriction, and control group patients were treated with fluid restriction and sodium restriction alone. The results showed that HSA could significantly increase the serum sodium level (124 ± 2 to 133 ± 6,

$P < 0.01$) [79]. In 2018, a prospective cohort study explored the effects of HSA on hyponatremia in liver cirrhosis [80]. Among this study, 1126 cirrhotic patients with hyponatremia were included, and 777 patients received HSA infusion with a median dosage of 225 g. The results showed that HSA infusion could significantly increase the resolution of hyponatremia (69% vs. 61%, $P = 0.008$), but had a higher 30-day mortality in the HSA group (16% vs. 8%, $P = 0.001$). Recently, a post-data analysis, based on the ATTIRE data set, also showed that HSA infusion could increase serum sodium level in hospitalized hyponatremic patients with cirrhosis, but this did not improve outcome [81].

7.6 Discussion

In the real world, a great number of HSA prescriptions are not supported by clinical evidence or guideline recommendations [82–84]. The indications of HSA for nutritional reasons or for the correction of hypoalbuminemia not accompanied by hypovolemia are examples of inappropriate use in various settings of general surgery, internal medicine, geriatrics, and oncology. Because it has been shown that the use of HSA is not associated with a real benefit for the patient [85]. The use of HSA for these inappropriate indications should be avoided, therefore, it is necessary to promote effective policies to control the appropriateness of prescription [85, 86]. In conclusion, HSA plays an important role in the management of liver cirrhosis-related complications, especially SBP, PPCD, and HRS. However, the evidence regarding the use of HSA in cirrhotic patients with ascites, HE, and hyponatremia remains insufficient, and high-quality RCTs are needed to further clarify its potential effects.

References

1. D'Amico G, Garcia-Tsao G, Pagliaro L. Natural history and prognostic indicators of survival in cirrhosis: a systematic review of 118 studies. J Hepatol. 2006;44:217–31.
2. Ginès P, Krag A, Abraldes JG, Solà E, Fabrellas N, Kamath PS. Liver cirrhosis. Lancet. 2021;398:1359–76.
3. Collaborators GBDC. The global, regional, and national burden of cirrhosis by cause in 195 countries and territories, 1990-2017: a systematic analysis for the global burden of disease study 2017. Lancet Gastroenterol Hepatol. 2020;5:245–66.
4. Pellicoro A, Ramachandran P, Iredale JP, Fallowfield JA. Liver fibrosis and repair: immune regulation of wound healing in a solid organ. Nat Rev Immunol. 2014;14:181–94.
5. Tsochatzis EA, Bosch J, Burroughs AK. Liver cirrhosis. Lancet. 2014;383:1749–61.
6. Engelmann C, Clària J, Szabo G, Bosch J, Bernardi M. Pathophysiology of decompensated cirrhosis: portal hypertension, circulatory dysfunction, inflammation, metabolism and mitochondrial dysfunction. J Hepatol. 2021;75:S49–66.
7. European Association for the Study of the Liver. EASL clinical practice guidelines for the management of patients with decompensated cirrhosis. J Hepatol. 2018;69:406–60.
8. Ge PS, Runyon BA. Treatment of patients with cirrhosis. N Engl J Med. 2016;375:767–77.
9. Bernardi M, Caraceni P. Novel perspectives in the management of decompensated cirrhosis. Nat Rev Gastroenterol Hepatol. 2018;15:753–64.

10. Caraceni P, Abraldes JG, Ginès P, Newsome PN, Sarin SK. The search for disease-modifying agents in decompensated cirrhosis: from drug repurposing to drug discovery. J Hepatol. 2021;75:S118–S34.
11. Caraceni P, Riggio O, Angeli P, et al. Long-term albumin administration in decompensated cirrhosis (ANSWER): an open-label randomised trial. Lancet. 2018;391:2417–29.
12. Solà E, Solé C, Simón-Talero M, et al. Midodrine and albumin for prevention of complications in patients with cirrhosis awaiting liver transplantation. A randomized placebo-controlled trial. J Hepatol. 2018;69:1250–9.
13. China L, Freemantle N, Forrest E, et al. A randomized trial of albumin infusions in hospitalized patients with cirrhosis. N Engl J Med. 2021;384:808–17.
14. Bai Z, Cheng G, Méndez-Sánchez N, Qi X. Human albumin infusion strategy in liver cirrhosis: liberal or restrictive? Ann Transl Med. 2021;9:1114.
15. Levitt DG, Levitt MD. Human serum albumin homeostasis: a new look at the roles of synthesis, catabolism, renal and gastrointestinal excretion, and the clinical value of serum albumin measurements. Int J Gen Med. 2016;9:229–55.
16. Fanali G, di Masi A, Trezza V, Marino M, Fasano M, Ascenzi P. Human serum albumin: from bench to bedside. Mol Asp Med. 2012;33:209–90.
17. Quinlan GJ, Martin GS, Evans TW. Albumin: biochemical properties and therapeutic potential. Hepatology. 2005;41:1211–9.
18. Dröge W. Aging-related changes in the thiol/disulfide redox state: implications for the use of thiol antioxidants. Exp Gerontol. 2002;37:1333–45.
19. Moman RN, Gupta N, Varacallo M. Physiology, Albumin. Treasure Island (FL): StatPearls; 2021.
20. De Simone G, di Masi A, Ascenzi P. Serum albumin: a multifaced enzyme. Int J Mol Sci. 2021;22
21. Garcia-Martinez R, Caraceni P, Bernardi M, Gines P, Arroyo V, Jalan R. Albumin: pathophysiologic basis of its role in the treatment of cirrhosis and its complications. Hepatology. 2013;58:1836–46.
22. Roche M, Rondeau P, Singh NR, Tarnus E, Bourdon E. The antioxidant properties of serum albumin. FEBS Lett. 2008;582:1783–7.
23. Carvalho JR, Verdelho MM. New insights about albumin and liver disease. Ann Hepatol. 2018;17:547–60.
24. Arroyo V, García-Martinez R, Salvatella X. Human serum albumin, systemic inflammation, and cirrhosis. J Hepatol. 2014;61:396–407.
25. Bosoi CR, Rose CF. Oxidative stress: a systemic factor implicated in the pathogenesis of hepatic encephalopathy. Metab Brain Dis. 2013;28:175–8.
26. Ruart M, Chavarria L, Campreciós G, et al. Impaired endothelial autophagy promotes liver fibrosis by aggravating the oxidative stress response during acute liver injury. J Hepatol. 2019;70:458–69.
27. Bajaj JS, O'Leary JG, Wong F, Kamath PS. Variations in albumin use in patients with cirrhosis: an AASLD members survey. Hepatology. 2015;62:1923–4.
28. Caraceni P, Pavesi M, Baldassarre M, Bernardi M, Arroyo V. The use of human albumin in patients with cirrhosis: a European survey. Expert Rev Gastroenterol Hepatol. 2018;12:625–32.
29. Runyon BA, Aasld. Introduction to the revised American association for the study of liver diseases practice guideline management of adult patients with ascites due to cirrhosis 2012. Hepatology. 2013;57:1651–3.
30. Møller S, Henriksen JH. Cirrhotic cardiomyopathy. J Hepatol. 2010;53:179–90.
31. Simonetto DA, Gines P, Kamath PS. Hepatorenal syndrome: pathophysiology, diagnosis, and management. BMJ. 2020;370:m2687.
32. Solé C, Solà E, Huelin P, et al. Characterization of inflammatory response in hepatorenal syndrome: relationship with kidney outcome and survival. Liver Int. 2019;39:1246–55.
33. Thabut D, Massard J, Gangloff A, et al. Model for end-stage liver disease score and systemic inflammatory response are major prognostic factors in patients with cirrhosis and acute functional renal failure. Hepatology. 2007;46:1872–82.

34. Aithal GP, Palaniyappan N, China L, et al. Guidelines on the management of ascites in cirrhosis. Gut. 2021;70:9–29.
35. Runyon BA, Committee APG. Management of adult patients with ascites due to cirrhosis: an update. Hepatology. 2009;49:2087–107.
36. Wong F, Pappas SC, Curry MP, et al. Terlipressin plus albumin for the treatment of type 1 Hepatorenal syndrome. N Engl J Med. 2021;384:818–28.
37. Sanyal AJ, Boyer TD, Frederick RT, et al. Reversal of hepatorenal syndrome type 1 with terlipressin plus albumin vs. placebo plus albumin in a pooled analysis of the OT-0401 and REVERSE randomised clinical studies. Aliment Pharmacol Ther. 2017;45:1390–402.
38. Boyer TD, Sanyal AJ, Wong F, et al. Terlipressin plus albumin is more effective than albumin alone in improving renal function in patients with cirrhosis and Hepatorenal syndrome type 1. Gastroenterology. 2016;150:1579–89 e2.
39. Best LM, Freeman SC, Sutton AJ, et al. Treatment for hepatorenal syndrome in people with decompensated liver cirrhosis: a network meta-analysis. Cochrane Database Syst Rev. 2019;9:CD013103.
40. Fernández J, Gustot T. Management of bacterial infections in cirrhosis. J Hepatol. 2012;56:S1–12.
41. Bajaj JS, Kamath PS, Reddy KR. The evolving challenge of infections in cirrhosis. N Engl J Med. 2021;384:2317–30.
42. Fernández J, Navasa M, Gómez J, et al. Bacterial infections in cirrhosis: epidemiological changes with invasive procedures and norfloxacin prophylaxis. Hepatology. 2002;35:140–8.
43. Fernández J, Acevedo J, Castro M, et al. Prevalence and risk factors of infections by multiresistant bacteria in cirrhosis: a prospective study. Hepatology. 2012;55:1551–61.
44. Bonnel AR, Bunchorntavakul C, Reddy KR. Immune dysfunction and infections in patients with cirrhosis. Clin Gastroenterol Hepatol. 2011;9:727–38.
45. Albillos A, Lario M, Álvarez-Mon M. Cirrhosis-associated immune dysfunction: distinctive features and clinical relevance. J Hepatol. 2014;61:1385–96.
46. O'Leary JG, Reddy KR, Wong F, et al. Long-term use of antibiotics and proton pump inhibitors predict development of infections in patients with cirrhosis. Clin Gastroenterol Hepatol. 2015;13:753–9 e1-2.
47. Fernandez J, Arroyo V. Bacterial infections in cirrhosis: a growing problem with significant implications. Clin Liver Dis (Hoboken). 2013;2:102–5.
48. Jalan R, Fernandez J, Wiest R, et al. Bacterial infections in cirrhosis: a position statement based on the EASL special conference 2013. J Hepatol. 2014;60:1310–24.
49. Evans LT, Kim WR, Poterucha JJ, Kamath PS. Spontaneous bacterial peritonitis in asymptomatic outpatients with cirrhotic ascites. Hepatology. 2003;37:897–901.
50. Piano S, Fasolato S, Salinas F, et al. The empirical antibiotic treatment of nosocomial spontaneous bacterial peritonitis: results of a randomized, controlled clinical trial. Hepatology. 2016;63:1299–309.
51. Sort P, Navasa M, Arroyo V, et al. Effect of intravenous albumin on renal impairment and mortality in patients with cirrhosis and spontaneous bacterial peritonitis. N Engl J Med. 1999;341:403–9.
52. Fernández J, Monteagudo J, Bargallo X, et al. A randomized unblinded pilot study comparing albumin versus hydroxyethyl starch in spontaneous bacterial peritonitis. Hepatology. 2005;42:627–34.
53. Guevara M, Terra C, Nazar A, et al. Albumin for bacterial infections other than spontaneous bacterial peritonitis in cirrhosis. A randomized, controlled study. J Hepatol. 2012;57:759–65.
54. Thévenot T, Bureau C, Oberti F, et al. Effect of albumin in cirrhotic patients with infection other than spontaneous bacterial peritonitis. A randomized trial. J Hepatol. 2015;62:822–30.
55. Fernández J, Angeli P, Trebicka J, et al. Efficacy of albumin treatment for patients with cirrhosis and infections unrelated to spontaneous bacterial peritonitis. Clin Gastroenterol Hepatol. 2020;18:963–73 e14.
56. Wilkinson P, Sherlock S. The effect of repeated albumin infusions in patients with cirrhosis. Lancet. 1962;2:1125–9.

57. Gentilini P, Casini-Raggi V, Di Fiore G, et al. Albumin improves the response to diuretics in patients with cirrhosis and ascites: results of a randomized, controlled trial. J Hepatol. 1999;30:639–45.
58. Hepatic encephalopathy in chronic liver disease: 2014 practice guideline by the European Association for the Study of the Liver and the American Association for the Study of Liver Diseases. J Hepatol. 2014;61:642–59.
59. Gluud LL, Vilstrup H, Morgan MY. Nonabsorbable disaccharides for hepatic encephalopathy: a systematic review and meta-analysis. Hepatology. 2016;64:908–22.
60. Bass NM, Mullen KD, Sanyal A, et al. Rifaximin treatment in hepatic encephalopathy. N Engl J Med. 2010;362:1071–81.
61. Kircheis G, Nilius R, Held C, et al. Therapeutic efficacy of L-ornithine-L-aspartate infusions in patients with cirrhosis and hepatic encephalopathy: results of a placebo-controlled, double-blind study. Hepatology. 1997;25:1351–60.
62. Brusilow SW, Koehler RC, Traystman RJ, Cooper AJ. Astrocyte glutamine synthetase: importance in hyperammonemic syndromes and potential target for therapy. Neurotherapeutics. 2010;7:452–70.
63. González-Usano A, Cauli O, Agustí A, Felipo V. Hyperammonemia alters the modulation by different neurosteroids of the glutamate-nitric oxide-cyclic GMP pathway through NMDA-GABAA - or sigma receptors in cerebellum in vivo. J Neurochem. 2013;125:133–43.
64. Jiang W, Desjardins P, Butterworth RF. Hypothermia attenuates oxidative/nitrosative stress, encephalopathy and brain edema in acute (ischemic) liver failure. Neurochem Int. 2009;55:124–8.
65. Duchini A, Govindarajan S, Santucci M, Zampi G, Hofman FM. Effects of tumor necrosis factor-alpha and interleukin-6 on fluid-phase permeability and ammonia diffusion in CNS-derived endothelial cells. J Investig Med. 1996;44:474–82.
66. Jain L, Sharma BC, Sharma P, Srivastava S, Agrawal A, Sarin SK. Serum endotoxin and inflammatory mediators in patients with cirrhosis and hepatic encephalopathy. Dig Liver Dis. 2012;44:1027–31.
67. Bai Z, Guo X, Tacke F, Li Y, Li H, Qi X. Association of serum albumin level with incidence and mortality of overt hepatic encephalopathy in cirrhosis during hospitalization. Ther Adv Gastroenterol. 2019;12:1756284819881302.
68. Simón-Talero M, García-Martínez R, Torrens M, et al. Effects of intravenous albumin in patients with cirrhosis and episodic hepatic encephalopathy: a randomized double-blind study. J Hepatol. 2013;59:1184–92.
69. Sharma BC, Singh J, Srivastava S, et al. Randomized controlled trial comparing lactulose plus albumin versus lactulose alone for treatment of hepatic encephalopathy. J Gastroenterol Hepatol. 2017;32:1234–9.
70. Bai Z, Bernardi M, Yoshida EM, et al. Albumin infusion may decrease the incidence and severity of overt hepatic encephalopathy in liver cirrhosis. Aging (Albany NY). 2019;11:8502–25.
71. Teh KB, Loo JH, Tam YC, Wong YJ. Efficacy and safety of albumin infusion for overt hepatic encephalopathy: a systematic review and meta-analysis. Dig Liver Dis. 2021;53:817–23.
72. Alukal JJ, John S, Thuluvath PJ. Hyponatremia in cirrhosis: an update. Am J Gastroenterol. 2020;115:1775–85.
73. Kim WR, Biggins SW, Kremers WK, et al. Hyponatremia and mortality among patients on the liver-transplant waiting list. N Engl J Med. 2008;359:1018–26.
74. Borroni G, Maggi A, Sangiovanni A, Cazzaniga M, Salerno F. Clinical relevance of hyponatraemia for the hospital outcome of cirrhotic patients. Dig Liver Dis. 2000;32:605–10.
75. Angeli P, Wong F, Watson H, Ginès P, Investigators C. Hyponatremia in cirrhosis: results of a patient population survey. Hepatology. 2006;44:1535–42.
76. Attar B. Approach to hyponatremia in cirrhosis. Clin Liver Dis (Hoboken). 2019;13:98–101.
77. Martell M, Coll M, Ezkurdia N, Raurell I, Genescà J. Physiopathology of splanchnic vasodilation in portal hypertension. World J Hepatol. 2010;2:208–20.
78. John S, Thuluvath PJ. Hyponatremia in cirrhosis: pathophysiology and management. World J Gastroenterol. 2015;21:3197–205.

79. Jalan R, Mookerjee R, Cheshire L, Williams R, Davies N. Albumin infusion for severe hyponatremia in patients with refractory ascites: a randomized clinical trial. J Hepatol. 2007;46:S95.
80. Bajaj JS, Tandon P, O'Leary JG, et al. The impact of albumin use on resolution of hyponatremia in hospitalized patients with cirrhosis. Am J Gastroenterol. 2018;113:1339.
81. China L, Freemantle N, Forrest E, et al. Targeted albumin therapy does not improve short-term outcome in Hyponatremic patients hospitalized with complications of cirrhosis: data from the ATTIRE trial. Am J Gastroenterol. 2021;116:2292–5.
82. Tarín Remohí MJ, Sánchez Arcos A, Santos Ramos B, Bautista Paloma J, Guerrero Aznar MD. Costs related to inappropriate use of albumin in Spain. Ann Pharmacother. 2000;34:1198–205.
83. Tanzi M, Gardner M, Megellas M, Lucio S, Restino M. Evaluation of the appropriate use of albumin in adult and pediatric patients. Am J Health Syst Pharm. 2003;60:1330–5.
84. Yazdani MS, Retter A, Maggs T, et al. Where does the albumin go? Human albumin solution usage following the implementation of a demand management programme. Transfus Med. 2017;27:192–9.
85. Caraceni P, Angeli P, Prati D, et al. AISF-SIMTI position paper on the appropriate use of albumin in patients with liver cirrhosis: a 2020 update. Blood Transfus. 2021;19:9–13.
86. Lanzoni M, Biffoli C, Candura F, Calizzani G, Vaglio S, Grazzini G. Plasma-derived medicinal products in Italy: information sources and flows. Blood Transfus. 2013;11:s13–7.

Non-selective Beta Blockers in Liver Cirrhosis

8

Mathias Jachs and Thomas Reiberger

Abstract

Non-selective beta blockers (NSBBs) are the cornerstone of medical therapy in the prophylaxis of variceal bleeding and rebleeding in patients with portal hypertension. Their efficacy in reducing portal pressure has been proven time and time again; however, their safety profile in advanced disease, such as in patients with refractory ascites, is still debated. Importantly, the recent landmark PREDESCI trial demonstrated that NSBBs are also able to prolong decompensation-free survival in portal hypertension, possibly owing to "non-hemodynamic" beneficial effects that have only recently been discovered. This chapter summarizes the current evidence on NSBB therapy in cirrhosis and portal hypertension.

Keywords

Portal hypertension · Variceal bleeding · Non-selective betablockers

8.1 Background

Two hallmarks of portal hypertension contribute to the elevation of portal pressure in patients with advanced chronic liver disease (ACLD), i.e. (i) increased intrahepatic (sinusoidal) vascular resistance and (ii) increased portal blood inflow. Portal

M. Jachs · T. Reiberger (✉)
Division of Gastroenterology and Hepatology, Department of Medicine III, Medical University of Vienna, Vienna, Austria

Vienna Hepatic Hemodynamic Laboratory, Division of Gastroenterology and Hepatology, Medical University of Vienna, Vienna, Austria

Christian Doppler Lab for Portal Hypertension and Liver Fibrosis, Medical University of Vienna, Vienna, Austria
e-mail: mathias.jachs@meduniwien.ac.at; thomas.reiberger@meduniwien.ac.at

X. Qi, Y. Yang (eds.), *Pharmacotherapy for Liver Cirrhosis and Its Complications*, https://doi.org/10.1007/978-981-19-2615-0_8

pressure rises as disease progresses, ultimately surpassing the critical threshold of ≥10 mmHg, marking the progression to clinically significant portal hypertension (CSPH) [1]. The development of CSPH often precedes the first decompensation, i.e., most commonly the occurrence of ascites, and—more rarely—hepatic encephalopathy or variceal hemorrhage [2].

Patients with CSPH show pronounced peripheral and splanchnic vasodilation that eventually lead to increased heart rate and cardiac output, which characterize the hyperdynamic circulatory state in advanced portal hypertension [3].

Most importantly, gastroesophageal varices (GEVs) exclusively occur in CSPH; however, CSPH might be present before GEVs can be detected during upper gastrointestinal endoscopy. Thus, the early diagnosis of CSPH and the quantification of portal pressure are crucial, as patients with CSPH without GEVs might benefit from earlier treatment initiation, and the risk for developing complications gradually increases with (invasively quantified) portal pressure [4]. Even though considerable efforts were made to find reliable surrogate markers that indicate the presence as well as the severity of CSPH, the invasive measurement of portal pressure, i.e. hepatic venous pressure gradient (HVPG) during liver vein catheterization remains the gold standard for the diagnosis of CSPH [5, 6]. Notably, the severity of CSPH determines the individual patient's risk for variceal bleeding, and (chronic or acute) changes in HVPG upon therapy or even etiological cure have demonstrated excellent prognostic merit [7].

Changes in the sympathetic nervous system (SNS) contribute significantly to the development of CSPH and the hyperdynamic circulatory state in portal hypertension [8]. Thus, blockade of beta-adrenergic receptors by non-selective beta blockers (NSBBs) efficiently reduces the portal pressure, thereby lowering the risk for variceal bleeding. NSBBs are therefore the mainstay of medical therapy for primary and secondary prophylaxis of variceal bleeding. Historically, only nadolol, timolol and, most importantly, propranolol were used. More recently, it was demonstrated that carvedilol, most likely owing to its inherent anti-alpha-1-adrenergic activity, had an even stronger effect on portal pressure and systemic vasodilation [9]. However, the role of carvedilol has been mostly studied in the setting of primary prophylaxis [10–12], while its use in patients with ascites [13–15] and/or a history of bleeding [16] remains controversial.

Traditionally, NSBBs had only been used for the prevention of variceal (re-) bleeding in patients that had already developed large varices or high-risk small varices [17–19]. However, recent evidence has indicated that the effects of NSBBs might not be limited to their efficient reduction of bleeding risk, but that NSBBs might also prevent (first) decompensation in patients with ACLD and CSPH [20]. The indications for NSBBs in liver cirrhosis might therefore be broadened in the near future. This chapter aims to comprehensively summarize current knowledge on NSBBs in liver cirrhosis, taking into account recent literature that gave valuable insight into their role in liver cirrhosis.

8.2 Diagnosis of CSPH

The gold standard for diagnosing CSPH is the invasive measurement of the HVPG that is thoroughly explained elsewhere [5]. The measurement of HVPG allows for a safe and reproducible assessment of the portal pressure, although dedicated infrastructure and training are obligatory. Importantly, the development of CSPH, i.e. an HVPG ≥10 mmHg, precedes the occurrence of clinical signs of portal hypertension (varices, portosystemic collaterals, and ascites) by definition. Therefore, a timely diagnosis of CSPH has prognostic and—as recently unveiled in the elegant PREDESCI trial [20]—maybe even therapeutic implications.

Non-invasive markers for the detection of CSPH have been extensively investigated in recent years [21]; however, most have failed to show a diagnostic accuracy that might compete with HVPG measurement. In fact, most investigated methods seem to be more suited for ruling-in/ruling-out the presence of CSPH or varices needing treatment (VNT) than for the diagnosis of CSPH—those include, among others, the measurement of liver [22] and spleen [23] stiffness via different elastography methods, spleen diameter [24], platelet count [24], and von Willebrand factor (VWF) [25]. In settings where the discussed advanced methods for the diagnosis of CSPH, including HVPG measurement, are not available, the most feasible and readily available tool for the assessment of the presence of CSPH is upper gastrointestinal endoscopy to detect varices.

8.3 Assessment of Hemodynamic Response to NSBB Therapy

Not all cirrhotic patients will respond to NSBB therapy, and thus, sequential HVPG measurements or i.v. propranolol studies remain the only means to directly assess chronic or acute response to NSBB therapy, respectively [7]. Chronic HVPG response was defined by the Baveno VI consensus as a reduction to absolute values ≤12 mmHg or a relative decrease by ≥10% or ≥ 20% in primary or secondary prophylaxis, respectively [18]. The 10% (to 12%) cut-off is also used in acute response assessment to i.v. propranolol [7]. Achievement of HVPG response is paralleled by marked reductions of bleeding risks and even a lower mortality risk in secondary prophylaxis [7]. Interestingly, both acute and chronic response are of prognostic value, even though there is no strong correlation between acute and chronic response [26]. Sequential HVPG response measurements, however, are resource-intensive, and therefore, access is limited to few academic centers. Moreover, HVPG response status is subject to bias from NSBB dose modification, alcohol intake [27], and natural history of the underlying etiology of ACLD [28]. Naturally, bias from those confounders will impact all sequentially measured biomarkers, and thus, HVPG response remains the only well-validated surrogate for benefit from NSBB therapy in patients with CSPH.

Intriguingly, surrogate (bio-)markers were also evaluated for the (non-invasive) monitoring of NSBB therapy, i.e. the assessment of hemodynamic response. Those "dynamic" surrogates for HVPG response include (i) changes in liver stiffness that correlated well with changes in HVPG in a small cohort of 23 patients [29], although this finding remains to be validated in a larger prospective study and (ii) changes in spleen stiffness—that might theoretically more accurately reflect dynamic changes in portal hypertension owing to their correlation with the portal venous inflow component of portal hypertension—that showed promising results in trials using transient elastography [23] and shear wave-elastography [30] methods. Using even more advanced methods, it has also been shown that MRI-based estimations of liver perfusions strongly correlated with HVPG [31, 32]; however, this method's clinical applicability is limited, and needs further validation.

Non-imaging-based surrogate markers for dynamic changes in HVPG were also evaluated. A free fatty acid [33] correlated well with the acute HVPG response to i.v. propranolol, as did serum levels of phosphatidylcholine [33] and RhoA-kinase (ROCK)2 and Ras homolog family member A (RhoA) transcription in the antrum mucosa [34]. All of those markers should be evaluated further.

In recent years, evidence was gathered that the effect of NSBBs might not solely comprise their hemodynamic effects, and the so-called non-hemodynamic beneficial effects of NSBB therapy were reported, including a reduction of surrogates of bacterial translocation via amelioration of the intestinal permeability [35], and a reduction of biomarkers of systemic inflammation in patients with acute-on-chronic-liver failure (ACLF) [36]. Additionally, in patients with stable ACLD, NSBB treatment led to a reduction of inflammatory biomarkers that—if a reduction of white blood cell count by ≥15% was achieved—translated into improved outcomes [37], and in patients with decompensated ACLD, even slight reductions in VWF had prognostic implications [38]. Overall, biomarkers of non-hemodynamic effects of NSBB deserve to be further evaluated as they support the previous notion that a larger proportion of patients than that achieving (chronic) hemodynamic response benefit from NSBBs therapy [39]. However, all those markers have yet to show reproducible and externally validated prognostic value in future trials. Ultimately, all mentioned biomarkers should be evaluated with regard to their prognostic value, possibly in comprehensive risk scores, to refine prognostication in patients with ACLD on NSBB therapy in a personalized manner.

8.4 Primary Prophylaxis

NSBBs are the mainstay of medical treatment in portal hypertension owing to their efficiency in reducing portal pressure and the risks of variceal bleeding and rebleeding. Importantly, NSBBs are the most efficient in reducing portal pressure in patients that have already developed CSPH, which was demonstrated in a Spanish mechanistical study [40]. The authors compared the effects of NSBBs in patients with subclinical portal hypertension, i.e., HVPG 6–9 mmHg, against their effect in patients with CSPH (HVPG ≥10 mmHg). Decreases in HVPG were significantly higher in patients that had already developed CSPH (−16% vs. -8%). This finding is most likely explained by the more advanced hyperdynamic circulatory state that is present in CSPH that, in turn, can be influenced by NSBBs. Thus, NSBB treatment is generally regarded ineffective in patients without CSPH, or—in settings where HVPG measurements are not available—that have not already developed clinical signs of CSPH, most importantly varices. Importantly, most landmark studies that addressed the role of NSBBs in cirrhosis included only patients with varices and/or an HVPG >12 mmHg [7], the threshold above which the risk of variceal bleeding vastly increases, explaining why an HVPG response can only be achieved in patients starting above 12 mmHg. Regardless of the definition, HVPG response guided therapy is the preferred setting for the prophylaxis of variceal bleeding, as NSBB treatment effects can be closely monitored and predicted, and the patients' outcome optimized [41].

Yet, the applicability of sequential measurements is limited, and thus, endoscopic screening for GEVs is most widely used today for the evaluation of the risk of variceal bleeding. In line, international guidelines by the European Association for the Study of the Liver (EASL) [17], the American Association for the Study of the Liver (AASLD) [19], and the Baveno VI consensus [18] have recommended the use of NSBBs for primary and secondary prophylaxis (in combination with endoscopic band ligation [EBL]) in cirrhotic patients according to the presence or absence of (high-risk) GEVs. The following overview is therefore structured in accordance with the existing recommendations.

8.4.1 Patients with No or Small Varices: A Shifting Paradigm

Generally, NSBB treatment seems to be ineffective in patients without varices. This was demonstrated in a study conducted by Groszmann and Garcia-Tsao et al. [42]. In their study involving patients with HVPG ≥6 mmHg without varices, patients were randomly assigned to timolol or placebo. After a median follow-up of 5 years, 40% in both treatment groups reached the composite endpoint of variceal bleeding or development of varices. And while the HVPG response rate was higher in the timolol group (53% vs. 38%), the authors also reported a considerable three times higher rate of adverse events in the NSBB treatment group. Therefore, there currently exists no evidence for the use of NSBBs in patients without CSPH and without varices.

Even in patients with small varices, conflicting data exists on the efficacy of NSBBs in preventing varix size progression and variceal bleeding [43, 44]. This was further highlighted by a meta-analysis showing no clear benefit of NSBB treatment in patients without large varices [45]. However, this might partly be influenced by the fact that this meta-analysis also included patients without any (i.e., small) varices and, more importantly, without CSPH. In line, another meta-analysis [46] that included only patients with small varices (i.e., CSPH) at baseline as well as results of an RCT that observed a lower risk for varix size progression upon carvedilol therapy [47] revealed a trend toward a lower risk for large varix development upon NSBB therapy in the fixed effect model.

Regardless of varix status, another recent landmark RCT has dealt with the effects of NSBB therapy in patients with known CSPH (i.e., HVPG ≥10 mmHg). The PREDESCI study by Villanueva et al. [20] included patients with a diagnosis of CSPH as detected during HVPG measurements regardless of varix status at baseline. Among the 201 patients that were included (carvedilol: $n = 33$, propranolol: $n = 67$, inactive treatment: $n = 101$), the primary endpoint comprising of ascites development, variceal bleeding, or hepatic encephalopathy occurred in 16% of patients in the NSBB group vs. 27% in the inactive treatment group. This was mostly driven by lower rates of ascites development, which is the most common first event of decompensation in cirrhosis. Ultimately, the PREDESCI trial has shown that in settings in which HVPG measurements are available, patients seem to profit from immediate initiation of NSBBs upon CSPH diagnosis, regardless of varix status. In settings where invasive HVPG measurement is not available, this might also extend to patients that have a very high probability of CSPH, e.g. patients that show a liver stiffness of ≥20–25 kPa; however, this has to be further evaluated in future trials. This might lead to a shift in the therapeutic paradigm in patients with CSPH, and might even instigate the repurposing of NSBBs in cirrhosis in general.

Most importantly, current international guidelines do not support the use of NSBBs in any of the mentioned indications (preprimary prophylaxis, prevention of varix size progression, and prevention of the first decompensation). While future trials will have to validate the mentioned findings, strong evidence already exists that might lead to a change in recommendations in the future.

8.4.2 Large or High-Risk Small Varices: Clear Indications for NSBBs

The detection of large or high-risk small varices represents a clear indication for NSBB therapy initiation to reduce the risk of bleeding. This is clearly stated in all current international guidelines [17–19], although slightly differing definitions exist for high-risk small varices: The EASL defines high-risk small varices as varices that are present in Child–Turcotte–Pugh C cirrhosis or that show red wale marks [17], while the AASLD definition comprises small varices also in patients with Child–Turcotte–Pugh B cirrhosis [19]. Nonetheless, NSBB therapy in primary prophylaxis leads to an absolute risk reduction of 10% (25% vs. 15% in inactive treatment) during a two-year follow-up, resulting in a comparably low number needed to treat (NNT) of 10 [48]. When only considering patients with large varices, the NNT decreases further to 6 [48].

Caution is warranted when using NSBBs for this indication in advanced cirrhosis, owing to results of a study that demonstrated increased risks of hepatorenal syndrome and mortality associated with propranolol therapy in advanced liver dysfunction [49], and other studies that have repeatedly shown that caution is warranted when using NSBBs in patients with refractory ascites. Still, there is an unmet need for studies specifically addressing the role of NSBBs in patients with small varices and advanced liver dysfunction.

When discussing the role of NSBBs in primary prophylaxis of variceal bleeding, their (dis-)advantages in comparison to EBL need to be addressed, since both treatment options are equally recommended as standalone therapy in primary prophylaxis. A large meta-analysis including 19 studies has demonstrated no difference in overall or bleeding-related mortality between the NSBB and the EBL treatment groups [50]. However, a more recent meta-analysis that included 32 RCTs and a total of 3362 patients found that patients with NSBB therapy exhibited a better safety profile and an improved overall survival in comparison to EBL [51]. Importantly, EBL is associated with fewer complications overall; however, EBL-related complications, such as post-banding ulcer bleeding, can be severe and potentially life threatening. Additionally, EBL, in contrast to NSBBs, does not influence the underlying portal pressure and has no hemodynamic and/or disease-modifying effects. Lastly, NSBB treatment is associated with higher cost efficiency and is not reliant on dedicated endoscopy units. However, EBL treatment can achieve variceal obliteration that might ease patients' anxiety, especially if they are at a high risk of bleeding and/or non-compliant to medication [52].

Still, the discussed results of the PREDESCI trial might likely extend to patients with high-risk or large varices and compensated disease (that were excluded from the study), indicating that those patients might as well benefit more from NSBB therapy and its disease-modifying effects.

In the end, both treatments are evidence-based and validated options for primary prophylaxis of variceal bleeding in patients with high-risk small or large varices. The decision should consider the patient's perspective as well as the other mentioned factors.

8.5 Secondary Prophylaxis

All current guidelines [17–19] support a combination of NSBBs plus EBL for the secondary prophylaxis of variceal bleeding based on two meta-analyses [53, 54]. Both analyses showed that combined medical and endoscopic therapy was associated with a tendency toward a lower risk of overall mortality as compared to EBL monotherapy. Of note, combination therapy did not improve overall survival as compared to NSBB monotherapy. Intriguingly, the impact of NSBBs on survival seems to be specific to patients in secondary prophylaxis [16], and it can be hypothesized that non-hemodynamic effects might contribute to this. If patients are intolerant to NSBB therapy, alternative treatment options, such as transjugular intrahepatic portosystemic shunt (TIPS), should be evaluated [17].

8.6 Carvedilol Versus Propranolol & Other Conventional NSBB

In comparison to the historically most widely used NSBB compounds that include propranolol, timolol, and nadolol, carvedilol has additional anti-alpha1-adrenergic activity, allowing for a more potent reduction of portal pressure as compared to propranolol [9]. This was supported by a recent meta-analysis [55]. The stronger effects on portal blood flow are paralleled by more adverse effects on systemic circulation, however, and it was found that carvedilol led to stronger reductions of mean arterial pressure in comparison to propranolol [55]. Therefore, carvedilol should not be used in doses higher than 12.5 mg/d, as higher doses do not seem to further impact on portal pressure.

Although no RCT directly compared carvedilol against propranolol in primary prophylaxis, an RCT by our group showed that carvedilol treatment led to hemodynamic response in 58% of patients who did not respond to propranolol therapy [12]. This was accompanied by lower bleeding and mortality rates in the carvedilol cohort vs. the propranolol and EBL cohort of the study. In summary, we recommend carvedilol for NSBB therapy in primary prophylaxis.

Importantly, no study has so far investigated the use of carvedilol plus EBL vs. conventional NSBB plus EBL in secondary prophylaxis, although its efficacy and safety as monotherapy were investigated by two RCTs [56, 57]. Nonetheless, the Baveno VI consensus did not recommend carvedilol therapy in the setting of secondary prophylaxis [18]. While carvedilol can still be a valid option in secondary prophylaxis in patients that are well compensated owing to its more potent reduction of portal pressure, its use should be carefully scrutinized in more advanced patients that are characterized by fragile circulatory homeostasis [13]. This is most relevant in patients with severe or refractory ascites, in which propranolol is thought to have less adverse effects on systemic hemodynamics, and is thus the compound of choice.

8.7 Dose Titration and Safety

The absence of HVPG measurement in most settings necessitates that NSBB therapy must be non-invasively monitored. Usually, NSBB doses are titrated a certain target heart rate (50–55 bpm) [17]. In theory, this could lead to the conclusion that more advanced patients, in whom worsening of liver function is paralleled by more pronounced activation of the SNS and who show a progressive hyperdynamic state, might need higher doses of treatment to achieve these target heart rates. This is challenged by the fact that especially in end-stage cirrhosis, i.e. refractory ascites, cardiac reserve is severely impaired, and NSBB therapy might have deleterious impact in this setting. Notably, in the study by Sérste et al. [13], almost half of the patients received high-dose propranolol treatment (i.e., 160 mg/d), a dose that would nowadays not be targeted in end-stage cirrhosis. A recent quasi-experimental, prospective proof-of-concept study by Téllez et al. confirmed that in patients with refractory ascites, high-dose propranolol therapy might in fact have negative impact on patients' circulatory homeostasis and kidney function, possibly worsening their prognosis [58]. However, a Danish nationwide study [59] found that NSBB therapy had differential impact on patients with spontaneous bacterial peritonitis (SBP), one of the most severe complications of ascites. In their study, the authors demonstrated that high-dose propranolol therapy (i.e., 160 mg/d) was associated with increased mortality after SBP, while doses of 80 mg or less per day were associated with reduced mortality after SBP. Two recent meta-analyses also confirmed that NSBB therapy is not generally harmful in patients with ascites, and that patients with ascites equally profit from the achievement of HVPG response [14, 15], even though patients with decompensated disease and impaired circulatory homeostasis seem to profit less from NSBBs [60].

In summary, careful dose titration under close clinical follow-up is warranted in patients with ascites, and further studies might elucidate target doses and titration schemes. NSBBs are a valid and impactful option for the prophylaxis of variceal (re-)bleeding in patients with or without ascites, although hemodynamic targets and maximum doses need to be considered in advanced disease. Current guidelines do not give recommendations on titration of NSBB doses, and this might be further investigated in future trials. In the absence of such recommendations, clinicians must make decisions according to risk/benefit considerations. Reduction or permanent cessation of therapy might be warranted in patients with signs of systemic circulatory dysfunction [61], hyponatremia [62], low cardiac output [63], and increasing levels of serum creatinine [64].

In line, Baveno VI consensus recommended that NSBB discontinuation be considered in patients with refractory ascites and (i) systolic arterial blood pressure < 90 mmHg, or (ii) serum creatinine >1.5 mg/dL, or (iii) hyponatremia <130 mmol/L [18].

8.8 Conclusion

NSBB therapy—where indicated—leads to a marked risk reduction of variceal bleeding in primary (NNT: 10) and secondary (NNT: 5) prophylaxis in comparison to inactive treatment [48]. Thus, all current guidelines strongly recommend their application for the prevention of variceal (re-)bleeding [17–19]. Of note, recent studies, most importantly the PREDESCI study, indicate that NSBB treatment might even be able to prevent the first decompensation in patients with CSPH, possibly broadening their indication in the future [20]. Nonetheless, a significant proportion of patients will not achieve chronic HVPG response to NSBB therapy, and therefore, clinicians need access to reliable means to evaluate the response to therapy [7]. Sequential HVPG measurements prior to and under stable NSBB intake will likely remain the most accurate tool for HVPG response assessment. The achievement of chronic HVPG response, i.e., a reduction of $\geq 10\%$ (primary prophylaxis) or $\geq 20\%$ (secondary prophylaxis), or to an absolute value ≤ 12 mmHg, is associated with a strong reduction of bleeding rates and increased survival in secondary prophylaxis [7]. It must be acknowledged, however, that this procedure is invasive, and clinical feasibility and availability are limited. While acute HVPG to response to i.v. propranolol might be a valid alternative [26], it still requires one invasive measurement. Non-invasive methods for the assessment of chronic HVPG response are under development, and some—such as spleen stiffness measurements before and after NSBB initiation [30]—have shown moderate correlations with HVPG dynamics. However, these findings need to be further validated before their application in clinical routine. Until then, HVPG guided therapy will remain the gold standard for NSBB therapy monitoring in portal hypertension.

In settings where portal hypertension can be only assessed by endoscopic screening for GEVs, NSBBs should be initiated in patients with medium to large sized or small high-risk varices according to the current guidelines. Patients without varices should undergo yearly screening endoscopies. In primary prophylaxis, NSBB therapy should be preferred over EBL in most patients; however, both are equally recommended options. The compound of choice in well compensated patients should be carvedilol owing to its higher potency to decrease portal pressure, as compared to conventional NSBB compounds, such as propranolol [9]. Treatment should be closely monitored in patients with hypotension, bradycardia, or signs of kidney dysfunction. In patients who show systolic arterial pressure of <90 mmHg, hyponatremia <130 mmol/L, or serum creatinine >1.5 mg/dL, switching to endoscopic therapy might be considered [18]. However, EBL has no effect on the underlying portal hypertensive syndrome, and thus, NSBBs should be continued whenever possible.

In secondary prophylaxis, combined endoscopic and medical therapy is recommended as the standard of care. In patients with advanced disease, i.e., patients with (refractory) ascites, carvedilol should be avoided and instead, propranolol should be used.

In patients who are very advanced, i.e., patients who are acutely decompensated or are diagnosed with ACLF, NSBB treatment should not be discontinued as long as the patient is hemodynamically stable, and in those in whom transient discontinuation is unavoidable, therapy should be reinitiated as soon as possible owing to potential disease-modifying effects of NSBBs [36].

Overall, NSBB therapy is highly recommended for patients with portal hypertension and varices. In the future, NSBBs might even be used for the prevention of the first decompensation in general. An individualized, patient-centered approach is warranted when applying NSBB therapy, considering the distinct stage of CSPH, a patient's individual HVPG level, endoscopic varix stage, possible adverse effects, and patient preference.

Disclosures MJ has nothing to declare. TR received grant support from AbbVie, Boehringer-Ingelheim, Gilead, MSD, Philips Healthcare, Gore; speaking honoraria from AbbVie, Gilead, Gore, Intercept, Roche, MSD; consulting/advisory board fee from AbbVie, Bayer, Boehringer-Ingelheim, Gilead, Intercept, MSD, Siemens; and travel support from Boehringer-Ingelheim, Gilead, and Roche.

References

1. Iwakiri Y. Pathophysiology of portal hypertension. Clin Liver Dis. 2014;18:281–91.
2. Ripoll C, Groszmann R, Garcia-Tsao G, et al. Hepatic venous pressure gradient predicts clinical decompensation in patients with compensated cirrhosis. Gastroenterology. 2007;133:481–8.
3. Bolognesi M, Di Pascoli M, Verardo A, et al. Splanchnic vasodilation and hyperdynamic circulatory syndrome in cirrhosis. World J Gastroenterol. 2014;20:2555–63.
4. Bosch J, Groszmann RJ, Shah VH. Evolution in the understanding of the pathophysiological basis of portal hypertension: how changes in paradigm are leading to successful new treatments. J Hepatol. 2015;62:S121–30.
5. Reiberger T, Schwabl P, Trauner M, et al. Measurement of the hepatic venous pressure gradient and Transjugular liver biopsy. J Vis Exp. 2020;(160). https://doi.org/10.3791/58819.
6. Bosch J, Abraldes JG, Berzigotti A, et al. The clinical use of HVPG measurements in chronic liver disease. Nature Rev Gastroenterol Hepatol. 2009;6:573–82.
7. Mandorfer M, Hernández-Gea V, Reiberger T, et al. Hepatic venous pressure gradient response in non-selective Beta-blocker treatment—is it worth measuring? Curr Hepatol Rep. 2019;18:174–86.
8. Reiberger T, Mandorfer M. Beta adrenergic blockade and decompensated cirrhosis. J Hepatol. 2017;66:849–59.
9. Bosch J. Carvedilol: the β-blocker of choice for portal hypertension? Gut. 2013;62:1529–30.
10. Schwarzer R, Kivaranovic D, Paternostro R, et al. Carvedilol for reducing portal pressure in primary prophylaxis of variceal bleeding: a dose-response study. Aliment Pharmacol Ther. 2018;47:1162–9.
11. Tripathi D, Ferguson JW, Kochar N, et al. Randomized controlled trial of carvedilol versus variceal band ligation for the prevention of the first variceal bleed. Hepatology. 2009;50:825–33.
12. Reiberger T, Ulbrich G, Ferlitsch A, et al. Carvedilol for primary prophylaxis of variceal bleeding in cirrhotic patients with haemodynamic non-response to propranolol. Gut. 2013;62:1634–41.
13. Serste T, Melot C, Francoz C, et al. Deleterious effects of beta-blockers on survival in patients with cirrhosis and refractory ascites. Hepatology. 2010;52:1017–22.
14. Chirapongsathorn S, Valentin N, Alahdab F, et al. Nonselective β-blockers and survival in patients with cirrhosis and ascites: a systematic review and meta-analysis. Clin Gastroenterol Hepatol. 2016;14:1096–1104.e9.
15. Turco L, Villanueva C, La Mura V, et al. Lowering portal pressure improves outcomes of patients with cirrhosis, with or without ascites: a meta-analysis. Clin Gastroenterol Hepatol. 2020;18:313–327.e6.
16. Pfisterer N, Dexheimer C, Fuchs E-M, et al. Betablockers do not increase efficacy of band ligation in primary prophylaxis but they improve survival in secondary prophylaxis of variceal bleeding. Aliment Pharmacol Ther. 2018;47:966–79.
17. EASL Clinical Practice Guidelines for the management of patients with decompensated cirrhosis. J Hepatol. 2018;69:406–60.
18. de Franchis R. Expanding consensus in portal hypertension: report of the Baveno VI consensus workshop: stratifying risk and individualizing care for portal hypertension. J Hepatol. 2015;63:743–52.
19. Garcia-Tsao G, Abraldes JG, Berzigotti A, et al. Portal hypertensive bleeding in cirrhosis: risk stratification, diagnosis, and management: 2016 practice guidance by the American association for the study of liver diseases. Hepatology. 2017;65:310–35.
20. Villanueva C, Albillos A, Genescà J, et al. β blockers to prevent decompensation of cirrhosis in patients with clinically significant portal hypertension (PREDESCI): a randomised, double-blind, placebo-controlled, multicentre trial. Lancet. 2019;393:1597–608.
21. Mandorfer M, Hernández-Gea V, García-Pagán JC, et al. Noninvasive diagnostics for portal hypertension: a comprehensive review. Semin Liver Dis. 2020;40:240–55.

22. Reiberger T, Ferlitsch A, Payer BA, et al. Noninvasive screening for liver fibrosis and portal hypertension by transient elastography–a large single center experience. Wien Klin Wochenschr. 2012;124:395–402.
23. Colecchia A, Montrone L, Scaioli E, et al. Measurement of spleen stiffness to evaluate portal hypertension and the presence of esophageal varices in patients with HCV-related cirrhosis. Gastroenterology. 2012;143:646–54.
24. Berzigotti A, Seijo S, Arena U, et al. Elastography, spleen size, and platelet count identify portal hypertension in patients with compensated cirrhosis. Gastroenterology. 2013;144:102–111.e1.
25. Ferlitsch M, Reiberger T, Hoke M, et al. Von Willebrand factor as new noninvasive predictor of portal hypertension, decompensation and mortality in patients with liver cirrhosis. Hepatology. 2012;56:1439–47.
26. Villanueva C, Aracil C, Colomo A, et al. Acute hemodynamic response to β-blockers and prediction of long-term outcome in primary prophylaxis of Variceal bleeding. Gastroenterology. 2009;137:119–28.
27. Villanueva C, López-Balaguer JM, Aracil C, et al. Maintenance of hemodynamic response to treatment for portal hypertension and influence on complications of cirrhosis. J Hepatol. 2004;40:757–65.
28. Merkel C, Bolognesi M, Berzigotti A, et al. Clinical significance of worsening portal hypertension during long-term medical treatment in patients with cirrhosis who had been classified as early good-responders on haemodynamic criteria. J Hepatol. 2010;52:45–53.
29. Choi S-Y, Jeong WK, Kim Y, et al. Shear-wave Elastography: a noninvasive tool for monitoring changing hepatic venous pressure gradients in patients with cirrhosis. Radiology. 2014;273:917–26.
30. Kim HY, So YH, Kim W, et al. Non-invasive response prediction in prophylactic carvedilol therapy for cirrhotic patients with esophageal varices. J Hepatol. 2019;70:412–22.
31. Palaniyappan N, Cox E, Bradley C, et al. Non-invasive assessment of portal hypertension using quantitative magnetic resonance imaging. J Hepatol. 2016;65:1131–9.
32. Danielsen KV, Hove JD, Nabilou P, et al. Using MR elastography to assess portal hypertension and response to beta-blockers in patients with cirrhosis. Liver Int. 2021;41:2149–58.
33. Reverter E, Lozano JJ, Alonso C, et al. Metabolomics discloses potential biomarkers to predict the acute HVPG response to propranolol in patients with cirrhosis. Liver Int. 2019;39:705–13.
34. Trebicka J, von Heydebrand M, Lehmann J, et al. Assessment of response to beta-blockers by expression of βArr2 and RhoA/ROCK2 in antrum mucosa in cirrhotic patients. J Hepatol. 2016;64:1265–73.
35. Reiberger T, Ferlitsch A, Payer BA, et al. Non-selective betablocker therapy decreases intestinal permeability and serum levels of LBP and IL-6 in patients with cirrhosis. J Hepatol. 2013;58:911–21.
36. Mookerjee RP, Pavesi M, Thomsen KL, et al. Treatment with non-selective beta blockers is associated with reduced severity of systemic inflammation and improved survival of patients with acute-on-chronic liver failure. J Hepatol. 2016;64:574–82.
37. Jachs M, Hartl L, Schaufler D, et al. Amelioration of systemic inflammation in advanced chronic liver disease upon beta-blocker therapy translates into improved clinical outcomes. Gut. 2021;70:1758–67.
38. Jachs M, Hartl L, Simbrunner B, et al. Decreasing VWF-levels upon NSBB-therapy indicate a decreased risk of further decompensation, ACLF, and death. Clin Gastroenterol Hepatol 2022;20:1362–73.e6.
39. Thalheimer U, Bosch J, Burroughs AK. How to prevent varices from bleeding: shades of grey–the case for nonselective beta blockers. Gastroenterology. 2007;133:2029–36.
40. Villanueva C, Albillos A, Genescà J, et al. Development of hyperdynamic circulation and response to β-blockers in compensated cirrhosis with portal hypertension: liver failure/cirrhosis/portal hypertension. Hepatology. 2016;63:197–206.
41. Villanueva C, Graupera I, Aracil C, et al. A randomized trial to assess whether portal pressure guided therapy to prevent variceal rebleeding improves survival in cirrhosis. Hepatology. 2017;65:1693–707.

42. Groszmann RJ, Garcia-Tsao G, Bosch J, et al. Beta-blockers to prevent gastroesophageal varices in patients with cirrhosis. N Engl J Med. 2005;353:2254–61.
43. Sarin SK, Mishra SR, Sharma P, et al. Early primary prophylaxis with beta-blockers does not prevent the growth of small esophageal varices in cirrhosis: a randomized controlled trial. Hepatol Int. 2013;7:248–56.
44. Merkel C, Marin R, Angeli P, et al. A placebo-controlled clinical trial of nadolol in the prophylaxis of growth of small esophageal varices in cirrhosis. Gastroenterology. 2004;127:476–84.
45. Qi XS. Nonselective beta-blockers in cirrhotic patients with no or small varices: a meta-analysis. World J Gastroenterol. 2015;21:3100.
46. Mandorfer M, Peck-Radosavljevic M, Reiberger T. Prevention of progression from small to large varices: are we there yet? An updated meta-analysis. Gut. 2017;66:1347–9.
47. Bhardwaj A, Kedarisetty CK, Vashishtha C, et al. Carvedilol delays the progression of small oesophageal varices in patients with cirrhosis: a randomised placebo-controlled trial. Gut. 2017;66:1838–43.
48. D'Amico G, Pagliaro L, Bosch J. Pharmacological treatment of portal hypertension: an evidence-based approach. Semin Liver Dis. 1999;19:475–505.
49. Kalambokis GN, Baltayiannis G, Christou L, et al. Red signs and not severity of cirrhosis should determine non-selective β-blocker treatment in child–Pugh C cirrhosis with small varices: increased risk of hepatorenal syndrome and death beyond 6 months of propranolol use. Gut. 2016;65:1228–30.
50. Gluud LL, Krag A. Banding ligation versus beta-blockers for primary prevention in oesophageal varices in adults. Cochrane Database Syst Rev. 2012;8:CD004544.
51. Sharma M, Singh S, Desai V, et al. Comparison of therapies for primary prevention of esophageal Variceal bleeding: a systematic review and network meta-analysis. Hepatology. 2019;69:1657–75.
52. Lo GH. Letter to the editor: Beta-blockers are preferable to banding ligation for primary prophylaxis of Variceal bleeding? Hepatology. 2019;70:1876.
53. Thiele M, Krag A, Rohde U, et al. Meta-analysis: banding ligation and medical interventions for the prevention of rebleeding from oesophageal varices. Aliment Pharmacol Ther. 2012;35:1155–65.
54. Puente A, Hernández-Gea V, Graupera I, et al. Drugs plus ligation to prevent rebleeding in cirrhosis: an updated systematic review. Liver Int. 2014;34:823–33.
55. Sinagra E, Perricone G, D'Amico M, et al. Systematic review with meta-analysis: the haemodynamic effects of carvedilol compared with propranolol for portal hypertension in cirrhosis. Aliment Pharmacol Ther. 2014;39:557–68.
56. Lo G-H, Chen W-C, Wang H-M, et al. Randomized, controlled trial of carvedilol versus nadolol plus isosorbide mononitrate for the prevention of variceal rebleeding: prevention of variceal rebleeding. J Gastroenterol Hepatol. 2012;27:1681–7.
57. Stanley AJ, Dickson S, Hayes PC, et al. Multicentre randomised controlled study comparing carvedilol with variceal band ligation in the prevention of variceal rebleeding. J Hepatol. 2014;61:1014–9.
58. Téllez L, Ibáñez-Samaniego L, Pérez del Villar C, et al. Non-selective beta-blockers impair global circulatory homeostasis and renal function in cirrhotic patients with refractory ascites. J Hepatol 2020:S0168827820303032.
59. Madsen BS, Nielsen KF, Fialla AD, et al. Keep the sick from harm in spontaneous bacterial peritonitis: dose of beta blockers matters. J Hepatol. 2016;64:1455–6.
60. Alvarado-Tapias E, Ardevol A, Garcia-Guix M, et al. Short-term hemodynamic effects of β-blockers influence survival of patients with decompensated cirrhosis. J Hepatol. 2020;73:829–41.
61. Llach J, Ginès P, Arroyo V, et al. Prognostic value of arterial pressure, endogenous vasoactive systems, and renal function in cirrhotic patients admitted to the hospital for the treatment of ascites. Gastroenterology. 1988;94:482–7.

62. Serste T, Gustot T, Rautou P-E, et al. Severe hyponatremia is a better predictor of mortality than MELDNa in patients with cirrhosis and refractory ascites. J Hepatol. 2012;57:274–80.
63. Krag A, Bendtsen F, Henriksen JH, et al. Low cardiac output predicts development of hepatorenal syndrome and survival in patients with cirrhosis and ascites. Gut. 2010;59:105–10.
64. Ruiz-del-Arbol L. Systemic, renal, and hepatic hemodynamic derangement in cirrhotic patients with spontaneous bacterial peritonitis. Hepatology. 2003;38:1210–8.

9 Somatostatin and Octreotide in Liver Cirrhosis

Arpan Mohanty

Abstract

Somatostatin and its synthetic counterpart, octreotide are commonly used for the management of portal hypertensive complications of cirrhosis, specifically acute variceal bleeding and hepatorenal syndrome. Somatostatin and octreotide reduce splanchnic blood flow and portal pressure without major systemic hemodynamic effects. Early initiation of somatostatin or octreotide is indicated in the management of acute variceal bleeding and is associated with improved outcomes. Octreotide in combination with midodrine, an α-receptor agonist, is used for the management of hepatorenal syndrome with modest effects. This chapter discussed the use of somatostatin and octreotide in management of acute variceal bleeding and hepatorenal syndrome.

Keywords

Somatostatin · Octreotide · Hepatorenal syndrome · Acute variceal bleeding

9.1 Introduction

Portal hypertension or increase in portal venous pressure is the main pathophysiological consequence of cirrhosis. It is the key mechanism for complications of cirrhosis, such as variceal bleeding, ascites, hepatorenal syndrome (HRS), and hepatic

A. Mohanty (✉)
Boston University School of Medicine, Boston, MA, USA

Boston Medical Center, Boston, MA, USA
e-mail: amohanty@bu.edu

X. Qi, Y. Yang (eds.), *Pharmacotherapy for Liver Cirrhosis and Its Complications*, https://doi.org/10.1007/978-981-19-2615-0_9

encephalopathy [1, 2]. Portal hypertension has two main components: increased intrahepatic vascular resistance and splanchnic vasodilation [3]. The increase in intrahepatic vascular resistance is due to progressive hepatic fibrosis (structural component) and increase in hepatic vascular tone due to imbalance in hepatic vasoconstrictors and vasodilators (dynamic component) [3]. Increase in intrahepatic vascular resistance leads to splanchnic vasodilation and diversion of blood flow through portosystemic collaterals, which further worsens portal hypertension. To counteract splanchnic vasodilation, splanchnic vasoconstrictors are commonly used as therapy for portal hypertension, primarily in acute variceal bleeding (AVB) and HRS [4]. Somatostatin and its analog octreotide and vasopressin and its analog terlipressin are splanchnic vasoconstrictors used for this purpose. As compared to vasopressin and terlipressin, somatostatin and octreotide have less severe side effects and are used more frequently. This chapter will summarize the use of somatostatin and octreotide in AVB and HRS.

9.2 Mechanisms of Action, Hemodynamic Effects, and Side Effects of Somatostatin and Octreotide

Somatostatin is found widely in the human body, including the hypothalamus, pancreatic islet cells, and intestinal epithelial cells. It exists as a 14 and 28 amino-acid peptide. It has many pharmacodynamic effects in the gastrointestinal system, including splanchnic vasoconstriction, inhibition of secretion of several endocrine and exocrine gastrointestinal peptides, inhibition of absorption of carbohydrates, inhibition of bile duct secretion and gall bladder contraction, and regulation of gastrointestinal motility and transport. Octreotide is a synthetic 8 amino acid peptide with greater potency and longer duration of action than somatostatin. In the USA, it has replaced somatostatin in management of portal hypertension, though its use remains off-label.

Somatostatin and octreotide cause splanchnic arterial vasoconstriction and reduction in portal blood flow. The mechanisms of action of somatostatin and octreotide are partially understood. They inhibit release of vasodilatory gut-mediated peptides, such as glucagon, and decrease splanchnic blood flow. They may have some direct vasoconstrictive effects on the mesenteric circulation, especially in the presence of other vasoconstrictors [5, 6]. Lastly, it is postulated that in AVB, somatostatin and octreotide prevent rebleeding by blunting postprandial splanchnic hyperemia response and resultant portal pressure rise [7–9].

The hemodynamic effects of somatostatin and octreotide are modest and transient. Decrease in portal pressure after bolus doses of somatostatin and octreotide lasts for about 5 min [10–12]. While some sustained reduction in portal pressure is noted with somatostatin at a higher dose infusion [12], this effect is not seen with octreotide, most likely due to tachyphylaxis. Both somatostatin and octreotide cause transient decrease in heart rate and cardiac output and mean increase in arterial and pulmonary artery pressure [7, 11, 12].

Somatostatin and octreotide have few side effects. Even though a more sustained decrease in portal pressure is seen with vasopressin and terlipressin, they are not commonly used due to their unfavorable side effect profile. Severe side effects, such as myocardial ischemia, mesenteric infarction, hyponatremia, hypertension, and peripheral ischemia that can be seen with vasopressin and terlipressin, are rarely seen with somatostatin and octreotide.

9.3 Indications for Use of Somatostatin and Octreotide

9.3.1 Acute Variceal Bleeding

AVB is a common and life-threatening complication of cirrhosis with high short-term mortality of 15–25% [13, 14]. Varices are commonly found in the esophagus though they may also be seen elsewhere like the stomach or small intestine. Increased blood flow in submucosal veins, lack of external tissue support that facilitates dilation, and VEGF mediated angiogenesis together make it conducive for formation of esophageal varices [3]. Management of AVB focuses on controlling of bleeding, preventing recurrent bleeding, and reducing 6-week mortality [4]. Splanchnic vasoconstrictors, such as somatostatin and octreotide, play a complementary but important role in the management of AVB, where the main interventions are variceal ligation and prevention of infection with antibiotics.

9.3.1.1 Use of Somatostatin and Octreotide in AVB

Somatostatin and octreotide are commonly used vasoactive peptides in AVB owing to their safety profile. They are used as intravenous infusions due to their short half-lives. Early initiation of vasoactive peptides, when variceal bleeding is suspected (prior to endoscopy), is associated with improved outcomes [15, 16] and is recommended by major guidelines [4, 17, 18]. Somatostatin, octreotide, or terlipressin (low dose) are comparable in safety profile and efficacy in preventing continued bleeding or early rebleeding within 5 days [19]. Octreotide, which is the only vasoactive drug available in the USA, is associated with significantly improved control of AVB [20]. Somatostatin and octreotide do not improve mortality in AVB [21]. It is not clear if these agents are useful in Child A cirrhosis [17].

Somatostatin is administered as an intravenous 250 μg bolus followed by infusion at 250–500 μg/hour. Octreotide is administered as a 50 μg intravenous bolus followed by infusion at 50 μg/hour. In each drug, the bolus can be repeated in the first hour, if bleeding is not controlled. The duration of treatment is typically 2–5 days [4, 17, 18], though further research is needed to determine the optimal, ideally shorter, time period [17].

9.3.2 Hepatorenal Syndrome

HRS is a form of kidney injury unique to patients with cirrhosis and ascites [22, 23]. Traditionally, HRS was considered to be solely a "functional" renal failure where splanchnic arterial vasodilation (as a result of portal hypertension) and decreased cardiac output (as a result of cirrhotic cardiomyopathy) caused a reduction in effective circulating volume and renal perfusion [22]. It is now recognized that "structural" or parenchymal renal injury is a component of HRS and is caused by systemic inflammation, oxidative stress, and bile salt-related tubular damage [23]. HRS represents a state of further decompensation in patients with decompensated cirrhosis (i.e., in those with uncomplicated ascites, encephalopathy, or history of variceal hemorrhage) and is associated with poor survival [18, 24]. Liver transplantation is the definitive therapy for HRS [18, 24]. The goal of pharmacologic therapy is HRS reversal (i.e. improvement in serum creatinine), and is typically used as a bridge to liver transplantation. There are two forms of HRS: (1) HRS-Acute Kidney Injury (AKI) (formerly known as type 1 HRS), which is a rapidly developing AKI; (2) HRS non-AKI (formerly known as type 2 HRS), a more chronic form of kidney injury [23]. Pharmacologic therapy is indicated in HRS-AKI. This chapter will focus on the use of octreotide in treatment of HRS-AKI. For convenience, HRS-AKI will be referred to as HRS in the rest of the chapter.

9.3.2.1 General Principles for Treating HRS

Vasoconstrictors and albumin are the mainstay treatment for HRS [18, 23, 24]. Vasoactive peptides—octreotide and terlipressin— and noradrenaline are three vasoconstrictors used in treatment of HRS. They cause splanchnic vasoconstriction, which in turn improves effective arterial volume and reduces activation of renal vasoconstrictors and thus increases renal perfusion. Octreotide is used in combination with midodrine, an α-adrenergic agonist which increases renal perfusion by increasing blood pressure. Albumin is an important adjunct to vasoconstrictor therapy that expands volume, diminishes endothelial dysfunction, and improves cardiac inotropic effect by binding to vasodilators like nitrous oxide and other deleterious cytokines [25–27]. As "structural" kidney damage often coexists with "functional" renal failure, the response to these agents is variable.

As soon as HRS is diagnosed, expedited transplant referral should be considered [18, 24], and pharmacologic therapy should be started. The goal of pharmacologic therapy is to reverse kidney injury before permanent damage sets in. The most important positive predictor of response to pharmacologic treatment is lower baseline creatinine [28, 29], and thus, treatment should start as soon as HRS is diagnosed. As the spectrum of kidney injury in HRS starts at lower creatinine levels, the older definition of HRS which included rise of serum creatinine >2.5 mg/dl has been changed. HRS is now defined as an increase in serum creatine by ≥0.3 mg/dl within 48 hours or ≥ 50% from baseline value and/or decrease in urinary output ≤0.5 ml/kg in ≥6 hours in patients with cirrhosis and ascites without other cause for AKI, such as shock or nephrotoxins [23].

9.3.2.2 A Note on Terlipressin

Terlipressin is the most investigated drug for HRS and is considered the first-line treatment [18]. Multiple clinical trials and meta-analyses have demonstrated the efficacy of terlipressin and albumin in HRS reversal (i.e., improvement in serum creatinine <1.5 mg/dl) [30–39]. The recent landmark CONFIRM trial demonstrated that terlipressin was more effective than placebo in reversing HRS [40]. Of note, this trial used the older definition of HRS (i.e., higher creatinine) as an inclusion criterion which means that many patients with HRS who had lower creatinine were excluded. As terlipressin was associated with serious adverse events, including respiratory failure, and in exploratory analyses, it was not associated with improved survival, it did not receive FDA approval for use in HRS. In the USA, octreotide remains the only vasoactive drug used for HRS, albeit off-label. Further studies are needed to understand the timing, safety, and efficacy of terlipressin in early HRS.

9.3.2.3 Use of Octreotide for HRS

Octreotide in combination with midodrine is commonly used for treatment of HRS. As compared to terlipressin, it is less effective in reversal of HRS [41]. In a small trial, it was noted to have similar efficacy as noradrenaline [42]. It is popular given its safety and the ease of administration via the oral/subcutaneous route in a non-intensive care setting (unlike noradrenaline and terlipressin) [43]. The use of octreotide alone is not effective in HRS and can worsen systemic hemodynamics and renal function [44]. The combination of midodrine and octreotide may improve renal function in HRS, but randomized controlled trials are lacking.

Octreotide is administered subcutaneously at 100–200 μg every 8 hours. Midodrine is given orally at a starting dose of 7.5 g three times a day and titrated up to a dose of 12.5 mg to achieve a 15 mm Hg increase in mean arterial blood pressure [23, 24].

9.4 Conclusion

Somatostatin and octreotide are important adjunctive therapies in management of AVB and HRS. Octreotide is the only available vasoactive agent used for these indications in the USA. In AVB, further research is needed to clarify the duration of treatment and their utility in patients with Child A cirrhosis. The understanding of HRS pathophysiology and management is evolving. Octreotide will continue to have its role in management of HRS while further investigations on more effective management strategies for HRS are underway.

References

1. Ripoll C, Groszmann R, Garcia-Tsao G, et al. Hepatic venous pressure gradient predicts clinical decompensation in patients with compensated cirrhosis. Gastroenterology. 2007;133:481–8.
2. Ripoll C, Groszmann RJ, Garcia-Tsao G, et al. Hepatic venous pressure gradient predicts development of hepatocellular carcinoma independently of severity of cirrhosis. J Hepatol. 2009;50:923–8.

3. Bosch J, Groszmann RJ, Shah VH. Evolution in the understanding of the pathophysiological basis of portal hypertension: how changes in paradigm are leading to successful new treatments. J Hepatol. 2015;62:S121–30.
4. Garcia-Tsao G, Abraldes JG, Berzigotti A, Bosch J. Portal hypertensive bleeding in cirrhosis: Risk stratification, diagnosis, and management: 2016 practice guidance by the American Association for the study of liver diseases. Hepatology. 2017;65:310–35.
5. Chatila R, Ferayorni L, Gupta T, Groszmann RJ. Local arterial vasoconstriction induced by octreotide in patients with cirrhosis. Hepatology. 2000;31:572–6.
6. Wiest R, Tsai MH, Groszmann RJ. Octreotide potentiates PKC-dependent vasoconstrictors in portal-hypertensive and control rats. Gastroenterology. 2001;120:975–83.
7. McCormick PA, Biagini MR, Dick R, et al. Octreotide inhibits the meal-induced increases in the portal venous pressure of cirrhotic patients with portal hypertension: a double-blind, placebo-controlled study. Hepatology. 1992;16:1180–6.
8. Albillos A, Rossi I, Iborra J, et al. Octreotide prevents postprandial splanchnic hyperemia in patients with portal hypertension. J Hepatol. 1994;21:88–94.
9. Villanueva C, Ortiz J, Miñana J, et al. Somatostatin treatment and risk stratification by continuous portal pressure monitoring during acute variceal bleeding. Gastroenterology. 2001;121:110–7.
10. Baik SK, Jeong PH, Ji SW, et al. Acute hemodynamic effects of octreotide and terlipressin in patients with cirrhosis: a randomized comparison. Am J Gastroenterol. 2005;100:631–5.
11. Escorsell A, Bandi JC, Andreu V, et al. Desensitization to the effects of intravenous octreotide in cirrhotic patients with portal hypertension. Gastroenterology. 2001;120:161–9.
12. Cirera I, Feu F, Luca A, et al. Effects of bolus injections and continuous infusions of somatostatin and placebo in patients with cirrhosis: a double-blind hemodynamic investigation. Hepatology. 1995;22:106–11.
13. Amitrano L, Guardascione MA, Manguso F, et al. The effectiveness of current acute variceal bleed treatments in unselected cirrhotic patients: refining short-term prognosis and risk factors. Am J Gastroenterol. 2012;107:1872–8.
14. Reverter E, Tandon P, Augustin S, et al. A MELD-based model to determine risk of mortality among patients with acute variceal bleeding. Gastroenterology. 2014;146:412–19.e3.
15. Avgerinos A, Nevens F, Raptis S, Fevery J. Early administration of somatostatin and efficacy of sclerotherapy in acute oesophageal variceal bleeds: the European acute bleeding oesophageal variceal episodes (ABOVE) randomised trial. Lancet. 1997;350:1495–9.
16. Calès P, Masliah C, Bernard B, et al. Early administration of vapreotide for variceal bleeding in patients with cirrhosis. N Engl J Med. 2001;344:23–8.
17. de Franchis R, Bosch J, Garcia-Tsao G, Reiberger T, Ripoll C, on behalf of the Baveno VII Faculty. Baveno VII - Renewing consensus in portal hypertension. J Hepatol. 2022;76:959–74.
18. European Association for the Study of the Liver. EASL Clinical Practice Guidelines for the management of patients with decompensated cirrhosis. J Hepatol. 2018;69:406–60.
19. Seo YS, Park SY, Kim MY, et al. Lack of difference among terlipressin, somatostatin, and octreotide in the control of acute gastroesophageal variceal hemorrhage. Hepatology. 2014;60:954–63.
20. Wells M, Chande N, Adams P, et al. Meta-analysis: vasoactive medications for the management of acute variceal bleeds. Aliment Pharmacol Ther. 2012;35:1267–78.
21. Bañares R, Albillos A, Rincón D, et al. Endoscopic treatment versus endoscopic plus pharmacologic treatment for acute variceal bleeding: a meta-analysis. Hepatology. 2002;35:609–15.
22. Arroyo V, Ginès P, Gerbes AL, et al. Definition and diagnostic criteria of refractory ascites and hepatorenal syndrome in cirrhosis. International ascites club. Hepatology. 1996;23:164–76.
23. Angeli P, Garcia-Tsao G, Nadim MK, Parikh CR. News in pathophysiology, definition and classification of hepatorenal syndrome: a step beyond the International Club of Ascites (ICA) consensus document. J Hepatol. 2019;71:811–22.
24. Runyon BA, AASLD. Introduction to the revised American Association for the Study of Liver Diseases practice guideline management of adult patients with ascites due to cirrhosis 2012. Hepatology. 2013;57:1651–3.

25. Krag A, Bendtsen F, Henriksen JH, Møller S. Low cardiac output predicts development of hepatorenal syndrome and survival in patients with cirrhosis and ascites. Gut. 2010;59:105–10.
26. Fernández J, Clària J, Amorós A, et al. Effects of albumin treatment on systemic and portal hemodynamics and systemic inflammation in patients with decompensated cirrhosis. Gastroenterology. 2019;157:149–62.
27. Garcia-Martinez R, Caraceni P, Bernardi M, Gines P, Arroyo V, Jalan R. Albumin: pathophysiologic basis of its role in the treatment of cirrhosis and its complications. Hepatology. 2013;58:1836–46.
28. Piano S, Schmidt HH, Ariza X, et al. Association between grade of acute on chronic liver failure and response to terlipressin and albumin in patients with hepatorenal syndrome. Clin Gastroenterol Hepatol. 2018;16:1792–800.e3.
29. Boyer TD, Sanyal AJ, Garcia-Tsao G, et al. Predictors of response to terlipressin plus albumin in hepatorenal syndrome (HRS) type 1: relationship of serum creatinine to hemodynamics. J Hepatol. 2011;55:315–21.
30. Sanyal AJ, Boyer TD, Frederick RT, et al. Reversal of hepatorenal syndrome type 1 with terlipressin plus albumin vs. placebo plus albumin in a pooled analysis of the OT-0401 and REVERSE randomised clinical studies. Aliment Pharmacol Ther. 2017;45:1390–402.
31. Uriz J, Ginès P, Cárdenas A, et al. Terlipressin plus albumin infusion: an effective and safe therapy of hepatorenal syndrome. J Hepatol. 2000;33:43–8.
32. Ortega R, Ginès P, Uriz J, et al. Terlipressin therapy with and without albumin for patients with hepatorenal syndrome: results of a prospective, nonrandomized study. Hepatology. 2002;36:941–8.
33. Martín-Llahí M, Pépin MN, Guevara M, et al. Terlipressin and albumin vs albumin in patients with cirrhosis and hepatorenal syndrome: a randomized study. Gastroenterology. 2008;134:1352–9.
34. Rodríguez E, Elia C, Solà E, et al. Terlipressin and albumin for type-1 hepatorenal syndrome associated with sepsis. J Hepatol. 2014;60:955–61.
35. Boyer TD, Sanyal AJ, Wong F, et al. Terlipressin plus albumin is more effective than albumin alone in improving renal function in patients with cirrhosis and hepatorenal syndrome type 1. Gastroenterology. 2016;150:1579–1589.e2.
36. Mattos Â, Mattos AA, Ribeiro RA. Terlipressin versus noradrenaline in the treatment of hepatorenal syndrome: systematic review with meta-analysis and full economic evaluation. Eur J Gastroenterol Hepatol. 2016;28:345–51.
37. Fabrizi F, Dixit V, Messa P, Martin P. Terlipressin for hepatorenal syndrome: a meta-analysis of randomized trials. Int J Artif Organs. 2009;32:133–40.
38. Facciorusso A, Chandar AK, Murad MH, et al. Comparative efficacy of pharmacological strategies for management of type 1 hepatorenal syndrome: a systematic review and network meta-analysis. Lancet Gastroenterol Hepatol. 2017;2:94–102.
39. Allegretti AS, Israelsen M, Krag A, et al. Terlipressin versus placebo or no intervention for people with cirrhosis and hepatorenal syndrome. Cochrane Database Syst Rev. 2017;6:CD005162.
40. Wong F, Pappas SC, Curry MP, et al. Terlipressin plus Albumin for the Treatment of Type 1 Hepatorenal Syndrome. N Engl J Med. 2021;384:818–28.
41. Cavallin M, Kamath PS, Merli M, et al. Terlipressin plus albumin versus midodrine and octreotide plus albumin in the treatment of hepatorenal syndrome: a randomized trial. Hepatology. 2015;62:567–74.
42. Tavakkoli H, Yazdanpanah K, Mansourian M. Noradrenalin versus the combination of midodrine and octreotide in patients with hepatorenal syndrome: randomized clinical trial. Int J Prev Med. 2012;3:764–9.
43. Angeli P, Volpin R, Gerunda G, et al. Reversal of type 1 hepatorenal syndrome with the administration of midodrine and octreotide. Hepatology. 1999;29:1690–7.
44. Kalambokis G, Economou M, Fotopoulos A, et al. The effects of chronic treatment with octreotide versus octreotide plus midodrine on systemic hemodynamics and renal hemodynamics and function in nonazotemic cirrhotic patients with ascites. Am J Gastroenterol. 2005;100:879–85.

Terlipressin in Liver Cirrhosis

10

Florence Wong and Tilman Sauerbruch

Abstract

Bleeding esophageal varices and acute kidney injury are the two most dreaded complications of decompensated cirrhosis, associated with high mortality if there is treatment failure. Portal hypertension and systemic inflammation play important pathogenetic roles in their development. Vasoconstrictors are essential in the management of these conditions, as they reduce portal pressure. Terlipressin is the most widely used vasoconstrictor worldwide. It is a vasopressin analogue, a prodrug of lysine vasopressin. It binds to the V_1 receptor in splanchnic vessels, decreasing portal inflow and therefore portal pressure. Terlipressin also reduces collateral blood flow, hence dropping blood flow and pressure in varices by 20–30%. Therefore, it is recommended as one of the first choices for treatment of acute bleeding varices. Terlipressin also causes an increase in systemic circulation, thereby raising the mean arterial pressure and hence the renal perfusion pressure. It is therefore also used in the treatment of hepatorenal syndrome, together with albumin for its volume expanding and anti-inflammatory effects. Terlipressin has been shown in 4 randomized controlled trials to be superior to placebo, in 5 trials to be equally efficacious as norepinephrine, and better than midodrine and octreotide in 1 trial in the treatment of hepatorenal syndrome.

F. Wong (✉)
Department of Medicine, University of Toronto, Toronto, ON, Canada
e-mail: florence.wong@utoronto.ca

T. Sauerbruch
Department of Internal Medicine, University of Bonn, Bonn, Germany
e-mail: tilman.sauerbruch@ukbonn.de

X. Qi, Y. Yang (eds.), *Pharmacotherapy for Liver Cirrhosis and Its Complications*, https://doi.org/10.1007/978-981-19-2615-0_10

Terlipressin can produce ischemic side effects in the susceptible patients, and careful monitoring is needed to avoid severe adverse events. Acute respiratory failure was also identified as a potential side effect of terlipressin in patients with baseline respiratory compromise when treated for hepatorenal syndrome. Judicious patient selection will ensure most efficacious use of terlipressin without significant side effects.

Keywords

Cirrhosis · Varices · Ascites · Vasoconstrictors · Acute kidney injury

Abbreviations

ACLF	acute-on-chronic liver failure
AKI	acute kidney injury
AVP	arginine vasopressin
DAMPs	damage-associated molecular patterns
HRS1	type 1 hepatorenal syndrome
HRS-AKI	hepatorenal syndrome-acute kidney injury
HVPG	hepatic venous pressure gradient
INR	international normalized ratio
LVP	lysine vasopressin
MELD	Model for End-Stage Liver Disease
OR	odds ratio
PAMPs	pathogen-associated molecular patterns
RCT	randomized controlled trial
sCr	serum creatinine

10.1 Introduction

The progression of chronic liver disease evolving into cirrhosis is associated with the increasing extent of fibrosis with distortion of liver architecture. Cirrhosis is also an inflammatory condition [1]. Failure to interrupt the inflammatory stimulus in chronic liver disease results in further progressive increase in intrahepatic outflow resistance, ultimately leading to the development of portal hypertension. With the increased blood pressure in the portal vein, there is an additional change in the hemodynamics of the splanchnic vessels, which increases the blood flow into the portal vein. This dynamic component outside the diseased liver then further increases the portal pressure. The presence of portal hypertension is associated with many complications and therefore has a negative impact on patient survival: the two most common ones are the development of varices along the gastrointestinal tract, and fluid retention leading to the formation of ascites. The hemodynamic changes accompanying the progression of cirrhosis, especially in patients with ascites, can lead to splanchnic and systemic arterial vasodilation, predisposing the patient to further complications, such as renal vasoconstriction [2], ultimately putting the patient at risk for the development of renal failure.

Terlipressin is a vasoconstrictor, acting on the vasopressin type 1 receptors located at vascular smooth muscle cells [3]. The vasoconstrictive action of terlipressin on the splanchnic circulation reduces portal inflow. Terlipressin has also been shown to dilate intrahepatic vessels, thereby reducing intrahepatic resistance to portal flow [4]. Therefore, terlipressin is useful in lowering portal pressure and potentially is an effective treatment for some of the complications of portal hypertension of advanced cirrhosis. Its actions on the systemic circulation improve the systemic hemodynamics, which can counteract the deleterious effects of systemic vasodilation. This chapter discusses firstly the properties of terlipressin as a vasoconstrictor and then the application of terlipressin in the management of variceal bleeding and renal dysfunction in cirrhosis.

10.2 Terlipressin

Terlipressin (tri-glycyl-8-lysine vasopressin) is a synthetic analogue of vasopressin. It is a 12 amino acid peptide, containing the nano-peptide sequence that constitutes lysine vasopressin (LVP) (Fig. 10.1), which only differs from arginine vasopressin (AVP) by having lysine instead of arginine at position 8 (Fig. 10.1). Terlipressin is a prodrug of LVP and is converted to LVP in the circulation by having the N-triglycyl residue cleaved by endothelial peptidases. Once the glycyl residues are cleaved, terlipressin disappears from the circulation at a mean time of 24 min [5]. The active metabolite LVP is gradually released over the course of several hours [5]. The effective half-life of terlipressin, mediated mostly by LVP, is 6 hours, which is much longer than that of 20 minutes of vasopressin, and therefore preferred over AVP in the management of patients who require vasoconstriction.

10.2.1 Vasopressin Receptors

Vasopressin and its analogues act on 3 subtypes of receptors: V_1, V_2, and V_3 (also known as V_{1b}) receptors. V_2 receptors are located in the renal collecting tubules, and are responsible for the insertion of aquaporin water channels and water reabsorption

Terlipressin	H-Gly-Gly-Gly-Cys-Tyr-Phe-Gln-Asn-Cys-Pro-Lys-Gly-NH_2
Lysine-vasopressin (LVP)	Cys-Tyr-Phe-Gln-Asn-Cys-Pro-Lys-Gly-NH_2
Arginine-vasopressin (AVP)	Cys-Tyr-Phe-Gln-Asn-Cys-Pro-Arg-Gly-NH_2

Fig. 10.1 The biochemical structures of arginine vasopressin, lysine vasopressin, and terlipressin. The 6 constant amino acids are indicated by the bracket

at that site. V_2 receptors mediate the most important physiological action of vasopressin, namely water homeostasis. V_1 receptors are located on vascular smooth muscle cells of mainly the systemic, splanchnic, renal, and coronary vessels. Activation of V_1 receptors leads to release of intracellular calcium, resulting in vasoconstriction [6]. At physiological concentrations of vasopressin, vasoconstriction is not a major action of vasopressin [6]. V_1 receptors are also present on platelets where its activation leads to thrombosis, and on myocardium where it mediates a weak inotropic effect of questionable clinical significance. V_{1b} receptors are predominantly located in the anterior pituitary, and involved in the secretion of adrenocorticotropic hormone, and hence cortisol secretion.

Terlipressin is a partial agonist of the V_1 receptor, but its metabolite LVP is a full agonist of the of the V_1 receptor [7]. In addition, the binding affinity of terlipressin to V_1 receptors is about 600-fold less than that of LVP. Therefore, the therapeutic effects of terlipressin are mediated mainly through its metabolite LVP. Both terlipressin and LVP bind to the V_1 receptors 6 times stronger than to the V_2 receptors. Because the biological effects of terlipressin can be maintained over several hours, it can effectively be used as bolus injections given every 4–6 h for its clinical effects.

10.2.2 Mechanism of Action of Terlipressin

Terlipressin has differential effects on various circulations. However, the overall effects are to improve the hemodynamics in decompensated cirrhosis. In the cardiovascular system, terlipressin causes systemic vasoconstriction, thereby increasing the peripheral vascular resistance and mean arterial pressure. Terlipressin also has a direct cardiac depressive effect; it slows the heart rate and reduces cardiac output [8–10]. The stroke volume is unaffected. In the splanchnic circulation, a 2 mg bolus dose of terlipressin causes splanchnic vasoconstriction, thereby reducing portal inflow by about 30% [11] together with a reduction in portal pressure. There is redistribution of some of the splanchnic volume to other circulatory beds, such as the central blood volume [4], including the thoracic blood volume [12]. This is supported by the vasodilatory effects of terlipressin on the pulmonary vasculature [13]. However, in the liver, terlipressin reduces hepatic arterial resistance, and this results in intrahepatic vasodilatation and a fall of the hepatic venous pressure gradient (a surrogate of the portal pressure) by at least 20% [14], an effect further contributing to the reduction in portal pressure. In the renal circulation, terlipressin also causes a reduction in the resistive index, related to an improved effective arterial blood volume, leading to a reduction in the activities of the renin-angiotensin system. Thus, the renal circulation improves, partly related to better renal perfusion pressure from an increased mean arterial pressure, and partly related to reduced activities of various systemic vasoconstrictor systems.

Because of terlipressin's pharmacological effects on the portal pressure and on the renal circulation, it is mainly used in the management of complications of portal hypertension and renal failure in patients with cirrhosis. Currently, it is approved for the treatment of acute variceal bleed and type 1 hepatorenal syndrome (HRS1).

10.3 Acute Variceal bleeding

It is believed that collateral vessels develop above a portal blood pressure threshold of 10 mmHg to allow blood flow to the right side of the heart. Of these collaterals, the vessels in the distal esophagus have the greatest risk of bleeding. Here, they are partially located directly below the mucosa [15]. In patients with compensated cirrhosis without esophageal varices, such collaterals develop at a rate of 7–8% per year [16]. The risk of bleeding depends on the blood pressure in the vessels. A potential risk of bleeding exists above a threshold of 12 mmHg of the hepatic venous pressure gradient (HVPG), which is an indirect measure for portal pressure. Besides the blood pressure in the vessels, the risk of bleeding is further determined by the diameter of the vessels, degree of liver dysfunction, and etiology of liver cirrhosis; i.e., patients with alcohol use disorder and decompensated cirrhosis have a particularly high risk of bleeding [17].

Acute variceal bleeding is a life-threatening event. The 6-week mortality has fallen within the last few decades but is still in the range of 10–20% for patients reaching the hospital [17]. It could be higher if patients who die outside the hospital are included [18]. Patients typically present with hematemesis and/or melena, often preceded by abdominal discomfort. Patients with clinical suspicion of variceal bleeding, e.g., hematemesis/melena together with ascites and or jaundice, should receive immediate resuscitation with adequate venous access upon arrival at the hospital. The patient's history and physical status have to be assessed in order to define etiology of disease and to determine the hemodynamic parameters. The need for airway management must be checked early. Blood needs to be drawn for typing, crossmatch, complete blood count, coagulation parameters, liver and kidney function tests, and glucose. Volume resuscitation using plasma expanders to maintain a systolic blood pressure of 100 mmHg is required. Blood transfusion should be restrictive not surpassing a target hemoglobin of 7–9 g/dL. A too liberal transfusion policy may increase the portal and variceal blood pressure and impair hemostasis. As soon as possible and prior to endoscopy, the patient should receive an intravenous vasoactive drug (terlipressin or octreotide) and antibiotics as per various guidelines [17, 19–22]. The terlipressin-induced reduction in the blood flow in the abdominal vessels extends into the collaterals that drain to the right side of the heart. This explains why both blood flow and blood pressure in esophageal varices decrease by 20–30% with terlipressin [23, 24]. Both effects are desirable in case of hemorrhage from these vessels and explain the hemostatic effect of terlipressin in acute variceal hemorrhage.

10.3.1 Clinical Studies, Efficacy, and Side Effects

Terlipressin, when given as an intravenous injection, causes a rapid reduction of the portal pressure of approximately 20% which is sustained for 4–6 h [9]. Compared with placebo, the administration of terlipressin alone improved hemostasis rates by at least 30% and reduced mortality. Adjuvant to endoscopic therapy, terlipressin still achieved a significant improvement in hemostasis rates and a slight but significant improvement in survival [25, 26].

As an alternative to terlipressin, somatostatin or its analogue octreotide have been used as vasoactive therapy for acute variceal hemorrhage. Somatostatin or its analogues reduce blood flow and pressure in the portal vein and varices but have no or much less continuous effect on blood pressure in the portal vein or varices [27, 28]. Nevertheless, several randomized trials have found no difference between terlipressin, somatostatin, or octreotide with respect to the endpoints of hemostasis rates and mortality when one or the other drug treatment was administered [25, 29–31].

A large multicenter study from Korea conducted in 780 patients compared the 5 day use of terlipressin (2 mg bolus followed by 1 mg every 6 hours intravenously), somatostatin (250 µg bolus followed by 250 µg/h by continuous infusion), or octreotide (50 µg bolus followed by 25 µg/h by continuous infusion) as initial vasoactive therapy followed by endoscopic therapy (mostly ligation) in the context of acute variceal hemorrhage in liver cirrhosis [32]. In the three-arm study, a nearly equal hemostasis rate, defined as stable hemoglobin and stable hemodynamics without the need for transfusion, was achieved (terlipressin 86%, somatostatin 83%, and octreotide 84%). Side effects were not different except for an increased rate of hyponatremia in the terlipressin regimen related to its slight affinity to the V2 receptor in the kidney. This finding is supported by a systematic review and meta-analysis finding no difference between terlipressin/vasopressin and octreotide/somatostatin in the prevention of early rebleeding after initial hemostasis in patients with acute variceal hemorrhage [33].

A meta-analysis consisting of 30 randomized controlled trials (RCTs) and 3111 patients assessing the role of vasoactive therapy overall in the treatment of variceal hemorrhage concluded that vasoactive treatment reduces all-cause mortality and transfusion requirements as well as improving hemostasis of variceal hemorrhage [34]. In a more recent meta-analysis consisting of 20 RCTs ($n = 1609$), terlipressin was superior to no treatment in terms of control of the acute bleed (odds ratio [OR], 2.94; $p = 0.0008$) and decreasing the in-hospital mortality (OR 0.31; $p = 0.008$) [35]. When compared to octreotide, terlipressin had a lower hemostasis rate (OR, 0.37; $p = 0.007$). Terlipressin also had a higher complication rate when compared to somatostatin (OR 2.44; $P = 0.04$) [35].

A recently published network analysis of 50 RCTs on the question of vasoconstrictive therapy for variceal hemorrhage found no significant difference in mortality and hemostasis rate between the respective regimens. Vasopressin or its analogue terlipressin was associated with a lower recurrent bleeding rate and fewer blood transfusions needed, but with more adverse events [36]. The slightly higher rate of adverse events during terlipressin treatment can be explained by its stronger vasoconstrictor effect and its direct effect on water reabsorption in the renal tubule. The rate of hyponatremia with terlipressin use ranged from 37% [37] to 67% [38]. Ischemic side effects include abdominal pain, diarrhea, or cardiovascular ischemia, which have been reported in 30–50% of patients [39].

10.3.2 Treatment Guidelines from the Various Academic Societies

The positive effect of vasopressin and its analogue terlipressin, as well as of somatostatin and its analogues, in the treatment of acute variceal hemorrhage, which has been demonstrated in a large number of randomized studies as shown above, is reflected in the therapeutic guidelines of various societies. There is evidence that continuous infusion of terlipressin (around 4 mg/24 h) lowers portal pressure more permanently and effectively [40] than bolus application while also having fewer side effects and improved survival [41]. However, these findings have not yet found their way into the guidelines.

The European practice guidelines recommend vasoactive treatment as soon as possible with terlipressin, somatostatin, or octreotide when variceal hemorrhage is suspected. This should be continued for 3–5 days in cases of endoscopically proven variceal hemorrhage. For terlipressin, a dose of 2 mg/4 h is recommended within the first 48 h and 1 mg/4 h thereafter until discontinuation [21].

Terlipressin is not available in North America, and therefore the American Association for the Study of the Liver recommends the use of octreotide for the management of acute variceal bleed at a dose of 50 μg as a bolus followed by an infusion of 50 μg/h for 2–5 days. However, they also concur with other academic societies the recommendation of using terlipressin where available [22].

The Asian Pacific Association for the Study of the Liver Disease recommends that pharmacotherapy should be initiated as soon as variceal hemorrhage is suspected. Terlipressin should be the first choice for pharmacological therapy when available, and there is no contraindication. However, where terlipressin is not available, somatostatin, octreotide, and vapreotide could be used. The dose of terlipressin is 2 mg every 4 h. The duration of treatment should be 2–5 days with the longer duration of treatment reserved for the difficult-to-treat patients or those with high severity score [42].

The Baveno VII symposium [43] summarizes pharmacological treatment for acute variceal bleed as follows:

- In suspected variceal bleeding, vasoactive drugs should be started as soon as possible, before endoscopy.
- Vasoactive drugs (terlipressin, somatostatin, and octreotide) should be used in combination with endoscopic therapy and continued for up to five days.
- Hyponatremia has been described in patients under terlipressin, especially in patients with preserved liver function. Therefore, sodium levels must be monitored.

Therefore, vasoactive pharmacotherapy is an integral part of the management of acute variceal bleed in cirrhosis. Together with endoscopic therapy, it has become the standard of care for this common complication of decompensated cirrhosis.

10.4 Hepatorenal Syndrome

HRS1 is one of the most serious complications in patients with decompensated cirrhosis. It is a condition whereby there is an acute deterioration in renal function with a doubling in serum creatinine (sCr) to a level > 2.5 mg/dL (233 μmol/L) in less than 2 weeks [44] (Table 10.1). It frequently occurs in the presence of other organ failures in a syndrome known as acute-on-chronic liver failure (ACLF) [46], although it can be a stand-alone organ failure in these patients. It is a condition associated with significant morbidity and is fatal within days to weeks if left untreated. The recent recognition that a sCr level of >2.5 mg/dL represents very advanced renal failure in cachectic cirrhotic patients has led to a change in the nomenclature and definition of renal failure in cirrhosis. Renal dysfunction in cirrhosis is now renamed acute kidney injury (AKI), in line with other patient populations [45]. AKI describes renal dysfunction of all severities and uses a dynamic change in sCr to define its occurrence [45] (Table 10.2). It also includes renal dysfunction of all etiologies, be it related to renal structural damage or functional

Table 10.1 Diagnostic criteria for type 1 hepatorenal syndrome as proposed by the International Club of Ascites in 2007

• Cirrhosis and ascites
• Doubling of serum creatinine >2.5 mg/dL (232 μmol/L) in <2 weeks
• No improvement of serum creatinine (decrease of creatinine to ≤232 μmol/L) after at least 48 hours of diuretic withdrawal and volume expansion with albumin (1 g/kg body weight/day for 2 days)
• Absence of hypovolemic shock or severe infection requiring vasoactive drugs to maintain arterial pressure
• No current or recent treatment with nephrotoxic drugs
• Proteinuria <500 mg/day and no microhematuria (<50 red blood cells/mL).

Adapted from reference [45]

Table 10.2 Diagnostic criteria for acute kidney injury in cirrhosis

Parameter	Definition
Baseline	Stable sCr in <3 months If not available, a stable sCr closest to the current one If no previous sCr at all, use the admission sCr
Definition of AKI	Either ↑ in sCr by 0.3 mg/dL (26.4 μmol/L) in <48 hours Or ↑ in sCr by 50% from baseline
Staging of AKI	Stage 1: ↑ in sCr ≥ 0.3 mg/dL (26.4 μmol/L) or ↑ in sCr ≥ 1.5 to 2.0 times from baseline Stage 2: ↑ in sCr > 2.0 to 3.0 times from baseline Stage 3: ↑ in sCr > 3.0 times from baseline or sCr ≥4 mg/dL (352 μmol/L) with an acute ↑ of ≥0.3 mg/dL (26.4 μmol/L) or the initiation of renal replacement therapy

AKI acute kidney injury, *sCr* serum creatinine
Adapted from reference [47]

changes in response to hemodynamic abnormalities that are typically seen in decompensated cirrhosis. HRS1 then becomes a special subtype of AKI, and has been renamed HRS-AKI, whereby a patient shows a doubling of sCr within 2 weeks from a stable baseline sCr, without regard for the final sCr, while fulfilling all other diagnostic criteria for HRS1 [47] (Table 10.3). It is also a diagnosis of exclusion after structural renal causes and pre-renal azotemia have been excluded.

The pathophysiology of HRS-AKI is complex (Fig. 10.2). Recent data suggest that both abnormal hemodynamics and excess inflammation in advanced cirrhosis contribute to the development of HRS-AKI. Splanchnic and systemic arterial vasodilatation is the hallmark of advanced cirrhosis, related to increased shear stress on the splanchnic blood vessels as a result of obstruction to portal flow, overproduction of splanchnic vasodilators, such as nitric oxide, carbon monoxide, and

Table 10.3 Diagnostic criteria for hepatorenal syndrome-acute kidney injury as proposed by the International Club of Ascites in 2015

• Cirrhosis and ascites
• Diagnosis of AKI according to International Ascites Club criteria (Table 10.2)
• No improvement of serum creatinine (decrease of creatinine to ≤232 μmol/L) after at least 48 hours of diuretic withdrawal and volume expansion with albumin (1 g/kg body weight/day for 2 days)
• Absence of hypovolemic shock or severe infection requiring vasoactive drugs to maintain arterial pressure
• No current or recent treatment with nephrotoxic drugs
• Proteinuria <500 mg/day and no microhematuria (<50 red blood cells/mL)

Adapted from reference [47]

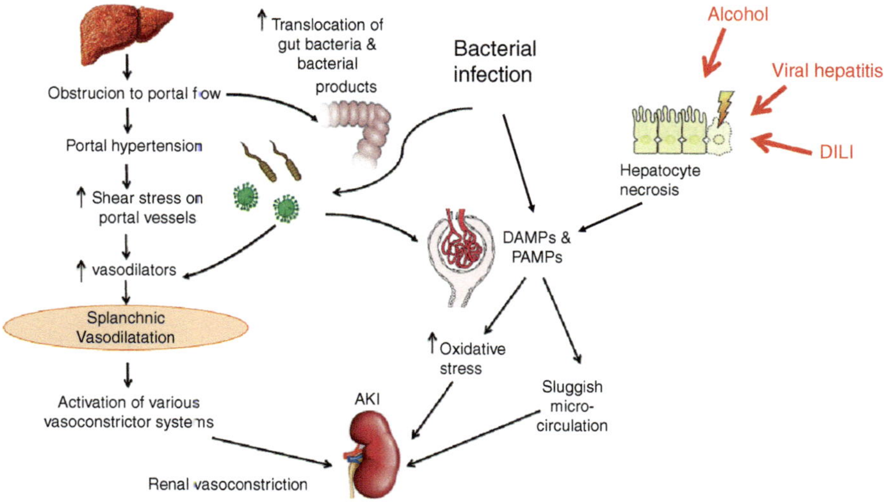

Fig. 10.2 The pathophysiology of hepatorenal syndrome indicating the abnormal hemodynamic changes on the left and inflammatory processes on the right. *AKI* acute kidney injury, *DAMPs* damage-associated molecular patterns, *DILI* drug induced liver injury, *PAMPs* pathogen-associated molecular patterns

endocannabinoids, and increased translocation of bacteria and bacterial products called pathogen-associated molecular patterns (PAMPs) from the gut lumen to the splanchnic circulation. Some of these PAMPs have vasodilatory properties and may induce an impaired response of vascular smooth muscle cells to vasoconstrictors [48, 49], adding to the vasodilatation of the splanchnic circulation [50]. A condition known as a reduction in the effective arterial blood volume then ensues, with further activation of various already activated vasoconstrictor systems as a physiological response. The renal circulation is particularly sensitive to the vasoconstrictive effects of these vasoconstrictors, and therefore is poised to undergo further vasoconstrictions [2].

The inflammation hypothesis proposes that in cirrhosis, inflammation can be induced by non-infective processes, such as ongoing hepatocyte death, be it from alcoholic hepatitis, a flare of viral hepatitis, or drug-induced liver injury, as well as from bacterial infections. The sterile inflammatory processes produce damage-associated molecular patterns (DAMPs), which, together with PAMPs, can stimulate the host's innate immune system to produce a series of chemokines and cytokines and reactive oxygen species, some of which can stimulate further production of vasodilators [51]. The reactive oxygen species can cause oxidative stress in end organs. Many of these chemokines and cytokines can directly damage renal tubules by forming microthrombi in the renal microcirculation through immunologic mechanisms and leukocyte/platelet activation [52], further compromising renal function.

10.4.1 Vasoconstrictors for HRS-AKI

Given the fact that underlying pathophysiology of HRS-AKI is one of splanchnic and systemic vasodilatation, it stands to reason that a vasoconstrictor should be used to treat the condition. Terlipressin has also been shown to ameliorate systemic inflammation by reducing bacterial translocation in decompensated cirrhosis and hence helps to reduce the extent of vasodilation in the presence of infection [53]. To date, all the RCTs that assessed the use of vasoconstrictors have used the older definition of HRS1 in their protocols. This is because HRS-AKI had not been defined either at the time of the study or the time of study design. Albumin is usually administered in conjunction with a vasoconstrictor, both for its volume expanding and anti-inflammatory properties [54]. However, albumin alone has been shown in multiple RCTs that it is ineffective in reversing HRS [55–58].

To date, terlipressin is the most commonly used vasoconstrictor for the treatment of HRS1 [59, 60]. It has been studied in many RCTs, either comparing to placebo [55–58] or to norepinephrine [61–65] or to midodrine and octreotide [66].

There are 4 RCTs comparing terlipressin versus placebo, both with albumin for the treatment of HRS, one from Spain and 3 from North America, totaling 654 patients, with 375 patients randomized to receive terlipressin and the remaining 279 patients receiving placebo. Terlipressin was given as bolus dosing of 0.5–2 mg every 4–6 h until either there has been a sustained reduction of sCr to <1.5 mg/dL

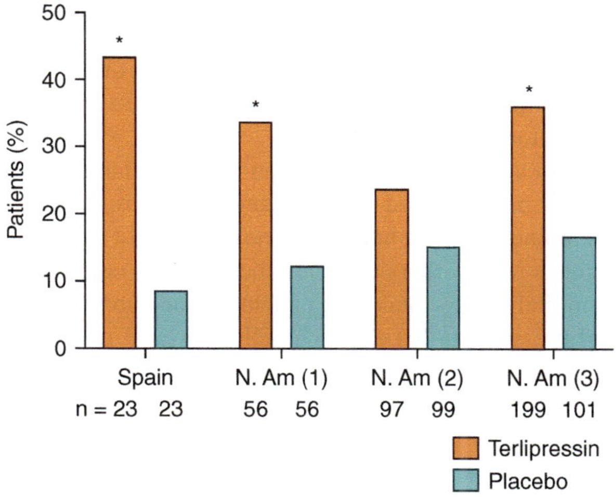

Fig. 10.3 Percentage of patients with reversal of hepatorenal syndrome in the 4 randomized controlled trials comparing terlipressin versus placebo, both with albumin. *N. Am* North America; * $p < 0.05$. Reprinted from Wong F. Latest treatment of acute kidney injury in cirrhosis. Curr Treat Options Gastro 2020;18:281–294 with permission

(133 μmol/L) or to a maximum of 14 days. The HRS reversal rate was 36–44% of patients, with 3 of the 4 studies showing a significant difference between the terlipressin and the placebo arms (Fig. 10.3). The difference in the response rates between the studies was attributed to the variations in the populations of patients studied, dosing regimens, or duration of treatment. Approximately 25% of patients included in the Spanish study had chronic or type 2 HRS. There was no difference in terms of the overall or transplant-free survival rate between the terlipressin and the placebo arms up to 90 days after completion of treatment. However, in patients who responded with reversal of HRS, there was a significant improvement in survival [67]. In fact, even a partial response with a > 20% reduction in sCr was associated with an improved survival [68]. The predictors of response to terlipressin include a pretreatment bilirubin of <10 mg/dL (170 μmol/L), a baseline sCr of <5 mg/dL (440 μmol/L) [69, 70], a lower stage of ACLF [71], and a sustained increase in the mean arterial pressure by 5–10 mmHg with treatment [72]. Patients with certain inflammatory conditions, such as alcoholic hepatitis or sepsis, seem to respond better to terlipressin and those with systemic inflammatory response syndrome [53, 58].

Terlipressin, by virtue of its mode of action, is associated with ischemic side effects. However, the side effects could be mitigated by using a continuous infusion rather than using bolus injections [40, 41, 65]. In the latest RCT, the CONFIRM study, one unexpected adverse event emerged. Significantly more patients in the terlipressin arm developed respiratory failure [58] when compared to the placebo arm. This was mostly observed in patients who had grade 3 ACLF as defined by the EASL-Chronic Liver Failure Consortium, 30% in those who received terlipressin versus none who received placebo [73]. This is felt to be related to the cardio-suppressive effects of terlipressin, together with the volume expansion brought about by albumin use in the treatment of these patients. Predictors of respiratory failure include several pretreatment parameters: a high international normalized ratio (INR), a high mean arterial blood pressure, and a low oxygen saturation of

<90% as measured on a pulse oximeter [73]. Therefore, it is recommended that in patients who have grade 3 ACLF that includes renal failure, careful consideration needs to be given before starting the patient on terlipressin. If a decision is made to use terlipressin, patients need to be monitored very carefully for the development of respiratory failure.

Given the fact that terlipressin is not available in North America, various investigators have studied the efficacy of other vasoconstrictors versus terlipressin. Norepinephrine (or noradrenaline) is the most studied comparator. These studies are rather small, with 4 out of 5 of these studies originating from India, and the last one from Italy. They totaled 96 patients in the norepinephrine arm and 99 patients in the terlipressin arm [61–65]. The HRS reversal rates ranged between 39% and 70%, with norepinephrine being equally efficacious as terlipressin [74–76]. In the context of ACLF, as defined by the Asian Pacific Association for the Study of the Liver ACLF Research Consortium, terlipressin was superior to norepinephrine in reversing HRS, observed as early as day 4, and continued to be so until end of treatment on day 14. However, their definition of ACLF was an INR of >1.5 and a serum bilirubin of >5 mg/dL (>85 μmol/L) together with the appearance of ascites with or without hepatic encephalopathy within 4 weeks. As this definition of ACLF suggests milder liver dysfunction, terlipressin may be more efficacious at an earlier stage of liver dysfunction. Terlipressin is definitely more efficacious than the combination of midodrine and octreotide for the treatment of HRS1 [66]. In fact, this particular trial was terminated after an interim analysis when the superiority of terlipressin over midodrine and octreotide was clearly demonstrated.

As all patients with HRS-AKI should be assessed for liver transplant, there is some controversy as to whether these patients should be treated with vasoconstrictors, as this lowers the Model for End-Stage Liver Disease (MELD) score, and therefore will lower their priority for liver transplantation. There is support for the pretreatment MELD score to be used for the prioritization of liver transplant [77]. Furthermore, the use of vasoconstrictors pre-liver transplant reduces the likelihood for pre- and post-transplant dialysis requirement [78] and is associated with improved survival post-liver transplant [79]. Therefore, vasoconstrictors should not be withheld from eligible patients because of concerns for delaying the definitive treatment for liver transplant.

10.4.2 Treatment Guidelines from Various Academic Societies

Vasoconstrictors are the mainstay of treatment for HRS1 in cirrhosis. However, with different availability issues around the world, various academic societies have laid down guidelines for the treatment of HRS1 based on the abovementioned studies.

The European Association for the Study of the Liver [21] recommends that:

- Terlipressin plus albumin should be considered as the first-line therapeutic option for the treatment of HRS-AKI.

- Terlipressin can be used by intravenous boluses at the initial dose of 1 mg every 4–6 h. However, a continuous intravenous infusion at an initial dose of 2 mg/day is able to reduce the total daily dose and, thus, potentially the incidence of its adverse effects.
- In case of non-response (decrease in sCr by less than 25% from the peak value) after two days, the dose of terlipressin should be increased in a stepwise manner to a maximum of 12 mg/day.
- Norepinephrine can be used as an alternative to terlipressin, but information is limited.

The American Association for the Study of the Liver Diseases has not been as clear cut as the European Association in recommending terlipressin as first-line treatment for HRS1 because of its unavailability commercially. It has been suggested that vasoconstrictors, either terlipressin or norepinephrine, in combination with albumin are effective in improving kidney function in patients with cirrhosis and HRS1 [80].

The Asian Pacific Association for the Study of the Liver has no formal guidelines for the treatment of HRS.

10.5 Conclusion

It has been widely accepted that terlipressin is the first-line treatment for acute variceal bleed and HRS1 in decompensated cirrhosis. Thus, if there is concomitant impaired renal function in esophageal variceal hemorrhage, terlipressin should be preferred over other vasoconstrictors if possible. Nevertheless, judicious patient selection is crucial to avoid the complications of terlipressin, especially in elderly patients who may have some underlying ischemic conditions, or the very ill patient with cirrhosis and multi-organ failure. Although we now have some predictors of response to terlipressin for HRS, the development of biomarkers that can more precisely predict response to terlipressin in HRS will improve its usefulness in this condition. There is some evidence that terlipressin may also be useful in the management in other complications of cirrhosis such as ascites, hepatic hydrothorax, paracentesis-induced circulatory dysfunction, or septic shock [81], the future direction for terlipressin will depend on the results of further well-designed RCTs to confirm these indications.

References

1. Arroyo V, Angeli P, Moreau R, Jalan R, Clària J, Trebicka J, Fernández J, et al. The systemic inflammation hypothesis: towards a new paradigm of acute decompensation and multiorgan failure in cirrhosis. J Hepatol. 2021;74:670–85.
2. Møller S, Bendtsen F. The pathophysiology of arterial vasodilatation and hyperdynamic circulation in cirrhosis. Liver Int. 2018;38:570–80.

3. Pesaturo AB, Jennings HR, Voils SA. Terlipressin: vasopressin analog and novel drug for septic shock. Ann Pharmacother. 2006;40:2170–7.
4. Kiszka-Kanewitz M, Henricksen JH, Hansen EF, Møller S, Bendtsen F. Effect of terlipressin on blood volume distribution in patients with cirrhosis. Scand J Gastroenterol. 2004;39:486–92.
5. Kam PCA, Williams S, Yoong FFY. Vasopressin and terlipressin: pharmacology and its clinical relevance. Anaesthesia. 2004;59:993–1001.
6. Holmes CL, Landry DW, Granton JT. Science review: vasopressin and the cardiovascular system part 1 – receptor physiology. Crit Care. 2003;7:427–34.
7. Jamil K, Pappas SC, Devarakonda KR. In vitro binding and receptor-mediated activity of terlipressin at vasopressin receptors V_1 and V_2. J Exp Pharmacol. 2017;10:1–7.
8. Israelsen M, Dahl EK, Madsen BS, Wiese S, Bendtsen F, Møller S, Fialla AD, et al. Dobutamine reverses the cardio-suppressive effects of terlipressin without improving renal function in cirrhosis and ascites: a randomized controlled trial. Am J Physiol Gastrointest Liver Physiol. 2020;318:G313–21.
9. Narahara Y, Kanazawa H, Taki Y, Kimura Y, Atsukawa M, Katakura T, Kidokoro H, et al. Effects of terlipressin on systemic, hepatic and renal hemodynamics in patients with cirrhosis. J Gastroenterol Hepatol. 2009;24:1791–7.
10. Krag A, Bendtsen F, Mortensen C, Henriksen JH, Møller S. Effects of a single terlipressin administration on cardiac function and perfusion in cirrhosis. Eur J Gastroenterol Hepatol. 2010;22:1085–92.
11. Møller S, Hansen EF, Becker U, Brinch K, Henriksen JH, Bendtsen F. Central and systemic haemodynamic effects of terlipressin in portal hypertensive patients. Liver. 2000;20:51–9.
12. Kalambokis GN, Pappas K, Tsianos EV. Differential effects of terlipressin on pulmonary and systemic hemodynamics in patients with cirrhosis and pulmonary hypertension: an echo study. Angiology. 2012;63:199–205.
13. Schultz J, Andersen A, Lyhne MD, Arcanjo DDR, Kjaergaard B, Simonsen U, Nielsen-Kudsk JE. Terlipressin increases systemic and lowers pulmonary arterial pressure in experimental acute pulmonary embolism. Crit Care Med. 2020;48:e308–15.
14. Villanueva C, Planella M, Aracil C, López-Balaguer JM, González B, Miñana J, Balanzó J. Hemodynamic effects of terlipressin and high somatostatin dose during acute variceal bleeding in non-responders to the usual somatostatin dose. Am J Gastroenterol. 2005;100:624–30.
15. Sauerbruch T, Wong F. Treatment of oesophageal varices in liver cirrhosis. Digestion. 2019;99:261–6.
16. D'Amico G, Morabito A, D'Amico M, Pasta L, Malizia G, Rebora P, Valsecchi MG. Clinical states of cirrhosis and competing risks. J Hepatol. 2018;68:563–76.
17. Sauerbruch T. Portal Hypertension and esophageal varices. In: Kuipers EJ, editor. Encyclopedia of gastroenterology, vol. 4. 2nd ed. Oxford: Academic Press; 2020. p. 237–46.
18. Schepke M, Kleber G, Nürnberg D, Willert J, Koch L, Veltzke-Schlieker W, Hellerbrand C, et al., German Study Group for the Primary Prophylaxis of Variceal Bleeding. Ligation versus propranolol for the primary prophylaxis of variceal bleeding in cirrhosis. Hepatology 2004;40:65–72.
19. Bosch J, Sauerbruch T. Esophageal varices: Stage-dependent treatment algorithm. J Hepatol. 2016;64:746–8.
20. Tripathi D, Stanley AJ, Hayes PC, Patch D, Millson C, Mehrzad H, Austin A, et al. Clinical Services and Standards Committee of the British Society of Gastroenterology. U.K. guidelines on the management of variceal haemorrhage in cirrhotic patients. Gut. 2015;64:1680–704.
21. European Association for the Study of the Liver. EASL Clinical Practice Guidelines for the management of patients with decompensated cirrhosis. J Hepatol. 2018;69:406–60.
22. Garcia-Tsao G, Abraldes JG, Berzigotti A, Bosch J. Portal hypertensive bleeding in cirrhosis: Risk stratification, diagnosis, and management: 2016 practice guidance by the American Association for the study of liver diseases. Hepatology. 2017;65:310–35.

23. Nevens F, Van Steenbergen W, Yap SH, Fevery J. Assessment of variceal pressure by continuous non-invasive endoscopic registration: a placebo-controlled evaluation of the effect of terlipressin and octreotide. Gut. 1996;38:129–34.
24. Cestari R, Braga M, Missale G, Ravelli P, Burroughs AK. Haemodynamic effect of triglycyl-lysine-vasopressin (glypressin) on intravascular oesophageal variceal pressure in patients with cirrhosis. A randomized placebo-controlled trial. J Hepatol. 1990;10:205–10.
25. Krag A, Borup T, Møller S, Bendtsen F. Efficacy and safety of terlipressin in cirrhotic patients with variceal bleeding or hepatorenal syndrome. Adv Ther. 2008;25:1105–40.
26. Ioannou G, Doust J, Rockey DC. Terlipressin for acute esophageal variceal hemorrhage. Cochrane Database Syst Rev. 2003;1:CD002147.
27. Abraldes JG, Bosch J. Somatostatin and analogues in portal hypertension. Hepatology. 2002;35:1305–12.
28. Kleber G, Sauerbruch T, Fischer G, Paumgartner G. Somatostatin does not reduce oesophageal variceal pressure in liver cirrhotics. Gut. 1988;29:153–6.
29. Walker S, Kreichgauer HP, Bode JC. Terlipressin vs. somatostatin in bleeding esophageal varices: a controlled, double-blind study. Hepatology. 1992;15:1023–30.
30. Feu F, Ruiz del Arbol L, Bañares R, Planas R, Bosch J. Double-blind randomised controlled trial comparing terlipressin and somatostatin for acute variceal hemorrhage variceal bleeding study group. Gastroenterology. 1996;111:1291–9.
31. Abid S, Jafri W, Hamid S, Salih M, Azam Z, Mumtaz K, Shah HA, et al. Terlipressin vs. octreotide in bleeding esophageal varices as an adjuvant therapy with endoscopic band ligation: a randomised double-blind placebo-controlled trial. Am J Gastroenterol. 2009;104:617–23.
32. Seo YS, Park SY, Kim MY, Kim JH, Park JY, Yim HJ, Jang BK, et al. Lack of difference among terlipressin, somatostatin, and octreotide in the control of acute gastroesophageal variceal hemorrhage. Hepatology. 2014;60:954–63.
33. Wang C, Han J, Xiao L, Jin CE, Li DJ, Yang Z. Efficacy of vasopressin/terlipressin and somatostatin/octreotide for the prevention of early variceal rebleeding after the initial control of bleeding: a systematic review and meta-analysis. Hepatol Int. 2015;9:120–9.
34. Wells M, Chande N, Adams P, Beaton M, Levstik M, Boyce E, Mrkobrada M. Meta-analysis: vasoactive medications for the management of acute variceal bleeds. Aliment Pharmacol Ther. 2012;35:1267–78.
35. Zhou X, Tripathi D, Song T, Shao LH, Han B, Zhu J, Han D, et al. Terlipressin for the treatment of acute variceal bleeding: a systematic review and meta-analysis of randomized controlled trials. Medicine. 2018;97:e13437.
36. Sridharan K, Sivaramakrishnan G. Vasoactive agents for the management of variceal bleeding: a mixed treatment comparison network meta-analysis and trial sequential analysis of randomized clinical trials. Drug Res (Stuttg). 2019;69:487–95.
37. Xu X, Lin S, Yang Y, Chen Y, Liu B, Li B, Wu Y, et al. Development of hyponatremia after terlipressin in cirrhotic patients with acute gastrointestinal bleeding: a retrospective multicenter observational study. Expert Opin Drug Saf. 2020;19:641–7.
38. Solà E, Lens S, Guevara M, Martín-Llahí M, Fagundes C, Pereira G, Pavesi M, et al. Hyponatremia in patients treated with terlipressin for severe gastrointestinal bleeding due to portal hypertension. Hepatology. 2010;52:1783–90.
39. Bunchorntavakul C, Reddy KR. Pharmacologic management of portal hypertension. Clin Liver Dis. 2019;23:713–36.
40. Ding C, Wu X, Fan X, He C, Li J. Hemodynamic effects of continuous versus bolus infusion of terlipressin for portal hypertension: a randomized comparison. J Gastroenterol Hepatol. 2013;28:1242–6.
41. Jha SK, Mishra M, Jha A, Dayal VM. Comparison of continuous versus intermittent infusions of terlipressin for the control of acute variceal bleeding in patients with portal hypertension: An open label randomized controlled trial. Indian J Gastroenterol. 2018;37:313–20.

42. Sarin SK, Kumar A, Angus PW, Baijal SS, Baik SK, Bayraktar Y, Chawla YK, et al. Asian Pacific Association for the Study of the Liver (APASL) Working Party on Portal Hypertension. Diagnosis and management of acute variceal bleeding: Asian Pacific Association for Study of the Liver recommendations. Hepatol Int. 2011;5:607–24.
43. de Franchis R, Bosch J, Garcia-Tsao G, Reiberger T, Ripoll C, on behalf of the Baveno VII Faculty. Baveno VII: Renewing consensus in portal hypertension. J Hepatol. 2022;76:959–74.
44. Salerno F, Gerbes A, Ginès P, Wong F, Arroyo V. Diagnosis, prevention and treatment of hepatorenal syndrome in cirrhosis. Gut. 2007;56:1310–8.
45. Wong F, Nadim MK, Kellum JA, Salerno F, Bellomo R, Gerbes A, Angeli P, et al. Working Party proposal for a revised classification system of renal dysfunction in patients with cirrhosis. Gut. 2011;60:702–9.
46. Zaccherini G, Weiss E, Moreau R. Acute-on-chronic liver failure: definitions, pathophysiology and principles of treatment. JHEP Rep. 2020;3:100176.
47. Angeli P, Gines P, Wong F, Bernardi M, Boyer TD, Gerbes A, Moreau R, et al. Diagnosis and management of acute kidney injury in patients with cirrhosis: revised consensus recommendations of the International Club of Ascites. Gut. 2015;64:531–17.
48. Schepke M, Heller J, Paschke S, Thomas J, Wolff M, Neef M, Malago M, et al. Contractile hypo-responsiveness of hepatic arteries in humans with cirrhosis: evidence for a receptor-specific mechanism. Hepatology. 2001;34:884–8.
49. Sauerbruch T, Hennenberg M, Trebicka J, Beuers U. Bile acids, liver cirrhosis, and extrahepatic vascular dysfunction. Front Physiol. 2021;12:718783.
50. Di Pascoli M, Sacerdoti D, Pontisso P, Angeli P, Bolognesi M. Molecular mechanisms leading to splanchnic vasodilation in liver cirrhosis. J Vasc Res. 2017;54:92–9.
51. Bernardi M, Moreau R, Angeli P, Schnabl B, Arroyo V. Mechanisms of decompensation and organ failure in cirrhosis: from peripheral arterial vasodilation to systemic inflammation hypothesis. J Hepatol. 2015;63:1272–84.
52. Gomez H, Ince C, De Backer D, Pickkers P, Payen D, Hotchkiss J, Kellum JA. A unified theory of sepsis-induced acute kidney injury: inflammation, microcirculatory dysfunction, bioenergetics, and the tubular cell adaptation to injury. Shock. 2014;41:3–11.
53. Wong F, Pappas SC, Boyer TD, Sanyal AJ, Bajaj JS, Escalante S, Jamil K, et al. Terlipressin improves renal function and reverses hepatorenal syndrome in patients with systemic inflammatory response syndrome. Clin Gastroenterol Hepatol. 2017;15:266-72.e1.
54. Bernardi M, Angeli P, Claria J, Moreau R, Gines P, Jalan R, Caraceni P, et al. Albumin in decompensated cirrhosis: new concepts and perspectives. Gut. 2020;69:1127–38.
55. Martín-Llahí M, Pépin MN, Guevara M, Díaz F, Torre A, Monescillo A, Soriano G, et al. Terlipressin and albumin vs albumin in patients with cirrhosis and hepatorenal syndrome: a randomized study. Gastroenterology. 2008;134:1352–9.
56. Sanyal AJ, Boyer T, Garcia-Tsao G, Regenstein F, Rossaro L, Appenrodt B, Blei A, et al. A randomized, prospective, double-blind, placebo-controlled trial of terlipressin for type 1 hepatorenal syndrome. Gastroenterology. 2008;134:1360–8.
57. Boyer TD, Sanyal AJ, Wong F, Frederick RT, Lake JR, O'Leary JG, Ganger D, et al. Terlipressin plus albumin is more effective than albumin alone in improving renal function in patients with cirrhosis and hepatorenal syndrome type 1. Gastroenterology. 2016;150:1579–89. e2
58. Wong F, Pappas SC, Curry MP, Reddy KR, Rubin RA, Porayko MK, Gonzalez SA, et al. Terlipressin plus albumin for the treatment of type 1 hepatorenal syndrome. N Engl J Med. 2021;384:818–28.
59. Facciorusso A, Chandar AK, Murad MH, Prokop LJ, Muscatiello N, Kamath PS, et al. Comparative efficacy of pharmacological strategies for management of type 1 hepatorenal syndrome: a systematic review and network meta-analysis. Lancet Gastroenterol Hepatol. 2017;2:94–102.
60. Belcher JM, Parada XV, Simonetto DA, Juncos LA, Karakala N, Wadei HM, Sharma P, et al. HRS-HARMONY Study Investigators. Terlipressin and the treatment of hepatorenal syndrome: how the CONFIRM trial moves the story forward. Am J Kidney Dis. 2022;79:737–45.

61. Sharma P, Kumar A, Shrama BC, Sarin SK. An open label, pilot, randomized controlled trial of noradrenaline versus terlipressin in the treatment of type 1 hepatorenal syndrome and predictors of response. Am J Gastroenterol. 2008;103:1689–97.
62. Alessandria C, Ottobrelli A, Debernardi-Venon W, Todros L, Cerenzia MT, Martini S, Falzola F, et al. Noradrenalin vs terlipressin in patients with hepatorenal syndrome: a prospective, randomized, unblinded, pilot study. J Hepatol. 2007;47:499–505.
63. Singh V, Ghosh S, Singh B, Kumar P, Sharma N, Bhalla A, Sharma AK, et al. Noradrenaline vs. terlipressin in the treatment of hepatorenal syndrome: a randomized study. J Hepatol. 2012;56:1293–8.
64. Goyal O, Sidhu SS, Sehgal N, Puri S. Noradrenaline is as effective as terlipressin in hepatorenal syndrome type 1: A prospective, randomized trial. J Assoc Physicians India. 2016;64:30–5.
65. Saif RU, Dar HA, Sofi SM, Andrabi MS, Javid G, Zargar SA. Noradrenaline versus terlipressin in the management of type 1 hepatorenal syndrome: a randomized controlled study. Indian J Gastroenterol. 2018;37:424–9.
66. Cavallin M, Kamath PS, Merli M, Fasolato S, Toniutto P, Salerno F, Bernardi M, et al. Terlipressin plus albumin versus midodrine and octreotide plus albumin in the treatment of hepatorenal syndrome: a randomized trial. Hepatology. 2015;62:567–74.
67. Cavallin M, Piano S, Romano A, Fasolato S, Frigo AC, Benetti G, Gola E, et al. Terlipressin given by continuous intravenous infusion versus intravenous boluses in the treatment of hepatorenal syndrome: a randomized controlled study. Hepatology. 2016;63:983–92.
68. Boyer TD, Wong F, Sanyal AJ, Pappas SC, Jamil K. Time for a new, more inclusive endpoint for treatment of type 1 hepatorenal syndrome (HRS-1)? Small changes in serum creatinine of >20% are equivalent to HRS reversal in predicting survival and need for renal replacement therapy during treatment of HRS-1 with terlipressin and albumin. [Abstract]. Hepatology. 2016;64:1030A–1031 1A.
69. Boyer TD, Sanyal AJ, Garcia-Tsao G, Blei A, Carl D, Bexon AS, Teuber P, et al. Predictors of response to terlipressin plus albumin in hepatorenal syndrome (HRS) type 1: relationship of serum creatinine to hemodynamics. J Hepatol. 2011;55:315–21.
70. Nazar A, Pereira GH, Guevara M, Martín-Llahi M, Pepin MN, Marinelli M, Solá E, et al. Predictors of response to therapy with terlipressin and albumin in patients with cirrhosis and type 1 hepatorenal syndrome. Hepatology. 2010;51:219–26.
71. Piano S, Schmidt HH, Ariza X, Amoros A, Romano A, Hüsing-Kabar A, Solà E, et al. Association between grade of acute on chronic liver failure and response to terlipressin and albumin in patients with hepatorenal syndrome. Clin Gastroenterol Hepatol. 2018;16:1792–800.e3.
72. Sanyal AJ, Boyer TD, Frederick RT, Wong F, Rossaro L, Araya V, Vargas HE, et al. Reversal of hepatorenal syndrome type 1 with terlipressin plus albumin vs. placebo plus albumin in a pooled analysis of the OT-0401 and REVERSE randomised clinical studies. Aliment Pharmacol Ther. 2017;45:1390–402.
73. Wong F, Pappas SC, Reddy KR, Vargas HE, Curry M, Jamil K, Sanyal A. Increased incidence of respiratory failure with terlipressin use in patients with hepatorenal syndrome type 1 and severe acute-on-chronic liver failure. [Abstract]. J Hepatol. 2021;75:S326.
74. Nassar Junior AP, Farias AQ, D'Albuquerque LA, Carillho FJ, Malbouisson LM. Terlipressin versus norepinephrine in the treatment of hepatorenal syndrome: a systematic review and meta-analysis. PLoS One. 2014;9:e107466.
75. Gilford FJ, Morling JR, Fallowfield JA. Systematic review with meta-analysis: vasoactive drugs for the treatment of hepatorenal syndrome type 1. Aliment Pharmacol Ther. 2017;45:593–603.
76. Best LM, Freeman SC, Sutton AJ, Cooper NJ, Tng EL, Csenar M, Hawkins N, et al. Treatment for hepatorenal syndrome in people with decompensated liver cirrhosis: a network meta-analysis. Cochrane Database Syst Rev. 2019;9:CD013103.
77. Angeli P, Gines P. Hepatorenal syndrome, MELD score and liver transplantation: an evolving issue with relevant implications for clinical practice. J Hepatol. 2012;57:1135–40.
78. Velez JCQ, Befeler A, Kurtz I, Gallegos-Orozco J, Vargas HE, Vierling JM, Pappas C, et al. Terlipressin improves renal replacement therapy-free survival inhepatorenal syndrome type 1. [Abstract]. J Hepatol. 2021;75:S327.

79. Piano S, Gambino C, Vettore E, Calvino V, Tonon M, Boccagni P, Gringeri E, et al. Response to terlipressin and albumin is associated with improved liver transplant outcomes in patients with hepatorenal syndrome. Hepatology. 2021;73:1909–19.
80. Biggins SW, Angeli P, Garcia-Tsao G, Ginès P, Ling SC, Nadim MK, Wong F, et al. Diagnosis, evaluation, and management of ascites, spontaneous bacterial peritonitis and hepatorenal syndrome: 2021 Practice Guidance by the American Association for the Study of Liver Diseases. Hepatology, 2021;74:1014–48.
81. Papaluca T, Gow P. Terlipressin: Current and emerging indications in chronic liver disease. J Gastroenterol Hepatol. 2018;33:591–8.

Diuretics in Cirrhotic Patients with Ascites

11

Ran Wang, Lu Chai, and Xiaozhong Guo

Abstract

Diuretics are widely used medications for the treatment of ascites in patients with cirrhosis. There are some different types of diuretics, such as aldosterone antagonists (i.e., spironolactone), loop diuretics (i.e., furosemide), and vasopressin V2 receptor antagonists (i.e., tolvaptan). Spironolactone is recommended for patients with first on-set of ascites or those with mild-moderate ascites. Furosemide is recommended for patients with moderate to severe ascites or those with a poor response to spironolactone alone. Tolvaptan is recommended for patients with poor response to conventional diuretics and those with hyponatremia. Diuretic regimens should be further explored to reach a better efficacy of diuretics and avoid adverse events in patients with cirrhosis. In the current chapter, we will briefly review commonly used diuretics for the treatment of ascites in cirrhotic patients.

Keywords

Diuretics · Liver cirrhosis · Ascites · Spironolactone · Tolvaptan

R. Wang (✉) · X. Guo
Department of Gastroenterology, General Hospital of Northern Theater Command, Shenyang, China

L. Chai
Department of Gastroenterology, General Hospital of Northern Theater Command, Shenyang, China

Postgraduate College, Shenyang Pharmaceutical University, Shenyang, China

X. Qi, Y. Yang (eds.), *Pharmacotherapy for Liver Cirrhosis and Its Complications*, https://doi.org/10.1007/978-981-19-2615-0_11

11.1 Introduction

Diuretics are defined as medications that can increase the flow of urine and the excretion of water from bodies. There are some different types of diuretics, mainly including aldosterone antagonists, loop diuretics, and vasopressin V2 receptor antagonists. Diuretics are commonly used for patients with edematous and some non-edematous diseases, including heart failure, hypertension, chronic kidney disease, and liver cirrhosis [1].

Liver cirrhosis is an end stage of multiple chronic liver diseases. Ascites is the most common complication of liver cirrhosis, and approximately 20% of patients with cirrhosis have ascites at their first presentations [2]. Ascites and its complications, including refractory ascites, spontaneous bacterial peritonitis, hepatorenal syndrome, and hernia, significantly worsen the patients' outcomes and reduce the quality of life [3, 4]. The 1- and 2-year mortality of patients with ascites is about 40% and 50%, respectively [5].

The pathogenesis of hepatic ascites is complex and still not completely understood. Portal hypertension is considered as the primary mechanism of ascites. In patients with cirrhosis, portal pressure is increased, leading to arterial splanchnic vasodilation and reduction of effective blood volume, which may activate the sympathetic nervous system and the renin–angiotensin system, resulting in water and sodium renal retention [5]. Furthermore, in patients with cirrhosis, impaired liver synthetic function leads to hypoproteinemia and generalized edema.

The management of ascites mainly includes bedrest, dietary salt restriction, diuretics, large-volume paracentesis, transjugular intrahepatic portosystemic shunting, and liver transplantation [5]. While paracentesis is the first choice treatment of severe ascites, diuretics are still the most important therapy for patients with ascites. In the current chapter, we will briefly review commonly used diuretics for the treatment of ascites in cirrhotic patients.

11.2 Diuretics

11.2.1 Aldosterone Antagonists

11.2.1.1 Spironolactone

Spironolactone, an aldosterone antagonist, is the most commonly used diuretic for patients with cirrhosis and ascites. Spironolactone competitively binds the receptors at the aldosterone-dependent sodium-potassium exchange site in the distal convoluted renal tubule, resulting in a potassium-sparing diuretic effect. Spironolactone is absorbed about 90% after oral administration, and can reach its peak plasma concentration in 2.6–3 h, and its activity persists for at least 24 h [6].

Spironolactone has been used for the treatment of ascites in patients with cirrhosis for a long time. In 1983, in a classical and well-recognized randomized comparative study by Pérez-Ayuso et al., a total of 40 nonazotemic cirrhotic patients were included and randomly assigned to spironolactone group ($n = 19$) and furosemide group ($n = 21$) [7]. In the spironolactone group, 94.73% (18/19) of patients responded to spironolactone, while only 52.38% (11/21) responded to furosemide. Spironolactone was more effective than furosemide.

Spironolactone monotherapy has been recommended as the first-line therapy for cirrhotic patients with moderate ascites according to several guidelines (Table 11.1) [5, 8–11]. In the latest Japanese Society of Hepatology guideline for liver cirrhosis, spironolactone is considered as the first-line therapy [3]. Consistently, in the guidelines on the management of ascites in cirrhosis by the British Society of Gastroenterology in collaboration with the British Association for the Study of the Liver, spironolactone monotherapy (starting dose 100 mg, increased to 400 mg) is recommended for patients with the first presentation of moderate ascites [9].

Common adverse events of spironolactone include electrolyte abnormalities, gynecomastia, renal failure, hepatic encephalopathy, nausea, vomiting, headache, rashes, and a decreased desire for sex. In particular, hyperkalemia is the most common complication of spironolactone in patients with ascites. Spironolactone can certainly lead to hyperkalemia by its anti-aldosterone mechanism. Further than that, a study found that the incidence of hyperkalemia may be associated with worsened liver function [12].

11.2.1.2 Eplerenone

Eplerenone, a highly selective aldosterone antagonist and potassium-sparing diuretic, is mostly used for the treatment of hypertension. Eplerenone can reach its peak plasma concentrations of approximately 1.5 h following oral administration. Eplerenone has little affinity to the androgen, progesterone, and glucocorticoid receptors. Compared with other aldosterone antagonist diuretics, eplerenone has a lower risk of gynecomastia and vaginal bleeding [13].

Eplerenone is considered as effective as spironolactone in cirrhotic patients with ascites [14]. In a randomized controlled trial study by Sehgal et al. [14], a total of 105 cirrhotic patients with ascites were included and randomly assigned to the spironolactone 100 mg group, eplerenone 100 mg group, and eplerenone 50 mg group. Patients who received eplerenone 50 mg/d had a significantly lower weight reduction compared with patients who received spironolactone 100 mg/d and eplerenone 100 mg/d ($p < 0.001$ and $p < 0.001$, respectively). There was no significant difference regarding mean weight reduction between patients who received spironolactone 100 mg/d and eplerenone 100 mg/d ($p = 0.964$). This study found that eplerenone and spironolactone are equally effective for the management of ascites in cirrhotic patients, but spironolactone has a better cost-effectiveness than eplerenone. Only the Sehgal's study investigates the efficacy of eplerenone in patients with cirrhosis, and further high-quality studies are required in this field, especially for patients with liver cirrhosis.

Table 11.1 Recommendations of different guidelines for the treatment of ascites

	Italian Association for the Study of the liver	Japanese Society of Gastroenterology and the Japan Society of Hepatology	British Society of Gastroenterology in collaboration with British Association for the Study of the Liver	Chinese guideline	Korean Association for the Study of the Liver	European Association for the Study of the Liver
Year of publication	**2021**	**2021**	**2021**	**2019**	**2018**	**2018**
Journal	**Digestive and Liver Disease**	**Journal of Gastroenterology**	**GUT**	**Hepatology International**	**Clinical and Molecular Hepatology**	**Journal of Hepatology**
Recommendations	***First on-set of ascites:*** Sodium restriction (4.5–7 g/d salt); anti-mineralocorticoid alone	***Grade 1 ascites:*** Sodium restriction (5–7 g/d salt); in some cases, diuretic	Sodium restriction (5–7 g/d salt)	***Grade 1 ascites:*** Sodium restriction (4–6 g/d salt); spironolactone alone (40–80 mg/d)	Sodium restriction (<5 g/d salt)	***Moderate, uncomplicated ascites:*** Sodium restriction (4.6–6.9 g/d salt)
	At least moderate ascites: Sodium restriction (4.5–7 g/d salt); anti-mineralocorticoid alone stepwise increasing dose of 100 mg every 72 h up to 400 mg/d	***Grade 2–3 ascites:*** Sodium restriction (5–7 g/d salt); spironolactone (25–50 mg/d)	***First presentation of moderate ascites:*** Spironolactone alone (100 mg/d, increased to 400 mg/d)	***Grade 2–3 ascites:*** Spironolactone alone (80–160 mg/d);furosemide (40–80 mg/d)	***Grade 2–3 ascites:*** Spironolactone at a starting dosage of 50–100 mg/d, increasing to 400 mg/d	***Grade 2 or moderate ascites:*** Anti-mineralocorticoid drugalone, at a starting 100 mg/d with stepwise increases every 72 h to a maximum of 400 mg/d
	In case of no response: A loop diuretic (furosemide or torasemide) should be added at an increasing stepwise dose (in case of furosemide: 25–50 mg every step to a maximum of 150–200 mg/d)	***In case of no response:*** Spironolactone (25–50 mg/d); furosemide (20–40 mg/d)	***Recurrent severe ascites, or faster diuresis is needed:*** Combination therapy, spironolactone (100–400 mg) and furosemide (40–160 mg)	***In case of no response:*** Tolvaptan 15 mg/d	***Need to increase the diuretic effect:*** Combination therapy,spironolactone and furosemide at a starting dosage of 50–100 mg/d, increasing to 400 mg/d	***In case of no response:*** Furosemide at an increasing stepwise dose from 40 mg/d to a maximum of 160 mg/d
	Moderate/large ascites: Low doses of loop diuretics (25–50 mg/d of furosemide or torasemide 10–20 mg/d) plus antimineralcorticoid	***Resistant to conventional diuretics:*** Tolvaptan 3.75–7.5 mg/d				***Grade 3 or large ascites:*** Large-volume paracentesis
	Refractory ascites: Long-term albumin administration	***Refractory ascites:*** Paracentesis or cell-free and concentrated ascites reinfusion therapy		***Refractory ascites:*** Repeated large-volume paracentesis plus albumin; transjugular intrahepatic portosystemic shunts; liver transplant	***Refractory ascites:***Liver transplantation; serial large-volume paracentesis; transjugular intrahepatic portosystemic shunt	***Refractory ascites:*** Repeated large-volume paracentesis plus albumin; Transjugular intrahepatic portosystemic shunts

11.2.2 Loop Diuretics

11.2.2.1 Furosemide

Furosemide, a loop diuretic, acts on the medullary loop of the ascending branch of the medulla, which can rapidly increase the excretion of water. Furosemide is rapidly but incompletely absorbed from the gut, its bioavailability being about 60% [15] can reach peak plasma concentration effect quickly within 1–2 h, and then diuretic effects end in 3–4 h after consumption [16]. Furosemide is the first-line medication in most people with edema caused by congestive heart failure.

In patients with cirrhosis, unlike spironolactone, furosemide has only been recommended when the efficacy of spironolactone monotherapy is inadequate or faster diuresis is needed [9, 10]. Furosemide alone for the management of cirrhotic patients with ascites has been rarely investigated, but there are studies exploring the efficacy of high-dose furosemide combined with hypertonic saline solutions for the management of cirrhosis patients with refractory ascites. In a randomized controlled study by Licata et al. [17], a total of 84 cirrhotic patients with refractory ascites were included and randomly assigned to group A: patients received intravenous furosemide injection (250 mg–1000 mg/bid) combined with hypertonic saline solutions; or to group B: patients received repeated paracentesis and standard diuretic treatment. This study found that compared with group B, group A had significantly higher diuresis and serum sodium levels ($p < 0.05$). The incidence of ascites at discharge was significantly lower in group A (23.3% vs. 45.8%, $p < 0.001$). Similarly, in a study by Yakar et al., high-dose oral furosemide with hypertonic saline solutions was considered as effective as repeated paracentesis in patients with refractory ascites [18].

Hypokalemia, hypotension, hyponatremia, and hepatic encephalopathy are common adverse events in cirrhotic patients who received furosemide. Skeletal muscle depletion, a common but less noticed complication of patients with cirrhosis, was considered to have a positive correlation with the use of loop diuretic [19]. A study found that muscle cramps, independently with muscle depletion, occurred in 51% of cirrhotic patients, and was significantly associated with the use of furosemide [20].

11.2.2.2 Torasemide

Torasemide, a loop diuretic, exerts its major diuretic activity on the Henle's loop to promote rapid and marked excretion of water. It was used for the treatment of fluid overload secondary to heart failure, kidney disease, and liver cirrhosis. Torasemide can be given in patients exhibiting a weak response to furosemide [5].

Gerbes et al. conducted a randomized controlled double-blind study [21], where a total of 28 patients were enrolled and randomly assigned to furosemide (80 mg) group and torasemide (20 mg) group. The drugs were alternated following a randomized double-blind cross-over design after a wash-out period of at least 2 days. This study found that in the first 6 h following oral administration, the natriuresis of torasemide and furosemide was comparable. However, torasemide had a significantly better natriuresis than furosemide in the 6–24 h interval (38 ± 11 vs. 17 ± 4 mmol/L, $p < 0.05$). The effects on urinary volume were significantly greater for patients who received torasemide than those who received furosemide. However, in a study by Fiaccadori et al., torasemide was found to have a similar effect with furosemide on body weight and urinary volume [22]. In this long-term randomized controlled trial, 28 patients were enrolled and randomly assigned to the torasemide 20 mg group ($n = 14$) and furosemide 50 mg group ($n = 14$). The results found that no significant body weight change was observed in both groups at the end of treatment. The urinary volume was increased in both groups, but the difference was not significant. In the torasemide group, 2 patients developed an episode of hepatic encephalopathy.

11.2.3 Vasopressin V2 Receptor Antagonist

11.2.3.1 Tolvaptan

Tolvaptan is a novel, orally effective, non-peptide vasopressin receptor antagonist, can selectively bind vasopressin V2 receptor of the renal collecting duct, inhibit reabsorption of water, and promote excretion of electrolyte-free water [23–25]. Compared with conventional diuretics, tolvaptan does not decrease serum sodium concentration and can be used for the treatment of hyponatremia. Tolvaptan is approved by the United States Food and Drug Administration for the treatment of hypervolemic hyponatremia secondary to liver cirrhosis, syndrome of inappropriate antidiuretic hormone secretion, and heart failure. Major adverse events of tolvaptan include thirst, dry mouth, polyuria, and fatigue, with an incidence of 3–10% [26, 27]. The United States Food and Drug Administration issued a warning on the potential risk of liver injury on tolvaptan in 2013. A clinical trial also reported that tolvaptan (120 mg/d for 3-year) had elevated serum liver-enzyme levels [28].

The optimal dosage of tolvaptan for the management of ascites in cirrhotic patients remains debated. Tolvaptan has been recommended in several guidelines for patients with refractory ascites and those with poor response to conventional doses of diuretics [8, 10, 29]. According to the guideline by the Japan Society of Hepatology, tolvaptan is recommended for patients with ascites with a dosage range from 3.75 mg–7.5 mg/d [10]. However, in the Chinese guidelines on the management of ascites and its related complications in cirrhosis, the initial dosage of tolvaptan is recommended at 15 mg/d [8]. In a randomized, double-blind, placebo-controlled trial by Okita et al. [30], a total of 101 patients were enrolled and randomly assigned to four groups receiving tolvaptan at 7.5 mg/d, 15 mg/d, or 30 mg/d, or placebo. The study population was primarily patients with hepatitis C virus related-cirrhosis (58.42%) and Child–Pugh B (56.43%). This study found that the largest reduction in body weight was observed in the 7.5 mg/d (mean change in body weight from baseline to day 7 was -2.31 ± 2.35 kg). There is no linear dosage response to change in body weight, but the urine volume showed a dose-dependent manner. Tang et al. designed a placebo-controlled, randomized, double-blinded, multicenter clinical trial for investigating the safety and efficacy of different dosages of tolvaptan for treating cirrhotic patients with ascites in China [31]. A total of 530 patients were enrolled and randomly assigned to groups receiving tolvaptan at

15 mg/d or 7.5 mg/d, or placebo. The study population was primarily patients with hepatitis B virus related-cirrhosis (66.04%) and Child–Pugh B (63.02%). Patients who received tolvaptan had a significantly decreased body weight and 24-h cumulative urine volume compared with placebo. This study found that the improvement of abdominal circumference was not significantly different between the 7.5 mg/d group and 15 mg/d group (−2.0). But considering that serum creatinine was higher in patients who received tolvaptan 15 mg/d, 7.5 mg/d is more recommended in this large study. Further studies need to confirm the optimal starting dosage of tolvaptan for the treatment of ascites in cirrhotic patients.

There is another therapeutic advantage over conventional diuretics that tolvaptan does not decrease serum sodium concentration, so it can be used for the treatment of hypervolemic hyponatremia in patients with cirrhosis [32]. Hyponatremia is common in patients with ascites secondary to cirrhosis and portal hypertension, and is characterized by excessive renal retention of water relative to sodium due to reduced solute-free water clearance. Cardenas et al. performed a study to explore the efficacy of tolvaptan for the treatment of hyponatremia in cirrhosis [26]. This is a sub-analysis of a prospective, multicenter, randomized, placebo-controlled, double-blind study where a total of 120 patients was enrolled and randomly assigned to the tolvaptan group ($n = 63$) and placebo group ($n = 57$). Serum sodium level was significantly higher in tolvaptan group compared with placebo group from baseline to day 4 ($p < 0.001$) and from baseline to day 30 ($p < 0.001$). Tolvaptan can increase serum sodium level better and faster than placebo. However, a real-life experience study by Pose et al. showed that only 22% of patients (2/9) had an increased serum sodium level that persisted throughout treatment [33]. The results suggest that efficacy of tolvaptan in patients with cirrhosis and severe hypervolemic hyponatremia seems to be limited. There are several possible reasons for different conclusions between these two studies, as follows: (1) in Cardenas' study, patients with a serum sodium <120 mmol/L were excluded, while in Pose's study, the range of serum sodium was 117-125 mmol/L; (2) in Cardenas's study, patients with hypovolemic hyponatremia were excluded; and (3) only 9 patients were enrolled in Pose's study.

The response to tolvaptan therapy may be a prognostic factor in patients with cirrhosis. In a recent meta-analysis study by Bellos et al. [34], where 9 studies and a total of 736 patients with ascites were included, patients who have a response to the tolvaptan treatment had a significantly improved survival (hazard ratio 0.42, 95% confidence Interval [0.31–0.58]). Similarly, in a multicenter prospective cohort study by Wang et al., a total of 230 cirrhotic patients with or without hyponatremia were enrolled into this study [35]. Patients were assigned to two groups according to receiving tolvaptan treatment or placebo. Compared with placebo, tolvaptan significantly improves serum sodium levels (63.8% vs. 36.2%, $P < 0.05$) and 6-month survival rate in patients with hyponatremia (89.94% vs. 68.97%, $P < 0.05$). Interestingly, this study found that in hyponatremia patients with a response to tolvaptan, the 6-month survival rate was significantly better than patients with no response. In a retrospectively study by Kanayama et al., long-term administration of tolvaptan was investigated in patients with cirrhosis and refractory ascites [36]. A total of 84 patients were enrolled. Responder to tolvaptan was defined as the one who had weight reduction of ≥1.5 kg in 7 days after the administration. The median overall survival time of responders and non-responders has no significant difference ($p = 0.86$, 14.9 months and 9.9 months, respectively). During long-term follow-up, approximately 50% of patients in this study showed re-exacerbation within 12 months. Furthermore, the responders without re-exacerbation within 3 months showed significantly longer overall survival than those with re-exacerbation within 3 months ($p < 0.01$).

Due to the heterogeneity among studies, there are still controversies regarding tolvaptan for the treatment of hypervolemic hyponatremia and the prognostic value of early response of tolvaptan [26, 33–35]. The sources of the heterogeneity are as follows: (1) different characteristics of the target population: patients with ascites or refractory ascites, patients with or without hepatocellular carcinoma, and patients with or without hyponatremia; (2) different definitions of responders: body weight loss ≥1.5 kg or 2 kg within first week, serum sodium changes; and (3) different study regions, sample size, and races.

Tolvaptan may not be effective for all patients. Sakaida et al. performed a post-hoc analysis, where a total of 152 patients were enrolled, and found that patients who had a heavier weight and lower blood urease nitrogen at baseline would have a better response to the treatment of tolvaptan [37]. The results suggest that 75% (114/152) of patients responded to the treatment of tolvaptan (a change in initial urine volume ≥ 500 mL). A stepwise multivariate regression analysis showed that baseline body weight (odds ratio 1.05; 95% confidence interval [1.01–1.09]; $P = 0.0143$) and BUN (odds ratio 0.95: 95% confidence interval [0.92–0.98]; $P = 0.0051$) were significantly associated with change in initial urine volume.

11.3 Other Medications

Other medications, including human albumin, midodrine, and terlipressin, are commonly used for the treatment of liver cirrhosis, may also improve the response to diuretics.

Human albumin infusion has been widely used for the treatment of post-paracentesis circulatory dysfunction, hepatorenal syndrome, and refractory ascites [38]. In a study by Gentilini et al., human albumin was used in combination with potassium canrenoate and/or furosemide [39]. Patients treated with albumin plus conventional diuretics had a significantly shorter hospital stay ($p < 0.05$) and higher cumulative rate of response to the treatment of ascites ($p < 0.05$).

Midodrine, a peripheral α-adrenergic agonist, was useful in the clinical management of patients with orthostatic hypotension. A randomized pilot study found that midodrine plus tolvaptan therapy has a significantly better control of ascites than midodrine or tolvaptan alone in the control of ascites ($p < 0.05$) at 3 months [40].

Terlipressin, a vasopressin derivative, has been widely used in patients with cirrhosis and variceal bleeding or hepatorenal syndrome. A meta-analysis found that terlipressin may be beneficial in cirrhosis with ascites and without hepatorenal syndrome [41].

11.4 Diuretic Regimens

Conventional diuretics, including spironolactone, furosemide, and torasemide, have been used in patients with ascites for a long time. The mechanisms of action of conventional diuretics have been deeply understood, but there are still debates regarding diuretic regimens for ascites. There is a board consensus that in patients with first presentation or mild ascites, spironolactone monotherapy is recommended as the first-line therapy [5, 9, 11]. However, there has been no consistent conclusion regarding diuretic regimens for patients with moderate/severe or refractory ascites. Whether loop diuretics should be added with spironolactone from the beginning of the treatment or added sequentially after spironolactone has long been debated [5].

Fogel et al. compared three diuretic regimens and found that spironolactone and furosemide combination therapy may the most potent regimen [42]. A total of 90 patients were randomly assigned to three treatment groups: Sequential group ($n = 30$), patients received spironolactone followed by furosemide if necessary; Combination group ($n = 31$), patients received both spironolactone and furosemide; Furosemide group ($n = 29$), patients received furosemide alone. The disappearance of ascites was comparable among three groups, while the combination group was the fastest. Similarly, a study by Angeli et al. concluded that the combined treatment was preferable because a shorter time was required to achieve an effective diuresis [43]. However, in a randomized controlled trial study by Santos et al., a total of 94 previously untreated patients with cirrhosis and ascites were included [44]. The results found the sequential treatment was more suitable for ascites, because it required less dose adjustment. All patients were randomly assigned to spironolactone monotherapy group ($n = 50$) and spironolactone combined with furosemide group ($n = 50$). The safety and effectiveness of spironolactone monotherapy were comparable with spironolactone associated with furosemide. Sequential treatment was recommended to be used on an outpatient basis.

Although the recommendations for diuretic regimens varied among studies, these diuretic regimens did not differ significantly in efficacy. In terms of the underlying pathogenesis, water retention in patients with cirrhosis and ascites is not an intrinsic abnormality of the kidneys, but rather to extra-renal mechanisms. At the early stages of ascites formation in cirrhotic patients, renal perfusion and glomerular filtration rate are well preserved, hyperaldosteronism is the principal pathogenic factor, and sodium retention mainly occurs at the distal nephron. Spironolactone is more recommended at this stage [7]. Once the glomerular filtration rate declines, proximal sodium reabsorption becomes prevalent, a loop diuretic may a necessary choice.

Newly developed vasopressin V2 receptor antagonist diuretics, tolvaptan, induces electrolyte-free water excretion without changing the total level of electrolyte excretion. Tolvaptan combined with conventional diuretics regimens showed a promising diuresis effect. In an observational study by Zhang et al., tolvaptan 15 mg/d was used with furosemide 40–80 mg/d and spironolactone 80–160 mg/d [45]. The results showed a significantly increased mean urine excretion volume after treatment ($p < 0.001$). Further high-quality study should explore the efficacy of tolvaptan combined with conventional diuretics regimens or sequentially after conventional diuretics.

11.5 Adverse Events

As discussed above, adverse events of diuretics mainly include electrolyte disturbances, muscle cramps, thirsty, decreased blood pressure, and hepatic encephalopathy. The prevalence of diuretic adverse events in patients with ascites ranged from 19–40% [43, 44, 46]. All adverse events should be carefully monitored when initiating diuretics in all patients. Hepatic encephalopathy occurs in approximately 25% of patients and is considered as the most common complication of diuretics, followed by renal dysfunction with a prevalence of 14–20% and hyponatremia with a prevalence of 8–30% [43, 47, 48].

11.6 Conclusion

Diuretics are the most important pharmacological therapy for patients with liver cirrhosis and ascites. Conventional diuretics, including spironolactone, furosemide, and torasemide, have been widely used in clinical practices over the last couple decades. Tolvaptan, a newly developed diuretic, has been used for patients with ascites and hyponatremia. Further high-quality studies should investigate different regimens of diuretics, including the combination of different diuretics, the appropriate sequence of diuretics, and the suitable dosage of diuretics.

References

1. Roush GC, Kaur R, Ernst ME. Diuretics: a review and update. J Cardiovasc Pharmacol Ther. 2014;19:5–13.
2. D'Amico G, et al. Competing risks and prognostic stages of cirrhosis: a 25-year inception cohort study of 494 patients. Aliment Pharmacol Ther. 2014;39:1180–93.
3. Wang R, et al. Association of umbilical hernia with volume of ascites in liver cirrhosis: a retrospective observational study. J Evid Based Med. 2016;9:170–80.
4. Wang R, Qi X, Guo X. Quantification of ascites based on abdomino-pelvic computed tomography scans for predicting the in-hospital mortality of liver cirrhosis. Exp Ther Med. 2017;14:5733–42.
5. European Association for the Study of the Liver. Electronic address, e.e.e. and L. European Association for the Study of the, EASL clinical practice guidelines for the management of patients with decompensated cirrhosis. J Hepatol. 2018;69:406–60.
6. National Center for Biotechnology Information (2021) PubChem compound summary for CID 5833, spironolactone. Retrieved December 22, 2021 from https://pubchem.ncbi.nlm.nih.gov/compound/Spironolactone.
7. Perez-Ayuso RM, et al. Randomized comparative study of efficacy of furosemide versus spironolactone in nonazotemic cirrhosis with ascites. Relationship between the diuretic response and the activity of the renin-aldosterone system. Gastroenterology. 1983;84:961–8.

8. Chinese Society of Hepatology, CMA, et al. Chinese guidelines on the management of ascites and its related complications in cirrhosis. Hepatol Int. 2019;13:1–21.
9. Aithal GP, et al. Guidelines on the management of ascites in cirrhosis. Gut. 2021;70:9–29.
10. Yoshiji H, et al. Evidence-based clinical practice guidelines for liver cirrhosis 2020. J Gastroenterol. 2021;56:593–619.
11. Italian Association for the Study of the, L. Portal hypertension and ascites: patient-and population-centered clinical practice guidelines by the Italian Association for the Study of the liver (AISF). Dig Liver Dis. 2021;53:1089–104.
12. Khan TU, et al. Risk factors for hyperkalemia in cirrhotic patients receiving spironolactone. Professional Med J. 2020;27:413–8.
13. Struthers A, Krum H, Williams GH. A comparison of the aldosterone-blocking agents eplerenone and spironolactone. Clin Cardiol. 2008;31:153–8.
14. Sehgal R, Singh H, Singh IP. Comparative study of spironolactone and eplerenone in management of ascites in patients of cirrhosis of liver. Eur J Gastroenterol Hepatol. 2020;32:535–9.
15. Laffi G, et al. Loop diuretic therapy in liver cirrhosis with ascites. J Cardiovasc Pharmacol. 1993;22:S51–8.
16. Zhu ZR, et al. Efficacy of furosemide for treatment of liver cirrhosis: a systematic review protocol of randomized controlled trial. Medicine (Baltimore). 2019;98:e15300.
17. Licata G, et al. Clinical trial: high-dose furosemide plus small-volume hypertonic saline solutions vs. repeated paracentesis as treatment of refractory ascites. Aliment Pharmacol Ther. 2009;30:227–35.
18. Yakar T, et al. High dose Oral furosemide with salt ingestion in the treatment of refractory ascites of liver cirrhosis. Clin Invest Med. 2016;39:27502.
19. Hanai T, et al. Effect of loop diuretics on skeletal muscle depletion in patients with liver cirrhosis. Hepatol Res. 2019;49:82–95.
20. Sawada Y, et al. Effect of furosemide on muscle cramps in patients with liver cirrhosis. J Gastroenterol Hepatol. 2020;35:76–81.
21. Gerbes AL, et al. Advantages of the new loop diuretic torasemide over furosemide in patients with cirrhosis and ascites. A randomized, double blind cross-over trial. J Hepatol. 1993;17:353–8.
22. Fiaccadori F, et al. Torasemide versus furosemide in cirrhosis: a long-term, double-blind, randomized clinical study. Clin Investig. 1993;71:579–84.
23. Yamamura Y, et al. OPC-41061, a highly potent human vasopressin V2-receptor antagonist: pharmacological profile and aquaretic effect by single and multiple oral dosing in rats. J Pharmacol Exp Ther. 1998;287:860–7.
24. Nakanishi H, et al. Urinary excretion of the water channel aquaporin 2 correlated with the pharmacological effect of tolvaptan in cirrhotic patients with ascites. J Gastroenterol. 2016;51:620–7.
25. Costello-Boerrigter LC, et al. Vasopressin-2-receptor antagonism augments water excretion without changes in renal hemodynamics or sodium and potassium excretion in human heart failure. Am J Physiol Renal Physiol. 2006;290:F273–8.
26. Cardenas A, et al. Tolvaptan, an oral vasopressin antagonist, in the treatment of hyponatremia in cirrhosis. J Hepatol. 2012;56:571–8.
27. Schrier RW, et al. Tolvaptan, a selective oral vasopressin V2-receptor antagonist, for hyponatremia. N Engl J Med. 2006;355:2099–112.
28. Torres VE, et al. Tolvaptan in patients with autosomal dominant polycystic kidney disease. N Engl J Med. 2012;367:2407–18.
29. Korean Association for the Study of the, L. KASL clinical practice guidelines for liver cirrhosis: ascites and related complications. Clin Mol Hepatol. 2018;24:230–77.
30. Okita K, et al. Dose-finding trial of tolvaptan in liver cirrhosis patients with hepatic edema: a randomized, double-blind, placebo-controlled trial. Hepatol Res. 2014;44:83–91.
31. Tang J, et al. Tolvaptan therapy of Chinese cirrhotic patients with ascites after insufficient diuretic routine medication responses: a phase III clinical trial. BMC Gastroenterol. 2020;20:391.

32. Alukal JJ, John S, Thuluvath PJ. Hyponatremia in cirrhosis: an update. Am J Gastroenterol. 2020;115:1775–85.
33. Pose E, et al. Limited efficacy of Tolvaptan in patients with cirrhosis and severe hyponatremia: real-life experience. Am J Med. 2017;130:372–5.
34. Bellos I, et al. Tolvaptan response improves overall survival in patients with refractory ascites: a meta-analysis. Dig Dis. 2020;38:320–8.
35. Wang S, et al. Tolvaptan treatment improves survival of cirrhotic patients with ascites and hyponatremia. BMC Gastroenterol. 2018;18:137.
36. Kanayama K, et al. Long-term administration of Tolvaptan to patients with decompensated cirrhosis. Int J Med Sci. 2020;17:874–80.
37. Sakaida I, et al. Predictive factors of the pharmacological action of tolvaptan in patients with liver cirrhosis: a post hoc analysis. J Gastroenterol. 2017;52:229–36.
38. Bai Z, et al. Albumin infusion may decrease the incidence and severity of overt hepatic encephalopathy in liver cirrhosis. Aging (Albany NY). 2019;11:8502–25.
39. Gentilini P, et al. Albumin improves the response to diuretics in patients with cirrhosis and ascites: results of a randomized, controlled trial. J Hepatol. 1999;30:639–45.
40. Rai N, et al. Midodrine and tolvaptan in patients with cirrhosis and refractory or recurrent ascites: a randomised pilot study. Liver Int. 2017;37:406–14.
41. Bai Z, et al. Role of Terlipressin in cirrhotic patients with ascites and without Hepatorenal syndrome: a systematic review of current evidence. Can J Gastroenterol Hepatol. 2020;2020:5106958.
42. Fogel MR, et al. Diuresis in the ascitic patient: a randomized controlled trial of three regimens. J Clin Gastroenterol. 1981;3:73–80.
43. Angeli P, et al. Combined versus sequential diuretic treatment of ascites in non-azotaemic patients with cirrhosis: results of an open randomised clinical trial. Gut. 2010;59:98–104.
44. Santos J, et al. Spironolactone alone or in combination with furosemide in the treatment of moderate ascites in nonazotemic cirrhosis. A randomized comparative study of efficacy and safety. J Hepatol. 2003;39:187–92.
45. Zhang X, et al. Clinical efficacy of tolvaptan for treatment of refractory ascites in liver cirrhosis patients. World J Gastroenterol. 2014;20:11400–5.
46. Lenaerts A, et al. Effects of clonidine on diuretic response in ascitic patients with cirrhosis and activation of sympathetic nervous system. Hepatology. 2006;44:844–9.
47. Sherlock S, et al. Complications of diuretic therapy in hepatic cirrhosis. Lancet. 1966;1:1049–52.
48. Arroyo V, et al. Definition and diagnostic criteria of refractory ascites and hepatorenal syndrome in cirrhosis. International Ascites Club. Hepatology. 1996;23:164–76.

Statins in Liver Cirrhosis

12

Alberto E. Muñoz, Mariano Cartier, and Ayelén B. Kisch

Abstract

A broad group of physicians is still afraid of administering statins because of the myth of statin toxicity and frequent statin-related nocebo effects. However, due to the statins cholesterol independent mechanism of action -pleiotropic effects, the focus on these drugs has shifted from harmful to helpful in patients with chronic liver disease. Recently, and most likely through these mentioned effects, statins were associated with significant clinical outcomes in these patients. Although only through experimental trials, this chapter describes the efficacy of statins in matter topics of Hepatology as portal hypertension, decompensated cirrhosis, and hepatocellular carcinoma. Finally, there is a discussion regarding the safety of statins in decompensated cirrhosis.

Keywords

Liver cirrhosis · Statins · Efficiency · Hypertension · Portal · Carcinoma · Hepatocellular · Safety · Adverse events

A. E. Muñoz (✉)
Sección Hepatología, Hospital Dr. Carlos Bonorino Udaondo, Facultad de Medicina, Universidad de Buenos Aires, Buenos Aires, Argentina

Instituto de Investigaciones en Salud Pública, Facultad de Odontología, Universidad de Buenos Aires, Ciudad Autónoma de Buenos Aires, Buenos Aires, Argentina
e-mail: aemunoz@intramed.net

M. Cartier · A. B. Kisch
Sección Hepatología, Hospital Dr. Carlos Bonorino Udaondo, Facultad de Medicina, Universidad de Buenos Aires, Buenos Aires, Argentina

X. Qi, Y. Yang (eds.), *Pharmacotherapy for Liver Cirrhosis and Its Complications*, https://doi.org/10.1007/978-981-19-2615-0_12

Abbreviations

ACLF	acute-on-chronic liver failure
ALT	serum alanine aminotransferase
AST	aspartate aminotransferase
BCLC	Barcelona Clinic Liver Cancer
BT	bacterial translocation
CAD	coronary artery disease
CK	serum creatine kinase
CVD	cardiovascular disease
eNOS	endothelial NO synthase
GTP	guanosine triphosphate
HCC	hepatocellular carcinoma
HMG-CoA	3-hydroxy-3-methyl-glutaril- coenzyme A reductase
HSCs	hepatic stellate cells
HVPG	hepatic venous pressure gradient
KLF2	Krüppel-like factor-2
LDL-C	low-density lipoprotein cholesterol
LSEC	liver sinusoidal endothelial cells
MELD	Model for End-stage Liver Disease
NO	nitric oxide
NSBB	non-selective β-blockers
OS	overall survival
PH	portal hypertension
PI3K/Akt	phosphatidylinositol 3-kinase/protein kinase Akt pathway
PVT	portal vein thrombosis
ROCK	Rho kinase
ROS	reactive oxygen species
RCT	randomized controlled trial
SVT20+RFX	simvastatin 20 mg/day plus rifaximin 1200 mg/day
SVT40+RFX	simvastatin 40 mg/day plus rifaximin 1200 mg/day
TP	time to progression
TACE	transcatether arterial embolization
VI	vascular invasion

12.1 Introduction

Statins: firstly antibiotics, then hypercholesterolemic and atherosclerotic cardiovascular disease therapy, and finally cirrhosis treatment: Until the 1950s, physicians were skeptical of any causal link between cholesterol and coronary artery disease (CAD) because most patients with heart disease have plasma cholesterol levels not much different from those of the average general population [1]. On the other hand, in the nineteenth century, many patients dying of occlusive vascular disease had their artery walls often thickened, with a non-uniform inner surface and coated with a yellowish fatty substance subsequently identified as cholesterol (after investigations carried out by Virchow). This pathological condition was termed atheroma. The objective of the Framingham study, considering these discrepant observations, was to examine the relationship between plasma cholesterol and other potential risk factors and death from CAD. This study established a strong relationship between high blood cholesterol and CAD mortality in the late 1950s [2]. Over the next several years, it was shown that low-density lipoprotein cholesterol (LDL-C) contributed to CAD mortality, whereas high-density lipoprotein cholesterol had an inverse correlation with CAD mortality [3]. These observations led to widespread attempts to develop new pharmacological therapies to improve CAD mortality through LDL-C reduction [3, 4].

A promising target for cholesterol reduction was the rate-limiting enzyme of cholesterol synthesis, 3-hydroxy-3-methyl-glutaril-coenzyme A (HMG-CoA) reductase. In this context, statins became the most significant output of microbiological research on a new target of antibacterial activity. On that subject, Endo et al. described a series of compounds affecting bacterial growth by inhibiting HMG-CoA reductase [5]. In the 1970s, during a search for antimicrobial agents they discovered the first HMG-CoA reductase inhibitor, compactin, in the fermentation broth of Penicillium citrinum [6, 7]. By 1978, Alberts et al. at the Merck Research Laboratories discovered another HMG-CoA reductase inhibitor, mevinolin -later called lovastatin, in the fermentation broth of Aspergillus terreus [8]. Due to concerns over potential adverse events, it was not until 1982 that lovastatin was tested in patients with familial hypercholesterolemia and shown a dramatic reduction of LDL-C with a favorable side-effect profile [9, 10]. Large-scale, randomized, double-blind trials started in 1984 and concluded with US FDA approval in 1987 of the first commercially available statin medication, lovastatin, to treat hypercholesterolemia [11–13]. However, up to that time point, the effects of lovastatin on vessel structure were few, since each trial included less than 800 patients –who were followed only for 2 years at most-, and limited safety information was obtained [14]. Then, in 1988, the Merck Research Laboratories derived a more powerful HMG-CoA inhibitor, later known as simvastatin that was trialed in a very well renowned study called "4S". The results from such a trial marked a turning point in medical thinking [15]. The study included more than 4,000 patients with CAD and high levels of total plasma cholesterol who were randomized in a double-blind trial administering simvastatin 20–40 mg once a day -or placebo- for 5 years. The most remarkable result was a 30% reduction in all-cause mortality due to a 42% reduction in coronary deaths. These effects on mortality were accompanied by a 34% reduction in major coronary events (nonfatal myocardial infarction plus CAD death) and a 37% reduction in revascularization procedures. In 1998, Bayer introduced cerivastatin, but it was shortly withdrawn from the market in 2001 due to reports of rhabdomyolysis, with more than 50 fatal cases [16]. Although regulatory agencies were careful to point out that their concern was specific to cerivastatin, its withdrawal shook the confidence of some physicians regarding the safety of statins in general. In this way, the prescription of these drugs decreased in many countries. This event was unfortunate because -even today- many high-risk patients still go untreated, and

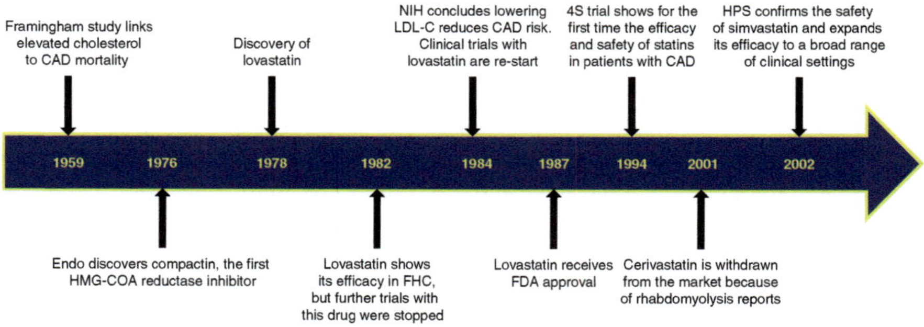

Fig. 12.1 The history of statins in Cardiology. *CAD* coronary artery disease; *HMG-CoA reductase* 3-hydroxy-3-methyl-glutaril-coenzyme A reductase, *FHC* familial hypercholesterolemia, *NIH* National Institutes of Health, *LDL-C* low-density lipoprotein cholesterol, *FDA* Food and Drug Administration, *4S trial* Scandinavian Simvastatin Survival Study, *HPS* Heart Protection Study

preventable major adverse cardiac events are not avoided [17]. Finally, in the Heart Protection Study (HPS) [18], over more than 20,000 patients for 5 years confirmed and expanded previous evidence upon "4S" results, establishing the benefit of simvastatin in women and its effectiveness for reducing the risk not only of CAD events but also of strokes. Likewise, significant reductions in the risk of major vascular events were observed in patients with diabetes without CAD, patients with cerebrovascular or peripheral vascular disease but no CAD, patients aged 70 or older, and patients with normal serum LDL-C at entry. These effects had not been previously reported for any statin. The safety of simvastatin was also confirmed since the incidence only of myopathy, including rhabdomyolysis, was <0.1%. This winding history of statins in Cardiology is depicted in Fig. 12.1.

The group led by Jaime Bosch of the Hepatic Hemodynamic Laboratory of Barcelona took the lead in the investigation of using simvastatin to reduce portal hypertension (PH), which is an almost unavoidable consequence of cirrhosis. Moreover, PH is directly or indirectly responsible for major clinical complications, such as variceal bleeding, a leading cause of death in cirrhotic patients [19].

Traditionally, PH is considered a mechanical consequence of disrupting the liver vascular architecture caused by the cirrhotic process. However, increased hepatic resistance is the first pathophysiological phenomenon that causes PH [20, 21]. Approximately 30% of the increase in portal pressure is due to this mechanism [20]. Therefore, modulation of intrahepatic vascular resistance has become a key therapeutic target of PH [22]. Studies in experimental cirrhosis suggest that increased hepatic resistance in cirrhosis would be because endothelial nitric oxide (NO) release is impaired in liver microvasculature [23–26]. In addition, such insufficient NO availability may explain the incapacity of the intrahepatic vasculature to relax in response to acute increases in portal blood flow, such as those induced by meals [27]. This impaired endothelium-dependent relaxation through NO production -endothelial dysfunction- may be worsened by postprandial hyperglycemia and hypertriglyceridemia [28]. In this regard, both unaltered [24, 25] and decreased [29] protein levels of endothelial NO synthase (eNOS) have been found in cirrhosis but decreased hepatic eNOS activity has been uniformly reported [23–26, 30]. This reduction has been attributed to complex posttranslational modifications of eNOS. Therefore, upregulating eNOS activity in the cirrhotic liver may constitute a new strategy to correct these patients' increased hepatic vascular tone [31, 32].

12.2 Rationale for the Use of Statins in Cirrhosis

Background for the Use of Statins in Cardiology Statins have been used in Cardiology for decades as the main drugs for treating CAD with or without hypercholesterolemia. In this regard, the rationale for using statins in Hepatology emerges from data obtained from cardiological research. This observation justifies a brief review of the background for the employment of statins in Cardiology.

Cardiovascular disease (CVD) is the leading cause of morbidity and mortality worldwide, with atherosclerosis being the main pathophysiological mechanism leading to CVD. Atherosclerosis, formerly considered a lipid deposition disease, is now regarded as a chronic low-grade inflammatory disease affecting the vascular wall. It begins with the sub-endothelial deposition of LDL-C in the artery wall, which may be modified by oxidation, promoting the infiltration of T cells and monocytes that increases free radical generation. This process leads to endothelial injury and dysfunction [33].

Considering that 60–70% of serum cholesterol comes from hepatic synthesis and HMG-CoA reductase is the crucial enzyme in the cholesterol synthesis pathway, inhibition of this enzyme by statins results in a marked reduction of circulating LDL-C (Fig. 12.2). Furthermore, the reduction of serum LDL-C leads to upregulation of the LDL-C receptor and increased hepatic clearance of LDL-C. Therefore, reducing serum LDL-C levels is the primary mechanism of statin therapy in CVD [34].

Statins, however, also exert cholesterol-independent or pleiotropic effects. By inhibiting the conversion of HMG-CoA to L-mevalonic acid, statins prevent the synthesis of essential isoprenoids, such as farnesylpyrophosphate and geranylgeranyl pyrophosphate, which are precursors of cholesterol synthesis [34] (Fig. 12.2). These intermediates are essential for the posttranslational modification of proteins through isoprenylation. This term refers to the posttranslational modification of proteins by adding a lipophilic isoprenyl group upon binding to isoprenoid intermediates. Isoprenylation enables subcellular localization and intracellular trafficking of membrane-associated proteins. Furthermore, the lipophilic isoprenyl group facilitates the covalent attachment to cell membranes, which is essential for biological functions in most situations. Important substrates for the isoprenylation are the small guanosine triphosphate (GTP)-binding proteins like Ras, and Ras-like proteins, such as Rho, Rab, Rac, Ral, or Rap [35, 36] (Fig. 12.2). In this regard, Rho proteins are involved in the expression of proinflammatory cytokines, mediated by its downstream effector Rho kinase (ROCK) [37]. Likewise, Rac proteins modulate reactive oxygen species (ROS) generation, while Ras proteins are involved in cell adhesion, cell proliferation, and apoptosis [38]. Because isoprenylated proteins can

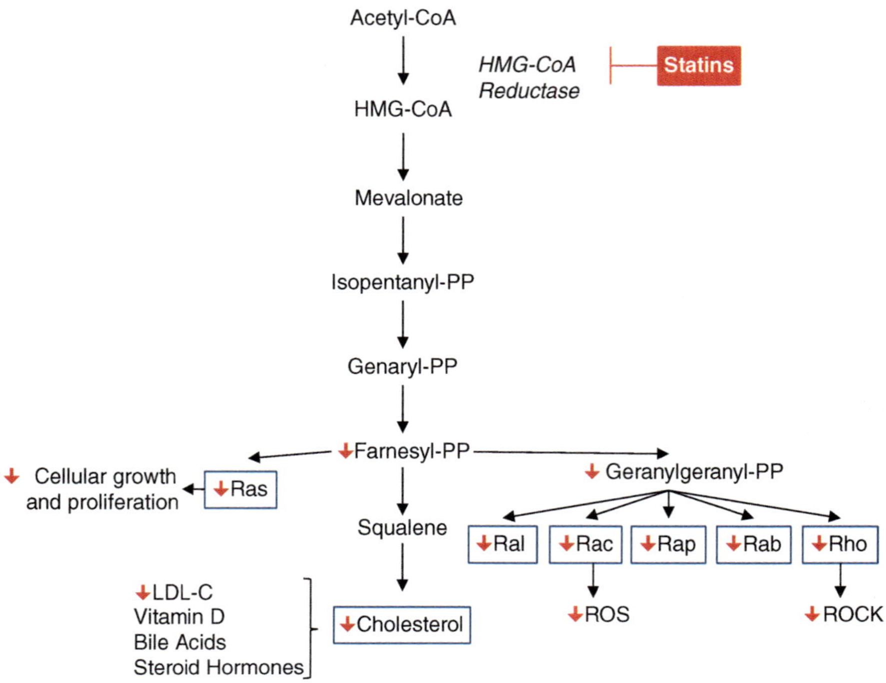

Fig. 12.2 Cholesterol biosynthesis pathway and the effects of statins. *HMG-CoA reductase* 3-hydroxy-3-methyl-glutaril-coenzyme A reductase, *LDL-C* low-density lipoprotein cholesterol, *PP* pyrophosphate, *GTP* guanosine triphosphate, *ROS* reactive oxygen species, *ROCK* Rho kinase

control diverse cellular functions, it is not surprising that statins may have additional effects beyond lipid lowering. Nevertheless, it is unclear whether statins exert pleiotropic effects independently of mevalonate synthesis inhibition or due to hepatic or non-hepatic isoprenylation inhibition [39].

In 1989, elevated serum cholesterol levels were shown to lead to endothelial dysfunction [40]. A further work from Harrison showed that the distinctive marker is the reduction of NO bioavailability [41]. The mechanism by which LDL-C causes endothelial dysfunction and decreases NO bioactivity involves the downregulation of eNOS expression, the decreased receptor-mediated NO release [42], and a decreased NO bioavailability due to increased ROS production [43].

Statins increase endothelial NO production, improving the expression and activity of eNOS due to pleiotropic effects [39]. The mechanism is consistent with the following steps: firstly, statins reduce caveolin-1 abundance; since caveolin-1 is an integral membrane protein, it binds to eNOS in caveolae and directly inhibits NO production [44]. Secondly, inhibition of the Rho/ROCK pathway activates the phosphatidylinositol 3-kinase/protein kinase Akt (PI3K/Akt) pathway [45]. Because Akt phosphorylates and activates eNOS, statins can also increase eNOS activity through the PI3K/Akt pathway [46, 47]. Third, due to inhibition of Rho geranylgeranylation, statins increase eNOS expression by prolonging its mRNA half-life [48]. Finally, statins induce Krüppel-like factor-2 (KLF2) mRNA in endothelial cells, which may be required for eNOS expression [49].

Background for the Use of Statins in Hepatology Several experimental trials demonstrate that pleiotropic effects are the rationale for using statins in Hepatology, as shown in Fig. 12.3.

Between 2007 and 2010, Trebicka and Martin [50–52] showed the slightly divergent effects of atorvastatin upon the different stages of chronic liver disease. During early fibrosis, it inhibits the translocation of Rho and ROCK activity; this, in turn, decreases the activation of hepatic stellate cells (HSCs) and collagen production. Furthermore, when reaching cirrhosis, it inhibits cytokine production and the proliferation and contraction of activated HSCs. Significantly, statins might induce senescence in activated HSCs, leading to a decreased turnover of these highly active cells [51–53]. Likewise, by inhibiting the translocation of Rho from the cytoplasm to plasma membrane and ROCK activity [51], statins improve endothelial dysfunction by increasing the activity of eNOS and the availability of NO [51, 54]. In this regard, simvastatin enhances NO production by increasing eNOS expression and Akt-dependent eNOS phosphorylation [54]. Additionally, it improves liver sinusoidal endothelial cells (LSEC) function through the upregulation of KLF2 expression, which induces the transcription of several vasoprotective genes on LSEC as eNOS and thrombomodulin [55]. Finally, statin-induced upregulation of eNOS mediated by KLF2 has been shown to decrease HSC contraction and lower portal pressure [55, 56].

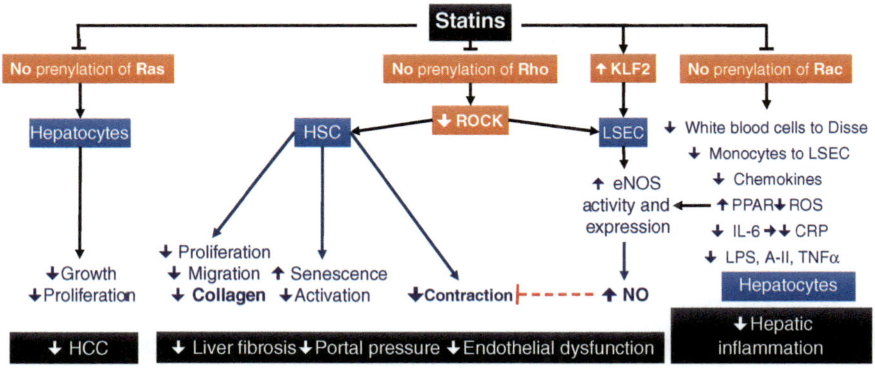

Fig. 12.3 Pleiotropic effects of statins on the small guanosine triphosphatase-binding proteins are the rationale for using in cirrhosis. *KLF-2* Krüppel-like factor-2, *HSC* hepatic stellate cells, *ROCK* Rho kinase, *LSEC* liver sinusoidal endothelial cells, *eNOS* endothelial NO synthase, *NO* nitric oxide, *PPAR* peroxisome proliferator-activated receptors, *ROS* reactive oxygen species, *IL6-* interleukin 6, *CRP* C-reactive protein, *LPS* lipopolysaccharides, *AII* angiotensin-II, *TNFα* tumor necrosis factor-alpha

Statins have exhibited anti-inflammatory effects in experimental models of chronic liver injury. These drugs exert anti-inflammatory effects via the inhibition of Rac prenylation and the decrease in downstream signaling [57]. In addition, statins reduce the production of chemokines, loosen monocyte adhesion to vascular endothelial cells, and lower the action of interleukin-6-induced C-reactive protein in human hepatocytes, mobilizing leukocytes into the subendothelial space [58]. Statins prevent endothelial dysfunction mediated by hepatic inflammation produced by lipopolysaccharides [59]. Statins also decrease interferon-γ-mediated induction of major histocompatibility complex II in endothelial cells, and therefore T-cell activation. Moreover, in rat liver, studies have shown the effect of atorvastatin in reducing the following: (a) angiotensin II, (b) the activation of κB factor, (c) the intercellular adhesion molecule-1 expression, (d) the secretion of interleukin-6, (e) the transforming growth factor β1, and (f) free radical production [58]. Statins also decrease oxidative stress by reducing the levels and oxidation of LDL-C and decreasing inducible NO production, thereby affecting reactive nitrogen species production [60, 61].

A significant effect would be that statins might exert anti malignant properties. Besides inhibiting proliferation in vitro, statins might also induce apoptosis of hepatocellular carcinoma (HCC) cells and inhibit intrahepatic angiogenesis. Reduced proliferation might be due to interferences with Ras prenylation and prevention of p21 and 27 breakdown in malignant cells, followed by induction of cell-cycle arrest. In addition, specific interference with integrins and ROCK expressed at the cell membrane reduced the proliferation and tumor cell adhesion in an in vitro HCC model [62].

Overall, this large body of evidence supports the favorable effect of statins on hepatic fibrosis, endothelial dysfunction, portal pressure, liver inflammation, and HCC.

So far, were discussed the results of experimental trials. From here on, to cover the outcomes of clinical trials. Between 2004 and 2009, two clinical trials in patients with cirrhosis and PH -carried out in the Hepatic Hemodynamic Laboratory of Barcelona- provided the rationale for using statins in Hepatology. In the first one, the acute administration of simvastatin significantly increased NO levels in hepatic venous blood and decreased hepatic sinusoidal resistance. Remarkably, systemic NO levels and hemodynamics were not modified [63]. In the second trial, a proof-of-concept study showed in a randomized clinical trial (RCT), that simvastatin lowers portal pressure in patients with cirrhosis and PH and that it has an excellent safety profile. Furthermore, simvastatin decreases portal pressure in those patients taking and patients not taking non-selective β-blockers (NSBB), suggesting that its effect on portal pressure is additive with these drugs. Finally, simvastatin improves quantitative liver function evaluated through indocyanine green clearance [64]. In summary, Fig. 12.4 shows the first steps of statins in Hepatology, from PH to decompensated cirrhosis.

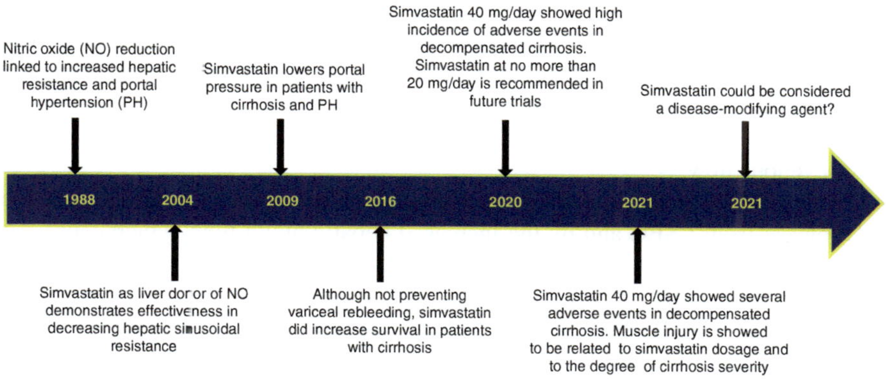

Fig. 12.4 The history of statins in Hepatology: the first steps

12.3 Efficacy of Statins in Hepatology

To date, many observational studies demonstrated the benefit of statins in patients with cirrhosis [65–74]. However, although many observational studies also showed the efficacy of statins in patients with non-hepatologic diseases, those results were not later confirmed in RCTs [75–81]. Therefore, in this last section of the chapter, we will rely on the experimental studies published to date to discuss the currently available clinical evidence on the efficacy and safety of statins in patients with cirrhosis.

12.3.1 Portal Hypertension

PH is a common clinical syndrome characterized by a pathologic increase of the portal pressure and the formation of portal-systemic collaterals that shunt part of the portal blood flow to the systemic circulation bypassing the liver [82]. PH usually is evaluated by catheterization of the hepatic vein. This procedure measures the hepatic venous pressure gradient (HVPG), rendering an indirect measure of portal pressure. HVPG results from the difference between the "wedged" hepatic venous pressure and the "free" hepatic venous pressure. The normal HVPG is between 1 and 5 mmHg [83]. The leading cause of PH is cirrhosis, a sinusoidal PH [19]. An HVPG ≥10 mm Hg defines clinically significant PH as varices, and decompensation can appear after reaching this threshold [84].

PH results from an increase in intrahepatic resistance and of the portal blood flow. The first event in PH development is the increase in intrahepatic vascular resistance that results from architectural distortion (fibrous tissue, regenerative nodules) and endothelial dysfunction [85]. Then, the systemic circulation is altered in cirrhosis, occurring after the development of PH, which is associated with a distinctive systemic circulatory abnormality known as the hyperkinetic syndrome. The latter is characterized by hypervolemia, increased cardiac index, hypotension, and decreased systemic vascular resistance [22]. The hyperkinetic syndrome contributes to the deterioration and the further increase of portal hypertension by raising the portal venous flow.

Groszmann et al. attributed the hepatic endothelial dysfunction to a deficit in the NO release from LSEC and by the increased hepatic blood flow, which causes an overproduction of NO in splanchnic and systemic vasculature. They named this situation "the paradox of NO in cirrhosis and PH", assuming that endothelial dysfunction in arteriosclerosis and cirrhosis could be physiopathological parallel [32].

Following Groszmann's line of thought, and as already described in the Introduction, Bosch's group considered that hepatic endothelial dysfunction was caused by the deficiency of NO and thought that statins could be used for treating PH of their hepatic NO donor capacity. Thus, they began in 2004 their clinical trials with simvastatin in patients with cirrhosis and PH [63].

The first multicenter RCT involving three university hospitals evaluated the effects of simvastatin on HVPG [64]. Simvastatin or placebo was administered for 1 month to patients with cirrhosis and severe PH. The decrease in HVPG was significantly greater in the simvastatin group than in the placebo group. This decrease was observed with any deleterious effect on the systemic hemodynamic circulation. This outcome was observed in both patients who received NSSB and those who did not; however, the portal pressure lowering effect was enhanced in patients receiving concomitant NSSB. Such reduction supports the additive effect of simvastatin and NSSB on portal pressure. On the other hand, the administration of simvastatin markedly increased indocyanine green clearance, fractional clearance, and intrinsic clearance, an effect not observed in the placebo group, suggesting that simvastatin increased effective hepatic perfusion and improved liver function. In summary, this proof-of-concept study showed that simvastatin reduces portal pressure in patients with cirrhosis and PH by reducing hepatic vascular resistance without effects on systemic circulation, suggesting that the hemodynamic effects of simvastatin are selective at the hepatic level. Simvastatin lowers HVPG, whether patients are on NSBB or not. In addition, simvastatin upgrades liver function and provides potential additional benefits to NSBB treatment.

The largest multicenter RCT evaluating the effects of statins in patients with decompensated cirrhosis was the Bleeding Prevention With Simvastatin (BLEPS) trial that included 158 cirrhotic patients decompensated by variceal bleeding [86]. The patients were randomized to receive simvastatin or placebo added to NSBB and endoscopic variceal ligation as standard secondary prophylaxis to prevent rebleeding for 2 years. A major secondary endpoint was rebleeding. The complication rate did not decrease significantly with the addition of simvastatin to standard therapy (25%) compared to placebo (28%). No beneficial effect was seen on other variables associated with PH, such as ascites, spontaneous bacterial peritonitis, hepatorenal syndrome, portal vein thrombosis (PVT), need for rescue transjugular intrahepatic portosystemic shunt, need for transfusion, liver transplantation, and Model for

End-Stage Liver Disease (MELD) score between the two groups. The BLEPS trial showed that adding simvastatin to standard therapy did not prevent variceal rebleeding nor reduced the rate of other cirrhosis complications.

Pollo-Flores et al. showed that simvastatin therapy was associated with a decrease in HVPG, whereas no change was observed in patients treated with placebo. In addition, in 55% of patients treated with simvastatin, the decrease in HVPG was greater than 20%, indicating a clinically significant reduction in portal pressure in these patients, versus no decrease in HVPG for patients with placebo ($P = 0.030$). Moreover, they observed a slight improvement in liver function by Child-Pugh (CTP) score, at baseline 6.6 versus at the end of the trial 6.2 ($P = 0.080$). Thus, they concluded that simvastatin lowers portal pressure and may improve liver function [87].

On the basis that statins can modulate the liver microvasculature in patients with cirrhosis, another study was carried out comparing atorvastatin associated with propranolol versus propranolol alone [88]. This study demonstrated that atorvastatin plus propranolol versus propranolol alone was associated with a more significant decrease in the mean HVPG and clinically significant HVPG reduction. On the other hand, no significant differences were observed between the two groups in the complications of cirrhosis and death after 1 year of follow-up. In conclusion, the combination of atorvastatin and NSSB significantly reduces portal pressure by reducing hepatic vascular resistance.

Another study was carried out in India to analyze the effect of statins in patients who did not respond to carvedilol to evaluate a rescue therapy [89]. They included 102 patients with cirrhosis and significant PH. HVPG was measured at baseline and after 3 months of treatment with carvedilol. Initially, 64 patients (63%) responded favorably to carvedilol. The other patients were classified as non-responders to carvedilol and were treated with simvastatin 20 mg daily for 2 weeks. Of this second group, 3 had adverse effects for which the statins had to be discontinued. The other 35 patients continued with the combination therapy carvedilol and simvastatin, now at a dose of 40 mg per day. After 1 month, HVPG was measured again, showing that 16 patients were responders (46%) and 19 were not, with a global response to carvedilol reaching 78%. Therefore, these results provide an excellent sequential strategy in the medical therapy of PH.

A more recent study evaluated the combination of carvedilol and simvastatin as the primary prophylaxis of variceal bleeding [90]. Patients were randomized into two groups: one treated only with carvedilol and the other with carvedilol plus simvastatin. The primary endpoint of the study was the reduction of HVPG, and the secondary endpoints were cirrhosis complications and death. The results were that primary and secondary endpoints were similar between the two groups. In conclusion, this combination therapy did not reduce primary variceal bleeding and other cirrhosis complications –including death.

A recent RCT evaluated the hemodynamic changes caused by NSSB plus simvastatin using Doppler ultrasound in patients with cirrhosis and PH [91]. They included 20 patients treated with NSBB and 20 patients treated with NSBB plus simvastatin. An ultrasound control was performed 30 days later: only the combination group showed a significant reduction in the hepatic artery resistance indexes and portal hypertension. However, the modified liver vascular index increased in patients of the combination group. Therefore, as a general conclusion, simvastatin was associated with a significant decrease in PH and a significant increase in liver perfusion.

12.3.2 Decompensated Cirrhosis

New Concepts The natural history of cirrhosis comprises two phases, the first stage being an asymptomatic and generally extended phase named "compensated cirrhosis", lately followed by a usually rapidly progressing stage known as "decompensated cirrhosis" resulting from the development of cirrhosis complications [92]. The change from the first stage to the second one leads to a poorer quality of life and a significant increase in mortality rate from 1% to 57% per year [92]. The current approach to managing patients with decompensated cirrhosis is supported by strategies aiming to prevent or treat each complication. However, although RCT have proven the effectiveness of this approach in managing specific complications, so far it has only had a scant impact on the overall natural history of cirrhosis [93]. The systemic inflammatory hypothesis proposes that cirrhosis decompensation, hepatorenal syndrome-acute kidney injury, and acute-on-chronic liver failure (ACLF) develop from a progressive systemic inflammatory process [94]. As shown in Fig. 12.5, the key event underlying this abnormality is abnormal bacterial translocation (BT) from the gut, defined as the migration of bacteria or bacterial products from the intestinal lumen to mesenteric lymph nodes or other extra-intestinal organs and sites [95]. By increasing intestinal permeability, PH is a major determinant of BT and contributes to quantitative and qualitative changes in the microbiome, impaired immune defense mechanisms in the intestinal wall, and regional lymph nodes [95]. The systemic spread of bacteria and pathogen-associated molecular patterns owing to BT and danger-associated molecular patterns from the diseased liver activate innate host immunity. The consequent release of proinflammatory cytokines and chemokines, and oxidative and nitrosative species, leads to circulatory dysfunction, to which splanchnic arterial vasodilation induced by PH contributes. The direct effects of systemic inflammation and circulatory abnormalities ultimately lead to multiorgan failure [94].

Thus arose the concept of disease-modifying treatment, based on the disease-modifying agents. They act on the key pathophysiological mechanisms of cirrhosis, regardless of the complications present, to stop or slow its progression and even to induce "recompensation" [93, 96]. PH, BT ("upstream" events), and the consequent systemic inflammation and circulatory dysfunction ("downstream" events) represent the main targets for mechanistic approaches [96]. Human albumin and statins, which can simultaneously target several downstream pathophysiological mechanisms, represent promising disease-modifying agents, as they have proved their efficacy in prospective randomized trials [96].

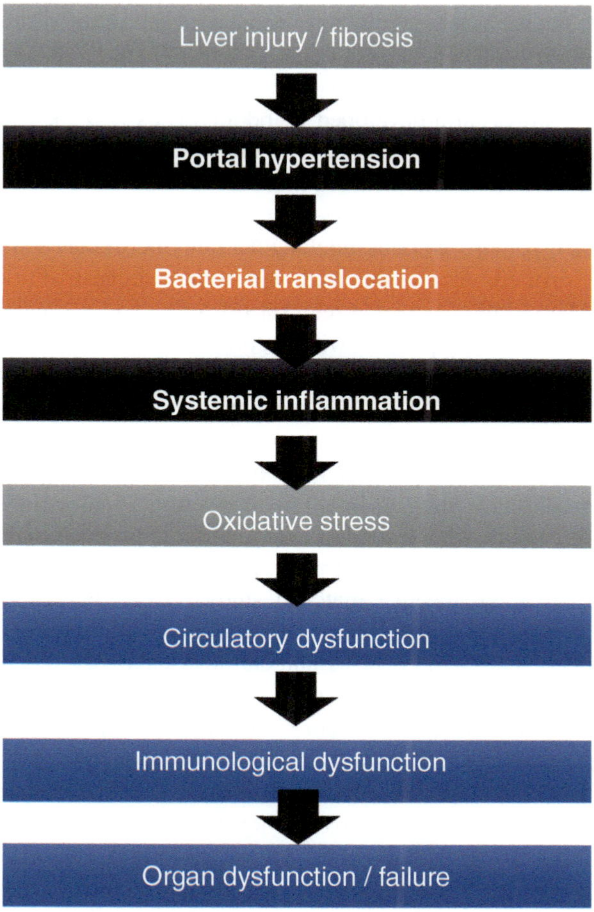

Fig. 12.5 The pathophysiological events of systemic inflammation hypothesis leading to multiorgan failure

Simvastatin Only three trials evaluated the survival of patients with decompensated cirrhosis after simvastatin administration for 1 year or more.

The BLEPS trial is the largest RCT that assessed the effects of statins in cirrhosis. In patients with variceal bleeding, simvastatin was added to standard prophylaxis to prevent rebleeding -NSBB and band ligation [86]. Patients were randomly assigned to receive simvastatin ($n = 69$) or placebo ($n = 78$) up to 2 years. The main endpoint was a composite of rebleeding or death. During a median follow-up of approximately 1 year, 30 out of 78 patients (39%) in the placebo group and 22 out of 69 patients (32%) in the simvastatin group reached the primary endpoint (hazard ratio [HR] = 0.82; $P = 0.420$). Nonetheless, when only death was evaluated, mortality was 22% in the placebo group compared to 9% in the simvastatin group (HR = 0.39; $P = 0.030$). Therefore, treatment with simvastatin was associated with a 61% reduction in the relative death risk than placebo. In a subgroup analysis, the effects of simvastatin on survival were quantitatively different in CTP class A/B patients from CTP class C patients. In CTP class A/B patients, an important outcome was a significant decrease in mortality with simvastatin, which was not observed in CTP class C patients (HR = 0.16; $P = 0.006$). There were no differences in the rate of cirrhosis complications between the two groups. Two out of 69 patients on simvastatin developed rhabdomyolysis (2.9%), which was a concerning issue considering an incidence of 0.009% to 0.1% in the general population [97]. The BLEPS trial demonstrated that adding simvastatin to the standard of care in patients who recover from an acute variceal bleeding episode improves survival in CTP class A/B patients without reducing the rate of cirrhosis complications.

An editorial of this trial, with a very suggestive title "Statins in Cirrhosis: The Magic Pill?," makes a relevant reflection and estimates the efficacy and safety of simvastatin in patients with decompensated cirrhosis [98]. First, they point out that the improvement in survival observed with the addition of simvastatin to the standard treatment of variceal bleeding was not related to reducing complications, further wondering if simvastatin would be associated with some improvement of an unknown liver function or mechanism. Alternatively, they also considered if it would have any anti-inflammatory action. Finally, they calculated that the number of patients who needed to treat in order to produce rhabdomyolysis was 25, and the number who needed to treat to prevent one death was 8.

In a retrospective, matched, study of cases (agreed to add simvastatin to standard treatment) and series (did not agree to add simvastatin), the survival of patients with decompensated cirrhosis and cardiovascular risk factors was evaluated [99]. Nine patients were included in each group and were matched 1:1 by age, gender, etiology, CTP score, and MELD score. The median survival in the case group was 107 months, whereas it was 20 months in the series group (HR = 0.14; $P < 0.0001$). This outcome was attributed to two findings, the first due to reducing the number of cirrhosis complications. In that regard, during the follow-up period, the mean interval between cirrhosis complications in the case group was 33.6 ± 19.9 months versus the series group, 9.4 ± 8.2 months, $P = 0.0065$. Secondly, there was a significant increase of cirrhosis severity at the end of the study versus baseline, evaluated through CTP and MELD scores in the series group while it was not affected in the case group. Thus, this study showed that the addition of simvastatin to the standard therapy in patients with decompensated cirrhosis and cardiovascular risk factors is clinically relevant compared to standard treatment since such intervention improved survival.

Simvastatin could be considered a disease-modifying agent from a recent publication presented in abstract form only [100]. After its administration to patients with decompensated cirrhosis, up to 1 year was demonstrated an improvement of quality of life, a reduction in hospital readmissions due to cirrhosis complications compared to the year before the study, a decrease in the burden on health care, and that no patient developed ACLF. Finally, the survival rate was 90%.

12.3.3 Hepatocellular Carcinoma

Hepatocellular carcinoma (HCC) is the most common worldwide type of liver cancer [101, 102], the sixth most common malignancy, and the third leading cause of cancer-related deaths [103]. Most HCC develops in patients with cirrhosis, and the most common etiologies are hepatitis B virus, hepatitis C virus, alcohol, and nonalcoholic fatty liver disease [101, 102].

So far, the best curative therapeutic option for HCC is surgery -resection or liver transplantation -EASL clinical practice guidelines: Management of hepatocellular carcinoma 2018, however, most patients are usually diagnosed with unresectable HCC due to advanced-stage disease, high-risk comorbidities, or limited resources. For these patients, systemic therapy is indicated [104] using sorafenib as first-line treatment and is currently widely used to treat patients with advanced HCC [105].

Two major phase III RCTs showed that sorafenib significantly increased overall survival (OS) and time to progression (TP) compared with placebo [106, 107]. These results allowed the approval of sorafenib as a standard treatment for patients with advanced HCC.

Lenvatinib is non-inferior to sorafenib in terms of OS benefit [103]; however, the median OS remains poor and limited in both therapeutic settings [103]. Considering that most patients have unresectable diseases and the clinical limitations of available drugs, there is an urgent need for more effective systemic treatments [104]. In this regard, drug combination strategies, when sorafenib is used, could be a promising approach [108].

The mevalonate pathway is an essential metabolic pathway that utilizes acetyl-CoA to produce sterols and isoprenoids essential for tumor growth and progression [107]. Since statins are inhibitors of HMG-CoA reductase, they block the production of mevalonate and its metabolites.

Chronic administration of statins is safe and effective for patients with hypercholesterolemia [15]. In addition, different studies showed there is an association between statin use and lower risk of developing colon, breast, esophageal, and prostate cancer [109].

Statins could even exert pleiotropic effects on HCC, including antiproliferative, antioxidant, anti-inflammatory, and antifibrotic effects [108]. In particular, pravastatin showed in vitro and in vivo inhibition of HCC growth via promoting tumor cells apoptosis [110, 111]. In addition, pravastatin is the only statin investigated in clinical trials that evaluated potential benefits over HCC. It was studied in association with sorafenib, transcatheter arterial embolization (TACE), and 5-fluorouracil.

The ESTAHEP (Efficacy and Safety of the Combination of Pravastatin and Sorafenib for the Treatment of Advanced Hepatocellular Carcinoma) study [112] evaluated the efficacy and safety of the combination of sorafenib and pravastatin on OS and PT in 31 patients with advanced HCC -of whom 77% were classified as Barcelona Clinic Liver Cancer (BCLC) stage C and CTP class A, and there were no differences in OS compared with placebo group. However, radiological TP was higher in patients treated with sorafenib associated with pravastatin compared with the control group (9.9 months versus 3.2 months; $P = 0.008$). Two independent variables were associated with lower OS: PVT (6.3 months versus 14.8 months) ($P = 0.026$) and vascular invasion (VI) (6.3 months versus 14.8 months) ($P = 0.041$).

The PRODIGE 21 study also evaluated the use of pravastatin alone or in combination with sorafenib in CTP class B patients. Patients were randomized to receive either sorafenib or pravastatin, the combination of both, or the best supportive care. The primary endpoint was TP, and the secondary endpoints were OS and safety. A total of 157 patients were included, of whom 86% were BCLC stage C, and 55% had a VI. Median TP was 3.5, 2.8, 2.0, and 2.2 months respectively, but the number of patients who died without radiological progression (59%) limited the analysis. Median OS was similar among the four groups: 3.8, 3.1, 4.0, and 3.5 months, respectively. The median OS was 4.0 months for all patients that received sorafenib in any form, compared with 2.9 months for patients that did not receive sorafenib. The trial concluded that neither sorafenib nor pravastatin provided significant benefit in terms of OS. As shown in other studies, VI is a variable associated with decreased survival rate [113].

Another investigation [114] -more or less in line with the PRODIGE 11 trial-evaluated the effect of sorafenib versus sorafenib plus pravastatin in a population with advanced HCC and CTP class A. The primary objective was OS, and the secondary one was progression-free survival. It showed to be a negative trial, as no differences in the objectives were observed between the two groups.

Regarding the trials using TACE, pravastatin was evaluated in CTP classes A and B patients undergoing TACE, followed by oral 5-fluorouracil 200 mg/day for 2 months. Patients were then randomly assigned to a control group (n = 42) or a pravastatin 40 mg/day group (n = 41). The primary endpoint was mortality from HCC progression. Pravastatin was administered for 16.5 ± 9.8 months. Median survival was 18 months in the pravastatin group and 9 months in controls ($P = 0.006$). Moreover, the multivariate analysis also demonstrated that pravastatin was associated with increased survival ($P = 0.005$), and the effect of VI in reducing survival. This observation suggests pravastatin would be useful as adjuvant therapy [115].

Subsequently, another prospective study included 183 patients with advanced HCC that were treated with TACE. Of the total, 52 patients were associated with pravastatin. The primary study objective was OS. Median survival was significantly increased in HCC patients treated with TACE and pravastatin (20.9 months) compared with patients treated with TACE alone (12.0 months) ($P = 0.003$). The results of this trial were encouraging; however, the study was limited in terms of the fact that it was not an RCT, nor was it double-blinded [116].

As already mentioned, pravastatin was associated with extending TP in patients with CTP class A [112]. In addition, the mevalonate pathway may mediate this result, associated with pro-apoptotic, antiproliferative, anti-inflammatory, and antifibrotic effects [108]. Indeed, it is known that simultaneous targeted inhibition of RAF/MEK/ERK with the combination of sorafenib and lovastatin demonstrated potent cytostatic/cytotoxic effects in tumor cell lines [117]. In addition, high doses of statins were associated with a reduction of HCC in patients with hepatitis C [118], which was mainly observed in patients with cirrhosis and others with diabetes mellitus [73].

Finally, a meta-analysis demonstrated that the use of statins is associated with a 37% HCC reduction risk in patients with liver disease. This chemoprotective association was primarily seen in the Asian and Western populations, where the most critical risk factors are the hepatitis B virus and the metabolic syndrome, respectively [119].

12.4 Safety

Over the population without liver disease, there were two aspects considered in terms of statin-associated adverse events, and these should also be carefully looked at in patients with chronic liver disease: hepatotoxicity and nocebo effect.

According to Bader, it is a myth that statins induce hepatotoxicity and that there is a legend supporting the fact that isolated serum alanine aminotransferase (ALT) elevation associated with statin therapy is harmful [120]. He also claims that this supposed fable arose from the 1978 Fogarty conference, where a three-fold increase in ALT value compared with normal (ULN) was considered "markedly abnormal" and should be used as an indicator for drug-induced liver injury. Sadly, there was little -if any- proof offered for this recommendation. Nevertheless, this arbitrary measure became a standard for monitoring drugs in clinical trials. In the 1980s, studies involving statins were just getting started, and since then, they have been observed to cause mild ALT elevations in up to 10% of recipients, and in 1–3% of patients, these increments are more than three times the ULN [121]. In this regard, a recent US nationwide survey of primary care physicians replied that they would be unlikely to prescribe statins to patients with proven indications if the subjects had elevated ALT values. In addition, these findings suggest that concern about hepatotoxicity may prevent and/or abbreviate the use of statins in cases where cardiovascular benefits could arise from these drugs [122]. It is essential to highlight that studies have demonstrated that statins would be safe in patients with hyperlipidemia and chronic liver disease and cirrhosis CTP class A [123] and could prevent cardiovascular events in non-alcoholic fatty liver disease [124].

The second aspect is the nocebo effect, a term coined in 1961 by Kennedy that denotes the counterpart of placebo [125]. This effect reflects changes in human psychobiology that affect the brain, body, and behavior rather than drug toxicity. Reports of statin-associated muscle adverse events could be due to negative press reports on using those drugs [126, 127], or confusing warnings regarding statin-associated side effects [128]. These adverse effects may lead to a poor treatment adherence -or even discontinuation of statins, and would also be associated with an increased risk of cardiovascular events and cardiovascular mortality [126, 127]. Therefore, physicians should be fully informed about possible nocebo effects and patients' knowledge or wrong perception of statin treatment and discuss with subjects the evidence about statin-associated muscle events. Finally, two trials demonstrate that the nocebo effect leads to risky discontinuation and underutilization of statins by patients with cardiovascular risk factors [129, 130].

Statins are safe drugs in patients with chronic liver disease and those with compensated cirrhosis, but there is little information on the safety of statins in patients with decompensated cirrhosis [131]. In addition, some authors have conjectured that they would be less safe because of altered metabolism due to liver failure [86].

The adverse events associated with statins over the general population are frequent, relatively mild, and transient. The most commonly reported are diarrhea, abdominal pain, meteorism, constipation, and headache [132]; however, others cause special concern, such as muscle damage, liver injury, and new-onset diabetes [133].

From the results of studies in Cardiology, statins are associated with a broad spectrum of muscle injury from asymptomatic elevations of serum creatine kinase (CK) to rhabdomyolysis [134], ranging from 1–5% in RCTs and 11–29% in observational studies [97].

In the European multicenter LIVERHOPE-SAFETY phase 2 RCT, patients with decompensated cirrhosis were randomly assigned to receive for 12 weeks either: simvastatin 40 mg/day plus rifaximin 1200 mg/day (SVT40 + RFX), simvastatin 20 mg/day plus rifaximin 1200 mg/day (SVT20 + RFX), or placebo of both drugs in a 1: 1: 1 ratio. Patients in the SVT40 + RFX group showed increased CK at the end of treatment compared with patients in the placebo group (1.060 IU/L vs. 106 IU/L, $P = 0.014$). No significant changes in CK levels were observed in the SVT20 + RFX group versus the placebo group. Three patients (19%) in the SVT40 + RFX group developed liver and muscle toxicity compatible with rhabdomyolysis [135]. Only in a prospective, open-label, uncontrolled, phase 2a trial, the safety of simvastatin was evaluated in 30 patients with decompensated cirrhosis (CTP class A [$n = 6$], CTP class B [$n = 22$], and CTP class C [$n = 2$]) receiving 40 mg/day up to one year. Muscle injury was observed in 36.7% of patients, and it was associated to a baseline MELD score > 12 ($P = 0.035$) and a baseline CTP class C ($P = 0.020$). The simvastatin was transiently reduced to 10 mg/day by myalgia in 23.4% of patients, and simvastatin was transiently discontinued in 13.3% of patients by myonecrosis. In conclusion, muscle injury is the only clinically significant adverse event because it required modification of simvastatin dosing. Furthermore, muscle injury was related to simvastatin dose, 40 mg/day, in agreement with the LIVERHOPE-SAFETY trial observation, and the severity degree of cirrhosis, with a MELD score > 12 and CTP class C [136].

The other major adverse event related to statin use is liver injury. The most common pattern of liver injury is hepatocellular—however, a mixed pattern with prolonged symptomatic cholestasis [137].

In the LIVERHOPE-SAFETY trial, due to data safety monitoring board recommendations, 10 patients were prematurely discontinued in the SVT40 + RFX group due to serious hepatic adverse events (grade 3) [135]. In addition, the SVT40 + RFX group showed a significant increase in aspartate aminotransferase (AST) and ALT compared with the SVT20 + RFX ($P = 0.025$) and placebo groups ($P = 0.0009$). At week 12, there were no significant differences observed in AST and ALT levels between the SVT20 + RFX and placebo groups. It is also to be noted that the number of patients who discontinued treatment due to adverse events was significantly higher in the SVT40 + RFX group (56%) compared with the other two groups (14%) ($P = 0.017$). In conclusion, in patients with decompensated cirrhosis, SVT40 + RFX was associated with a significant increase in adverse events, specifically liver and muscle toxicity, requiring discontinuation of treatment compared with SVT20 + RFX and placebo. On the other hand, in the other safety study, no patient developed a liver injury. Conversely, when comparing values at the end of the trial with values at baseline, AST was slightly decreased, serum ALT was markedly decreased (32 ± 16 versus 39 ± 20 IU/L, respectively; $P = 0.090$), and serum alkaline phosphatase was significantly decreased (119 ± 48 versus 147 ± 67 IU/L, respectively; $P = 0.020$) [136]. In summary, due to the muscle and liver adverse events related to simvastatin 40 mg/day, both safety studies recommend the administration of simvastatin at no more than 20 mg/day in future clinical trials involving patients with decompensated cirrhosis [135, 136].

12.5 Summary and Conclusions

Initially, statins were assessed as liver-specific NO-donors to decrease PH, and as such, they were deemed as a sequential strategy when carvedilol does not reduce HVPG. However, it came out as an important observation that statins alone did not prevent variceal rebleeding.

Statins reduce portal pressure by reducing hepatic vascular resistance with or without the administration of NSBB and could improve liver function. The largest RCT in patients with decompensated cirrhosis (BLEPS trial) demonstrated that the addition of simvastatin to standard therapy did not reduce variceal rebleeding but increased survival. According to the systemic inflammation hypothesis, experimental and clinical trials suggested that statins could be disease-modifying drugs in decompensated cirrhosis, and a recent study published in abstract form would confirm this outcome. Statins could be helpful in the prevention of early stages of HCC in patients with various chronic liver diseases, as well as being associated with other therapeutic procedures in advanced HCC stages. In patients with cirrhosis, the most clinically significant adverse event is statin-related myopathy, and this may be related to high serum statin concentrations in the setting of severely impaired liver function. In agreement with the LIVERHOPE-SAFETY trial findings, patients with decompensated cirrhosis should be administered with simvastatin up to 20 mg/day. Likewise, based on a safety trial, it is advised not to prescribe a simvastatin dose of 40 mg/day in patients with cirrhosis CTP class C and/or MELD score > 12 due to potential severe muscle injury.

The road of statins in Cardiology was challenging; however, the rationale and background for their use in Hepatology arose from here. Unfortunately, the use of statins in Hepatology will continue to be hampered due to the scarcity and poor quality of research in this matter: for these reasons, further RCTs should be performed over a more significant number of patients, with hard clinical endpoints, and using different statins and dosage [138, 139]. These outcomes will enable the safe and effective endorsement of statins in patients with hepatic diseases to prevent liver-related morbidity and mortality.

Conflict of Interest The authors declare no conflicts of interest.

Financial Support No funding was received to design and undertake this study and to write this manuscript. In most cases, when research and studies are initiated and conducted in Argentina by the researchers, there is no funding from any public or private institution as they are made with financial contributions from the researchers.

References

1. Steinberg D, Gotto AM Jr. Preventing coronary artery disease by lowering cholesterol levels: fifty years from bench to bedside. JAMA. 1999;82:2043–50.
2. Dawber TR, Kannel WB, Revotskie N, et al. Some factors associated with the development of coronary heart disease. Six years' follow-up experience in the Framingham study. Am J Public Health Nations Health. 1959;49:1349–56.
3. Tobert JA. Lovastatin and beyond: the history of the HMG-COA reductase inhibitors. Nat Rev Drug Discov. 2003;2:517–26.
4. Kirby TJ. Cataracts produced by triparanol. Trans Am Ophthalmol Soc. 1967;65:494–543.
5. Endo A, Kuroda M, Tsujita Y. ML-236A, ML-236B, and ML-236C, new inhibitors of cholesterogenesis produced by penicillium citrinium. J Antibiot. 1976;29:1346–8.
6. Endo A, Kuroda M, Tanzawa K. Competitive inhibition of 3-hydroxy-3-methylglutaryl coenzyme a reductase by ML-236a and ML-236b fungal metabolites, having hypocholesterolemic activity. FEBS Lett. 1976;72:323–6.
7. Endo A, Tsujita Y, Kuroda M, et al. Inhibition of cholesterol synthesis in vitro and in vivo by ML-236A and ML-236B, competitive inhibitors of 3-hydroxy-3methylglutaryl-coenzyme a reductase. Eur J Biochem. 1977;77:31–6.
8. Alberts AW, Chen J, Kuron G, Hunt V, et al. Mevinolin: a highly potent competitive inhibitor of hydroxymethylglutaryl-coenzyme a reductase and a cholesterol-lowering agent. Proc Natl Acad Sci U S A. 1980;77:3957–61.
9. Bilheimer DW, Grundy SM, Brown MS, et al. Mevinolin and colestipol stimulate receptor-mediated clearance of low density lipoprotein from plasma in familial hypercholesterolemia heterozygotes. Proc Natl Acad Sci U S A. 1983;80:4124–8.
10. Illingworth DR, Sexton GJ. Hypocholesterolemic effects of mevinolin in patients with heterozygous familial hypercholesterolemia. J Clin Invest. 1984;74:1972–8.
11. Lovastatin Study Group II. Therapeutic response to lovastatin (mevinolin) in nonfamilial hypercholesterolemia. A multicenter study. JAMA. 1986;256:2829–34.
12. Lovastatin Study Group III. A multicenter comparison of lovastatin and cholestyramine therapy for severe primary hypercholesterolemia. JAMA. 1989;260:359–66.
13. Lovastatin Study Group IV. A multicenter comparison of lovastatin and probucol for the treatment of severe primary hypercholesterolemia. Am J Cardiol. 1990;66:22B–30B.
14. Tobert JA, Shear CL, Chremos AN, et al. Clinical experience with lovastatin. Am J Cardiol. 1990;65:23F–6F.
15. Scandinavian Simvastatin Survival Study Group. Randomised trial of cholesterol lowering in 4444 patients with coronary heart disease: the Scandinavian simvastatin survival study (4S). Lancet. 1994;344:1383–9.
16. Bolego C, Baetta R, Bellosta S, et al. Safety considerations for statins. Curr Opin Lipidol. 2002;13:637–44.
17. Ballantyne CM, Corsini A, Davidson MH, et al. Risk for myopathy with statin therapy in high-risk patients. Arch Intern Med. 2003;163:553–64.
18. Heart Protection Study Collaborative Group. MRC/BHF heart protection study of cholesterol lowering with simvastatin in 20.536 high-risk individuals: a randomized placebo-controlled trial. Lancet. 2002;360:7–22.
19. Bosch J. Vascular deterioration in cirrhosis. The big picture. J Clin Gastroenterol. 2007;41:S247–53.

20. Bhathal PS, Grossman HJ. Reduction of the increased portal vascular resistance of the isolated perfused cirrhotic rat liver by vasodilators. J Hepatol. 1985;1:325–37.
21. Marteau P, Ballet F, Chazouilleres O, et al. Effect of vasodilators on hepatic microcirculation in cirrhosis: a study in the isolated perfused rat liver. Hepatology. 1989;9:820–3.
22. Bosch J, Abraldes JG, Groszmann RJ. Current management of portal hypertension. J Hepatol. 2003;38:S54–68.
23. Gupta TK, Toruner M, Chung MK, et al. Endothelial dysfunction and decreased production of nitric oxide in the intrahepatic microcirculation of cirrhotic rats. Hepatology. 1998;28:926–31.
24. Rockey DC, Chung JJ. Reduced nitric oxide production by endothelial cells in cirrhotic rat liver: endothelial dysfunction in portal hypertension. Gastroenterology. 1998;114:344–51.
25. Shah V, Toruner M, Haddad F, et al. Impaired endothelial nitric oxide synthase activity associated with enhanced caveolin binding in experimental cirrhosis in the rat. Gastroenterology. 1999;117:1222–8.
26. Shah V, Cao S, Hendrickson H, et al. Regulation of hepatic eNOS by caveolin and calmodulin after bile duct ligation in rats. Am J Physiol Gastrointest Liver Physiol. 2001;280:G1209–16.
27. Bellis L, Berzigotti A, Abraldes JG, et al. Low doses of isosorbide mononitrate attenuate the postprandial increase in portal pressure in patients with cirrhosis. Hepatology. 2003;37:378–84.
28. Ceriello A, Taboga C, Tonutti L, et al. Evidence for an independent and cumulative effect of postprandial hypertriglyceridemia and hyperglycemia on endothelial dysfunction and oxidative stress generation: effects of short- and long-term simvastatin treatment. Circulation. 2002;106:1211–8.
29. Van de Casteele M, Omasta A, Janssens S, et al. In vivo gene transfer of endothelial nitric oxide synthase decreases portal pressure in anaesthetised carbon tetrachloride cirrhotic rats. Gut. 2002;51:440–5.
30. Sarela AI, Mihaimeed FM, Batten JJ, et al. Hepatic and splanchnic nitric oxide activity in patients with cirrhosis. Gut. 1999;44:749–53.
31. Shah V. Cellular and molecular basis of portal hypertension. Clin Liver Dis. 2001;5:629–44.
32. Wiest R, Groszmann RJ. The paradox of nitric oxide in cirrhosis and portal hypertension: too much, not enough. Hepatology. 2002;35:478–91.
33. Russell R. Atherosclerosis - an inflammatory disease. N Engl J Med. 1999;340:115–26.
34. Goldstein JL, Brown MS. Regulation of the mevalonate pathway. Nature. 1990;343:425–30.
35. Van Aelst L, D'Souza-Schorey C. Rho GTPases and signaling networks. Genes Dev. 1997;11:2295–322.
36. Hall A. Rho GTPases and the actin cytoskeleton. Science. 1998;279:509–14.
37. Shimizu T, Liao JK. Rho kinases and cardiac remodeling. Circ J. 2016;80:1491–8.
38. Wolfrum S, Jensen KS, Liao JK. Endothelium-dependent effects of statins. Arterioscler Thromb Vasc Biol. 2003;23:729–36.
39. Oesterle A, Laufs U, Liao JK. Pleiotropic effects of statins on the cardiovascular system. Circ Res. 2017;120:229–43.
40. Steinberg D, Parthasarathy S, Carew TE, et al. Beyond cholesterol. Modifications of low-density lipoprotein that increase its atherogenicity. N Engl J Med. 1989;320:915–24.
41. Harrison DG. Perspective series: nitric oxide and nitric oxide synthases cellular and molecular. Mechanisms of endothelial cell dysfunction. J Clin Invest. 1997;100:2153–7.
42. Liao JK. Inhibition of Gi proteins by low density lipoprotein attenuates bradykinin-stimulated release of endothelial-derived nitric oxide. J Biol Chem. 1994;269:12987–92.
43. Alderson LM, Endemann G, Lindsey S, et al. LDL enhances monocyte adhesion to endothelial cells in vitro. Am J Pathol. 1986;123:334–42.
44. Plenz GAM, Oliver Hofnagel O, Robenek H. Differential modulation of caveolin-1 expression in cells of the vasculature by statins. Circulation. 2004;109:e7–8.
45. Kureishi Y, Luo Z, Shiojima I, Bialik A, et al. The HMG-CoA reductase inhibitor simvastatin activates the protein kinase Akt and promotes angiogenesis in normocholesterolemic animals. Nat Med. 2000;6:1004–10.

46. Dimmeler S, Fleming I, Fisslthaler B, et al. Activation of nitric oxide synthase in endothelial cells by Akt-dependent phosphorylation. Nature. 1999;399:601–5.
47. Wolfrum S, Dendorfer A, Rikitake Y, et al. Inhibition of rho-kinase leads to rapid activation of phosphatidylinositol 3-kinase/protein kinase Akt and cardiovascular protection. Arterioscler Thromb Vasc Biol. 2004;24:1842–7.
48. Laufs U, Liao JK. Post-transcriptional regulation of endothelial nitric oxide synthase mRNA stability by rho GTPase. J Biol Chem. 1998;273:24266–71.
49. Sen-Banerjee S, Mir S, Lin Z, et al. Kruppel-like factor 2 as a novel mediator of statin effects in endothelial cells. Circulation. 2005;112:720–6.
50. Martin JE, Cavanaugh TM, Trumbull L, et al. Incidence of adverse events with HMG-CoA reductase inhibitors in liver transplant patients. Clin Transpl. 2008;22:113–9.
51. Trebicka J, Hennenberg M, Laleman W, et al. Atorvastatin lowers portal pressure in cirrhotic rats by inhibition of RhoA/Rho-kinase and activation of endothelial nitric oxide synthase. Hepatology. 2007;46:242–53.
52. Trebicka J, Hennenberg M, Odenthal M, et al. Atorvastatin attenuates hepatic fibrosis in rats after bile duct ligation via decreased turnover of hepatic stellate cells. J Hepatol. 2010;53:702–12.
53. Klein S, Klosel J, Schierwagen R, et al. Atorvastatin inhibits proliferation and apoptosis, but induces senescence in hepatic myofibroblasts and thereby attenuates hepatic fibrosis in rats. Lab Investig. 2012;92:1440–50.
54. Abraldes JG, Rodriguez-Vilarrupla A, Graupera M, et al. Simvastatin treatment improves liver sinusoidal endothelial dysfunction in CCl4 cirrhotic rats. J Hepatol. 2007;46:1040–6.
55. Marrone G, Russo L, Rosado E, et al. The transcription factor KLF2 mediates hepatic endothelial protection and paracrine endothelial-stellate cell deactivation induced by statins. J Hepatol. 2013;58:98–103.
56. Marrone G, Maeso-Diaz R, Garcia-Cardena G, et al. KLF2 exerts antifibrotic and vasoprotective effects in cirrhotic rat livers: behind the molecular mechanisms of statins. Gut. 2015;64:1434–43.
57. Schierwagen R, Maybüchen L, Hittatiya K, et al. Statins improve NASH via inhibition of RhoA and Ras. Am J Physiol Gastrointest Liver Physiol. 2016;311:G724–33.
58. Jain MK, Ridker PM. Anti-inflammatory effects of statins: clinical evidence and basic mechanisms. Nat Rev Drug Discov. 2005;4:977–87.
59. La Mura V, Pasarin M, Meireles CZ, et al. Effects of simvastatin administration on rodents with lipopolysaccharide-induced liver microvascular dysfunction. Hepatology. 2013;57:1172–81.
60. Wagner AH, Schwabe O, Hecker M. Atorvastatin inhibition of cytokine inducible nitric oxide synthase expression in native endothelial cells in situ. Br J Pharmacol. 2002;136:143–9.
61. Huang KC, Chen CW, Chen JC, et al. HMG-CoA reductase inhibitors inhibit inducible nitric oxide synthase gene expression in macrophages. J Biomed Sci. 2003;10:396–405.
62. Relja B, Meder F, Wang M, et al. Simvastatin modulates the adhesion and growth of hepatocellular carcinoma cells via decrease of integrin expression and ROCK. Int J Oncol. 2011;38:879–85.
63. Zafra C, Abraldes JG, Turnes J, et al. Simvastatin enhances hepatic nitric oxide production and decreases the hepatic vascular tone in patients with cirrhosis. Gastroenterology. 2004;126:749–55.
64. Abraldes JG, Albillos A, Bañares R, et al. Simvastatin lowers portal pressure in patients with cirrhosis and portal hypertension: a randomized controlled trial. Gastroenterology. 2009;136:1651–8.
65. Motzkus-Feagans C, Pakyz AL, Ratliff SM, et al. Statin use and infections in veterans with cirrhosis. Aliment Pharmacol Ther. 2013;38:611–8.
66. Kumar S, Grace ND, Qamar AA. Statin use in patients with cirrhosis: a retrospective cohort study. Dig Dis Sci. 2014;59:1958–65.
67. Simon TG, King LY, Zheng H, et al. Statin use is associated with a reduced risk of fibrosis progression in chronic hepatitis C. J Hepatol. 2015;62:18–23.

68. Yang YH, Chen WC, Tsan YT, et al. Statin use and the risk of cirrhosis development in patients with hepatitis C virus infection. J Hepatol. 2015;63:1111–7.
69. Hsiang JC, Wong GLH, Tse YK, et al. Statin and the risk of hepatocellular carcinoma and death in a hospital-based hepatitis B-infected population: a propensity score landmark analysis. J Hepatol. 2015;63:1190–7.
70. Mohanty A, Tate JP, Garcia-Tsao G. Statins are associated with a decreased risk of decompensation and death in veterans with hepatitis C-related compensated cirrhosis. Gastroenterology. 2016;150:430–40.e1.
71. Bang UC, Benfield T, Bendtsen F. Reduced risk of decompensation and death associated with use of statins in patients with alcoholic cirrhosis. A nationwide case-cohort study. Aliment Pharmacol Ther. 2017;46:673–80.
72. Chang FM, Wang YP, Lang HC, et al. Statins decrease the risk of decompensation in hepatitis B virus- and hepatitis C virus-related cirrhosis: a population-based study. Hepatology. 2017;66:896–907.
73. Kim G, Jang SY, Nam CM, et al. Statin use and the risk of hepatocellular carcinoma in patients at high risk: a nationwide nested case-control study. J Hepatol. 2018;68:476–84.
74. Kaplan DE, Serper MA, Mehta R, et al. Effects of hypercholesterolemia and statin exposure on survival in a large national cohort of patients with cirrhosis. Gastroenterology. 2019;156:1693–1706.e12.
75. Sano M, Bell KL, Galasko D, et al. A randomized, double-blind, placebo-controlled trial of simvastatin to treat Alzheimer disease. Neurology. 2011;77:556–63.
76. Papazian L, Roch A, Charles PE, et al. Effect of statin therapy on mortality in patients with ventilator associated pneumonia: a randomized clinical trial. JAMA. 2013;310:1692–700.
77. McAuley DF, Laffey JG, O'Kane CM, et al. Simvastatin in the acute respiratory distress syndrome. N Engl J Med. 2014;371:1695–703.
78. Kamm CP, El-Koussy M, Humpert S, et al. Atorvastatin added to interferon beta for relapsing multiple sclerosis: 12-month treatment extension of the randomized multicenter SWABIMS trial. PLoS One. 2014;9:e86663.
79. Kim ST, Kang JH, Lee J, et al. Simvastatin plus capecitabine-cisplatin versus placebo plus capecitabine cisplatin in patients with previously untreated advanced gastric cancer: a double-blind randomised phase 3 study. Eur J Cancer. 2014;50:2822–30.
80. Dhamija P, Hota D, Kochhar R, et al. Randomized clinical trial: atorvastatin versus placebo in patients with acute exacerbation of mild to moderate ulcerative colitis. Indian J Gastroenterol. 2014;33:151–6.
81. John ME, Cockcroft JR, McKeever TM, et al. Cardiovascular and inflammatory effects of simvastatin therapy in patients with COPD: a randomized controlled trial. Int J Chron Obstruct Pulm Dis. 2015;10:211–21.
82. Garcia-Pagan JC, Groszmann RJ, Bosch J. Portal hypertension. In: Weinstein WM, Hawkey CJ, Bosch J, editors. Clinical gastroenterology and hepatology, vol. 2005. Philadelphia: Elsevier Mosby; 2005. p. 707–16.
83. Berzigotti A, Seijo S, Reverter E, et al. Assessing portal hypertension in liver diseases. Rev Gastroenterol Hepatol. 2013;7:141–55.
84. Ripoll C, Groszmann R, Garcia-Tsao G, et al. Hepatic venous pressure gradient predicts clinical decompensation in patients with compensated cirrhosis. Gastroenterology. 2007;133:481–8.
85. Cadelina G, Shah V, Choo K, et al. Elevated portal pressure in mice with targeted disruption of the gene for endothelial nitric oxide synthase. Hepatology. 2002;32:A12.
86. Abraldes JG, Villanueva C, Aracil C, et al. Addition of simvastatin to standard therapy for the prevention of variceal rebleeding does not reduce rebleeding but increases survival in patients with cirrhosis. Gastroenterology. 2016;150:1160–70.e3.
87. Pollo-Flores P, Soldan M, Santos U, et al. Three months of simvastatin therapy vs. placebo for severe portal hypertension in cirrhosis: a randomized controlled trial. Dig Liver Dis. 2015;47:957–63.

88. Bishnu S, Ahammed SM, Sarkar A, et al. Effects of atorvastatin on portal hemodynamics and clinical outcomes in patients with cirrhosis with portal hypertension: a proof of concept study. Eur J Gastroenterol Hepatol. 2018;30:54–9.
89. Wani ZA, Mohapatra S, Khan AA. Addition of simvastatin to carvedilol non responders: a new pharmacological therapy for treatment of portal hypertension. World J Hepatol. 2017;9:270–7.
90. Vijayaraghavan R, Jindal A, Arora V, et al. Hemodynamic effects of adding simvastatin to carvedilol for primary prophylaxis of variceal bleeding: a randomized controlled trial. Am J Gastroenterol. 2020;115:729–37.
91. Elwan N, Salah R, Hamisa M, et al. Evaluation of portal pressure by doppler ultrasound in patients with cirrhosis before and after simvastatin administration - a randomized controlled trial. F1000Res. 2018;7:256.
92. D'Amico G, Garcia-Tsao G, Pagliaro L. Natural history and prognostic indicators of survival in cirrhosis: a systematic review of 118 studies. J Hepatol. 2006;44:217–31.
93. Caraceni P, Abraldes JG, Gines P, et al. The search for disease-modifying agents in decompensated cirrhosis: from drug repurposing to drug discovery. J Hepatol. 2021;75:S118–34.
94. Bernardi M, Moreau R, Angeli P, et al. Mechanisms of decompensation and organ failure in cirrhosis: from peripheral arterial vasodilation to systemic inflammation hypothesis. J Hepatol. 2015;63:1272–84.
95. Wiest R, Lawson M, Geuking M. Pathological bacterial translocation in liver cirrhosis. J Hepatol. 2014;60:197–209.
96. Bernardi M, Caraceni P. Novel perspectives in the management of decompensated cirrhosis. Nat Rev Gastroenterol Hepatol. 2018;15:753–64.
97. Thompson PD, Panza G, Zaleski A, et al. Statin-associated side effects. J Am Coll Cardiol. 2016;67:2395–410.
98. Malizia G, D'Amico G. Statins in cirrhosis: the magic pill? Hepatology. 2016;63:2047–9.
99. Muñoz AE, Taddey W, Salgado P. Addition of simvastatin to the standard therapy increases survival and is safe in patients with decompensated cirrhosis. Gastroenterol Hepatol. 2019;4:1–5.
100. Muñoz AE, Pollarsky F, Marino M, et al. Further analysis of simvastatin safety trial in patients with decompensated cirrhosis provides promising information about improving liver function and reducing cirrhosis severity. J Hepatol. 2021;75:S346.
101. Baecker A, Liu X, La Vecchia C, et al. Worldwide incidence of hepatocellular carcinoma cases attributable to major risk factors. Eur J Cancer Prev. 2018;27:205–12.
102. Yang JD, Hainaut P, Gores GJ, et al. A global view of hepatocellular carcinoma: trends, risk, prevention and management. Nat Rev Gastroenterol Hepatol. 2019;16:589–604.
103. Forner A, Reig M, Bruix J. Hepatocellular carcinoma. Lancet. 2018;391:1301–14.
104. Saffo S, Taddei TH. Systemic management for advanced hepatocellular carcinoma: a review of the molecular pathways of carcinogenesis, current and emerging therapies, and novel treatment strategies. Dig Dis Sci. 2019;64:1016–29.
105. Villanueva A. Hepatocellular carcinoma. N Engl J Med. 2019;380:1450–62.
106. Llovet JM, Ricci S, Mazzaferro V, et al. Sorafenib in advanced hepatocellular carcinoma. N Engl J Med. 2008;359:378–90.
107. Cheng AL, Kang YK, Chen Z, et al. Efficacy and safety of sorafenib in patients in the Asia-Pacific region with advanced hepatocellular carcinoma: a phase III randomised, double-blind, placebo-controlled trial. Lancet Oncol. 2009;10:25–34.
108. Kim G, Kang ES. Prevention of hepatocellular carcinoma by statins: clinical evidence and plausible mechanisms. Semin Liver Dis. 2019;39:141–52.
109. Kubatka P, Kruzliak P, Rotrekl V, et al. Statins in oncological research: from experimental studies to clinical practice. Crit Rev Oncol Hematol. 2014;92:296–311.
110. Sutter AP, Maaser K, Hopfner M, et al. Cell cycle arrest and apoptosis induction in hepatocellular carcinoma cells by HMG-CoA reductase inhibitors. Synergistic antiproliferative action with ligands of the peripheral benzodiazepine receptor. J Hepatol. 2005;43:808–16.

111. Hijona E, Banales JM, Hijona L, et al. Pravastatin inhibits cell proliferation and increased MAT1A expression in hepatocarcinoma cells and in vivo models. Cancer Cell Int. 2012;12:5.
112. Riaño I, Martin L, Varela M, et al. Efficacy and safety of the combination of pravastatin and sorafenib for the treatment of advanced hepatocellular carcinoma (ESTAHEP clinical trial). Cancers (Basel). 2020;12:1900.
113. Blanc JF, Khemissa F, Bronowicki JP, et al. Phase 2 trial comparing sorafenib, pravastatin, their combination or supportive care in HCC with Child-Pugh B cirrhosis. Hepatol Int. 2021;15:93–104.
114. Jouve JL, Lecomte T, Bouché O, et al. Pravastatin combination with sorafenib does not improve survival in advanced hepatocellular carcinoma. J Hepatol. 2019;71:516–22.
115. Kawata S, Yamasaki E, Nagase T, et al. Effect of pravastatin on survival in patients with advanced hepatocellular carcinoma. A randomized controlled trial. Br J Cancer. 2001;84:886–91.
116. Graf H, Jungst C, Straub G, et al. Chemoembolization combined with pravastatin improves survival in patients with hepatocellular carcinoma. Digestion. 2008;78:34–8.
117. Bil J, Zapala L, Nowis D, et al. Statins potentiate cytostatic/cytotoxic activity of sorafenib but not sunitinib against tumor cell lines in vitro. Cancer Lett. 2010;288:57–67.
118. Tsan YT, Lee CH, Ho WC, et al. Statins and the risk of hepatocellular carcinoma in patients with hepatitis C virus infection. J Clin Oncol. 2013;31:1514–21.
119. Kamal S, Khan MA, Seth A, et al. Beneficial effects of statins on the rates of hepatic fibrosis, hepatic decompensation, and mortality in chronic liver disease: a systematic review and meta-analysis. Am J Gastroenterol. 2017;112:1495–505.
120. Bader T. The myth of statin-induced hepatotoxicity. Am J Gastroenterol. 2010;105:978–80.
121. Tolman KG. The liver and lovastatin. Am J Cardiol. 2002;89:1374–80.
122. Rzouq FS, Volk ML, Hatoum HH, et al. Hepatotoxicity fears contribute to underutilization of statin medications by primary care physicians. Am J Med Sci. 2010;340:89–93.
123. Lewis JH, Mortensen ME, Zweig S, et al. Efficacy and safety of high-dose pravastatin in hypercholesterolemic patients with well-compensated chronic liver disease: results of a prospective, randomized, double-blind, placebo-controlled, multicenter trial. Hepatology. 2007;46:1453–63.
124. Athyros VG, Tziomalos K, Gossios TD, et al. Safety and efficacy of long-term statin treatment for cardiovascular events in patients with coronary heart disease and abnormal liver tests in the Greek atorvastatin and coronary heart disease evaluation (GREACE) study: a posthoc analysis. Lancet. 2010;376:1916–22.
125. Kennedy WP. The nocebo reaction. Med. WORLD. 1961;95:203–5.
126. Matthew A, Herrett E, Gasparrini A, et al. Impact of statin related media coverage on use of statins: interrupted time series analysis with UK primary care data. BMJ. 2016;353:i3283.
127. Nielsen SF, Nordestgaard BG. Negative statin-related news stories decrease statin persistence and increase myocardial infarction and cardiovascular mortality: a nationwide prospective cohort study. Eur Heart J. 2016;37:908–16.
128. Webster RK, Weinman J, Rubin GJ. A systematic review of factors that contribute to nocebo effects. Health Psychol. 2016;35:1334–55.
129. Gupta A, Thompson D, Whitehouse A, et al. Adverse events associated with unblinded, but not with blinded, statin therapy in the Anglo-Scandinavian cardiac outcomes trial-lipid-lowering arm (ASCOT-LLA): a randomised double-blind placebo-controlled trial and its non-randomised non-blind extension phase. Lancet. 2017;389:2473–81.
130. Goldacre B, van Staa T, MacDonald TM, et al. Statin treatment and muscle symptoms: series of randomised, placebo controlled n-of-1 trials. BMJ. 2021;372:n135.
131. Rosenson R, Baker S, Jacobson T, et al. An assessment by the statin muscle safety task force: 2014 update. J Clin Lipidol. 2014;8:S58–71.
132. Boccuzzi S, Bocanegra T, Walker F, et al. Long-term safety and efficacy of simvastatin. Am J Cardiol. 1991;68:1127–31.
133. Collins R, Reith C, Emberson J, et al. Interpretation of the evidence for the efficacy and safety of statin therapy. Lancet. 2016;388:2532–61.

134. More V, Cheng Q, Donepudi A, et al. Alcohol cirrhosis alters nuclear receptor and drug transporter expression in human liver. Drug Metab Dispos. 2013;41:1148–55.
135. Pose E, Napoleone L, Amin A, et al. Safety of two different doses of simvastatin plus rifaximin in decompensated cirrhosis (LIVERHOPE-SAFETY): a randomised, double-blind, placebo-controlled, phase 2 trial. Lancet Gastroenterol Hepatol. 2020;5:31–41.
136. Muñoz AE, Pollarsky F, Marino M, et al. Safety of chronic simvastatin treatment in patients with decompensated cirrhosis: many adverse events but no liver injury. Dig Dis Sci. 2021;66:3199–208.
137. Russo MW, Scobey M, Bonkovsky HL. Drug-induced liver injury associated with statins. Semin Liver Dis. 2009;29:412–22.
138. Tsochatzis EA, Bosch J. Statins in cirrhosis-ready for prime time. Hepatology. 2017;66:697–9.
139. Moctezuma-Velazquez C, Abraldes JG, Montano-Loza AJ. The use of statins in patients with chronic liver disease and cirrhosis. Curr Treat Options Gastroenterol. 2018;16:226–40.

L-Ornithine L-Aspartate for the Prevention and Treatment of Liver Cirrhosis and its Complications

13

Roger F. Butterworth

Abstract

This chapter documents, in an evidence-based manner, current knowledge on the importance of L-ornithine L-aspartate (LOLA) for the prevention and treatment of cirrhosis and its complications. Electronic and manual searches of established databases using appropriate keywords revealed a wealth of pertinent data, including three high-quality recently published systematic reviews, each with meta-analysis detailing the results of randomized controlled trials (RCTs) on the efficacy of LOLA. Results confirmed that LOLA significantly lowered circulating ammonia with concomitant improvements of mental state in patients with minimal hepatic encephalopathy (MHE), overt hepatic encephalopathy (OHE), and episodic OHE where, in all cases, intravenous and oral formulations of LOLA functioned effectively. Combination therapy with LOLA, lactulose, and rifaximin led to more rapid improvement of OHE grade, rapid recovery of mental state, and decreased mortality compared to the lactulose/rifaximin combination alone. LOLA is also effective for the treatment of muscle wasting (sarcopenia) in cirrhosis. Improvements in liver function tests and MELD scores also occur following treatment with LOLA consistent with a hepatoprotective property where possible mechanisms include LOLA-induced synthesis of the antioxidant glutathione and of nitric oxide leading to improved hepatic microcirculation. A new dimension for LOLA in relation to cirrhosis is heralded by results of RCTs demonstrating its efficacy for the prevention of OHE resulting from a range of presentations, including OHE associated with variceal bleeding (primary prophylaxis), prevention of repeat episodes of OHE (secondary prophylaxis), post-TIPSS OHE prophylaxis as well as prevention of the deterioration of MHE to OHE in cirrhosis.

R. F. Butterworth (✉)
Department of Medicine, University of Montreal, Montreal, Canada
e-mail: rb@enceph.com

X. Qi, Y. Yang (eds.), *Pharmacotherapy for Liver Cirrhosis and Its Complications*, https://doi.org/10.1007/978-981-19-2615-0_13

Keywords

L-ornithine L-aspartate · Cirrhosis · Hyperammonemia · Sarcopenia · Hepatoprotection · Hepatic encephalopathy · Treatment · Prophylaxis · Combination therapy

13.1 Introduction

A key function of the liver is the effective removal of blood-borne ammonia generated from intestinal protein digestion and carried to the liver via the portal vein. Ammonia removal by the liver takes place by two distinct mechanisms and cellular systems located differentially in the liver acinus [1]. Periportal hepatocytes are equipped with molecular and metabolic components necessary for the incorporation of ammonia into the molecule of urea (the urea cycle). Any residual ammonia is then incorporated into the molecule of glutamine by perivenous hepatocytes that express the gene coding for the enzyme glutamine synthetase (GS), a process identified as ammonia scavenging. The localization of the key steps and their selective anatomical locations are depicted in Fig. 13.1 in a simplified manner in relation to inter-organ trafficking of ammonia in normal individuals compared to patients with cirrhosis.

The loss of hepatic parenchyma in cirrhosis leads to increases in vascular resistance resulting in portal hypertension and portal-systemic shunting of venous blood. The concomitant loss (up to 85%) of functional perivenous and periportal hepatocytes represents a major impairment in capacity for hepatic ammonia removal.

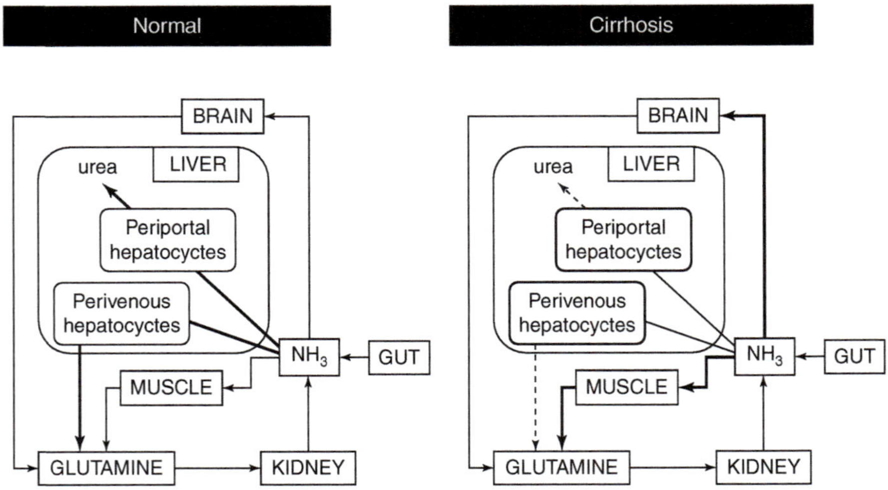

Fig. 13.1 Key steps in multiple organs involved in inter-organ trafficking of ammonia between the gut, liver, muscle, kidney, and brain in a healthy subject compared to a patient with cirrhosis

13.2 Efficacy of L-Ornithine L-Aspartate [LOLA] for the Treatment of Hyperammonemia in Cirrhosis

LOLA is a 1:1 stable salt of two naturally-occurring amino acids, L-ornithine and L-aspartic acid. Studies in isolated hepatocytes reveal that urea synthesis from ammonia is limited by the supply of L-ornithine and that L-ornithine requirements are dependent upon the supply of ammonia [2].

Based upon evidence derived from the results of randomized controlled clinical trials (RCTs) as well as systematic reviews with meta-analyses of the results of these trials, there is now strong support for the use of LOLA for the lowering of blood-borne ammonia in patients with cirrhosis. Results are shown in the form of forest plots in Fig. 13.2.

The primary mechanism whereby LOLA results in the reduction of circulating ammonia in cirrhosis relates to the consequences of activation or optimization of key metabolic processes responsible for the incorporation of ammonia into the molecules of urea or glutamine by residual periportal and perivenous hepatocytes, respectively (Fig. 13.1). Both L-ornithine and L-aspartate are metabolic substrates for the urea cycle, where they act at distinct enzymic steps, as shown in Fig. 13.3a. Thus, L-ornithine stimulates flux via ornithine transcarbamylase, whereas L-aspartate has the potential to contribute a second nitrogen donor to the cycle at the position indicated in Fig. 13.3a.

In addition to stimulation of urea synthesis, beneficial effects of the two amino acid components of LOLA participate in the process of ammonia removal by supplying increased concentrations of glutamate, the obligate substrate for the enzyme GS and they achieve this by displacement of transaminase equilibria as shown in Fig. 13.3b. By so doing, one molecule of LOLA gives rise to three molecules of glutamate for ammonia removal by incorporation into glutamine in perivenous hepatocytes, skeletal muscle, and brain [4].

Given its activation of ammonia removal by residual hepatocytes in patients with cirrhosis, LOLA is considered as a "metabolic ammonia scavenger" [5]. It is

	LOLA			Control				Mean Difference	
Study or subgroup	Mean	SD	Total	Mean	SD	Total	Weight	IV, Random, 95% CI	Year
Kircheis et al	−17.3	37.2	57	−6.4	32.5	60	16.1%	−10.90 [−23.58, 1.78]	1997
Stauch et al	−27	56	33	−24	73	30	6.8%	−3.00 [−35.36, 29.36]	1998
Chen et al	−132	60	45	−69.5	58	40	9.3%	−62.50 [−87.61, −37.39]	2005
Schmid et al	−15	40.1	20	11.1	36.6	20	9.9%	−26.10 [−49.89, −2.31]	2010
Abid et al	−9.6	9.3	32	−0.5	7.8	31	20.6%	−9.10 [−13.33, −4.87]	2011
Mittal et al	−18.8	53.3	60	−8.7	85	60	9.2%	−10.10 −35.49, 15.29]	2011
Alvares de Silva et al	5	24	28	8.5	26.7	35	16.1%	−3.50 [−16.04, 9.04]	2014
Sidhu et al	−69.8	65.5	80	−38.4	60.4	78	11.9%	−31.40 [−51.04, −11.76]	2018
Total (95% CI)			**355**			**354**	**100.0%**	**−17.50 [−27.73, −7.26]**	

Heterogeneity: $Tau^2 = 128.00$; $Chi^2 = 24.24$, df = 7 (P = 0.001); $I^2 = 71\%$

Test for overall effect: Z = 3.35 (P = 0.0008)

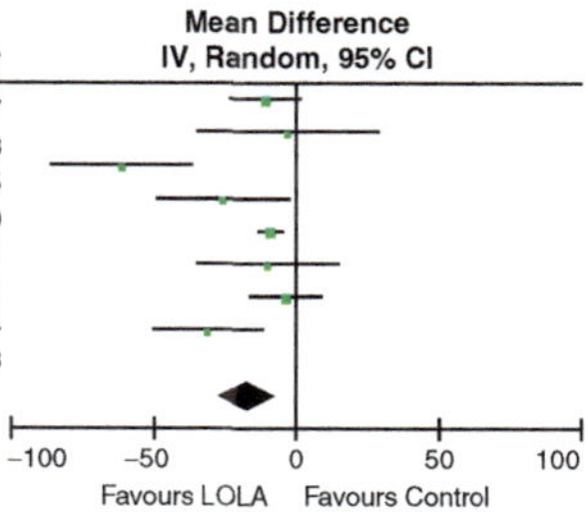

Fig. 13.2 Pooled effect of LOLA versus placebo/no intervention for the lowering of circulating ammonia. Data presented in the form of forest plot from RCTs identified by the first author and year with full citation in references [3]

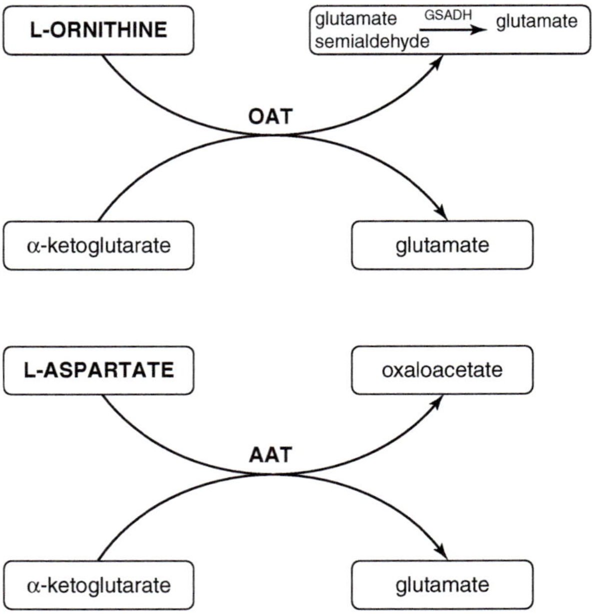

Fig. 13.3 Displacement of transaminase equilibria by LOLA. *OAT* ornithine aminotransferase, *AAT* aspartate aminotransferase, *GSADH* glutamate semialdehyde dehydrogenase (adapted from [4])

interesting in this regard that a recent review article provides new insights into a group of such scavenger molecules that specifically target ammonia for the prevention and treatment of HE in adults with cirrhosis [6]. The agents selected include compounds with demonstrated ammonia-lowering potential for the treatment of patients with inherited urea cycle enzymopathies and include sodium benzoate (3 trials), analogs of phenylbutyrate (1 trial), or phenylacetate (2 trials), a carbon fiber absorbent AST-120 (2 trials), and polyethylene glycol (3 trials). The authors of this systematic review concluded that there was insufficient evidence to determine the effects of these pharmacotherapies on the prevention and treatment of HE in adults with cirrhosis. A subsequent review of the evidence for the efficacy of metabolic ammonia scavengers for the treatment of HE in cirrhosis that included LOLA and branched-chain amino acids (BCAAs) in addition to the ones listed above concluded that only LOLA and glycerol phenylbutyrate were effective both for lowering ammonia and improving mental state [5].

13.3 Hepatoprotective Properties of LOLA in Cirrhosis

There is a growing body of evidence in support of the notion that LOLA may have hepatoprotective properties in patients with cirrhosis. Improvements in liver enzymes and total bilirubin were reported in a cohort of 314 patients with cirrhosis [7]. The findings were subsequently confirmed in three independent RCTs, in which improvements in prothrombin time [8], Child-Pugh score [9], and Model of End

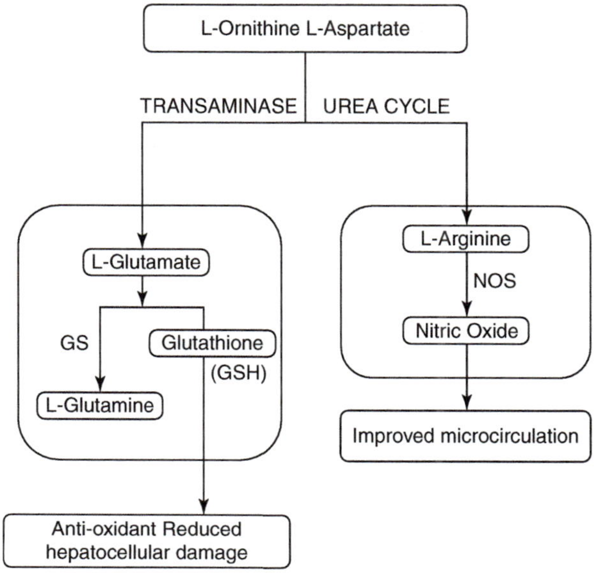

Fig. 13.4 Possible mechanisms related to hepatoprotective properties of LOLA [11]

Stage Liver Disease [MELD] score [9, 10] give support to hepatoprotection by LOLA from a clinical perspective.

In a review of possible mechanisms responsible for the apparent hepatoprotective effects of LOLA in cirrhosis, it was proposed that the diversion of L-ornithine towards the production of nitric oxide could lead to improved hepatic microcirculation. Additionally, L-ornithine and L-aspartate are converted via transaminases to glutamate, resulting in increased synthesis of antioxidants, such as glutamine and glutathione (Fig. 13.4), with the ability to prevent oxidative stress-related hepatocellular damage [11].

13.4 Potential for the Use of LOLA for the Treatment of Sarcopenia in Cirrhosis

It is well established that, as cirrhosis progresses, skeletal muscle increasingly takes over from the failing liver for the removal of blood-borne ammonia (Fig. 13.1) but, unlike the liver, this occurs exclusively via glutamine synthesis since muscle cells do not express the constituent enzymes of the urea cycle. Evidence for this transfer from liver to muscle is provided by studies of A-V differences for ammonia and glutamine across the forearm of patients with cirrhosis and hyperammonemia [12] and in a study using ^{13}N-ammonia [13]. Molecular biological studies in an animal model of chronic liver failure demonstrate that the trigger for increasing the use of skeletal muscle for ammonia removal in cirrhosis is due to the post-translational up-regulation of the GS gene [14].

Severe muscle wasting (sarcopenia) is a common complication of cirrhosis with negative impact on patient's health-related quality of life (HRQOL) as well as their post-transplant outcomes and survival [15].

Given the role of muscle as the principal backup system for removal of ammonia in cirrhosis, it is evident that the presence of any degree of sarcopenia would likely jeopardize this system leading to worsening of hyperammonemia and, indeed, such is the case [12, 16]. Moreover, results of recent in vitro and preclinical studies suggest that sarcopenia is caused by exposure of muscle to ammonia per se. Exposure of differentiated myotubes to millimolar concentrations of ammonia results in decreases of myotubular diameter together with decreased protein synthesis and increased expression of autophagic markers [16]. Moving to a well-validated animal model of chronic liver failure, the end-to-side portacaval-shunted rat, the investigators went on to demonstrate that 1-week post-shunt, animals manifested significant reductions in muscle mass, grip strength, and muscle fiber diameter compared to pair-fed controls with concomitant increases of both blood and muscle ammonia concentrations. These findings of hyperammonemia-mediated autophagy of skeletal muscle were subsequently confirmed in patients with cirrhosis [17].

Treatment of portacaval-shunted animals with LOLA and an antibiotic resulted in significant improvements in lean body mass, skeletal muscle mass, grip strength, and muscle diameter together with marked reductions of circulating and muscle ammonia levels [16]. Moreover, protein synthesis rates in gastrocnemius muscle that had been reduced by the shunt procedure were improved by LOLA. It has been proposed that the worsening of hyperammonemia due to the presence of sarcopenia in cirrhosis represents a vicious cycle [18], and that LOLA has the potential to tame the cycle by mechanisms summarized schematically in Fig. 13.5.

In order to evaluate the relevance of these mechanisms to the phenomenon of sarcopenia in patients with cirrhosis and to possible beneficial effects of LOLA, relevant clinical studies have been undertaken. In the first such study, 16 patients with alcoholic cirrhosis and sarcopenia were randomized to receive LOLA (40 g/d at 5 g/h for 8 h) or placebo for 7 days. All patients received nutritional supplements in accordance with daily requirements. After each 4 h fasting or fed period, protein synthesis rates were measured in percutaneous biopsies of *anterior tibalis* muscle. Whereas patients in the placebo group manifested a reduction in muscle protein synthesis, those in the LOLA group showed significant increases over baseline [19]. In a subsequent study, 34 patients with cirrhosis were randomized to receive LOLA or placebo and markers of muscle function, including handgrip strength and biceps skinfold thickness, were recorded. A significant gain of 1.5 mm was noted in the latter parameter in the LOLA treatment group compared to a loss of 1.0 mm in the placebo group [20].

It is evident that, given the now well-established role of skeletal muscle as a key factor of the control of hyperammonemia in cirrhosis, it is conceivable that the ammonia-lowering properties of LOLA discussed above result to a significant degree from LOLA's beneficial effects for the control of sarcopenia.

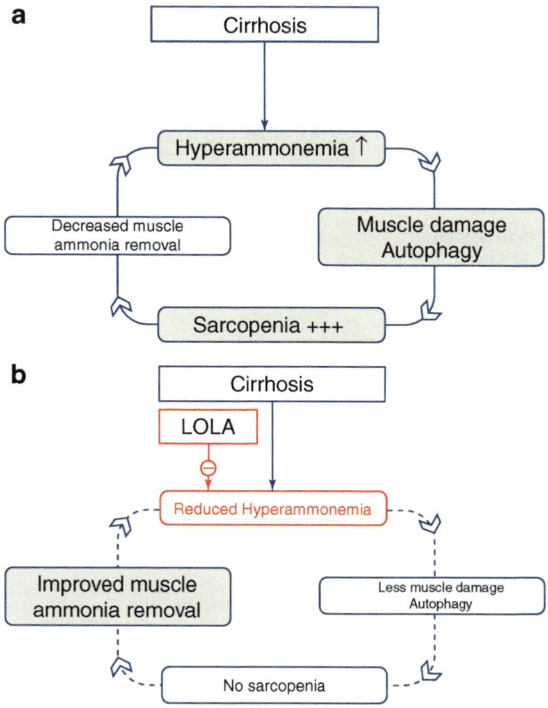

Fig. 13.5 (**a**) Schematic representation of key steps linking hyperammonemia to sarcopenia leading to a vicious cycle [18]. (**b**) Slowing of the vicious cycle resulting in improved muscle function due to the effect of LOLA in reducing hyperammonemia [18]

The benefits of LOLA for the prevention of sarcopenia and associated beneficial effects on MELD scores have the potential to lead to improvements in liver transplantation priority and outcomes in patients with cirrhosis [21].

13.5 Efficacy of LOLA for the Treatment of the Multiple Forms of HE in Cirrhosis

Agents with the proven ability to cause lowering of blood ammonia are the mainstay for the management of HE in cirrhosis; LOLA is one such agent. Results of a systematic review with meta-analysis of 10 RCTs were recently published relating to the efficacy of LOLA (intravenous or oral formulations) for improvement of mental state in 919 patients with cirrhosis. Trial quality and risk of bias assessment were evaluated using a novel Jadad/Cochrane paradigm developed by the authors [22]. Pooled data from 9 of the trials in which modifications of mental state were assessed by West-Haven criteria for overt hepatic encephalopathy (OHE) or psychometric testing for minimal hepatic encephalopathy (MHE) were included. In all cases, a significant benefit was noted using the random-effects model for data analysis with risk ratio (RR): 1.36 95% CI: 1.10–1.69, test for overall effect, $Z = 2.82$, $p = 0.005$. Findings in the form of a forest plot are shown in Fig. 13.6a.

a

Study or subgroup	LOLA Events	LOLA Total	Control Events	Control Total	Weight	Risk Ratio M-H, Random, 95% CI	Year
Kircheis et al	37	63	20	63	11.2%	1.85 [1.22, 2.81]	1997
Stauch et al	17	34	8	32	6.5%	2.00 [1.01, 3.98]	1998
Chen et al	43	45	33	40	17.4%	1.16 [0.99, 1.35]	2005
Ahmad et al	37	40	31	40	16.7%	1.19 [0.99, 1.44]	2008
Abid et al	55	60	47	60	17.5%	1.17 [1.00, 1.36]	2011
Mittal et al	14	40	4	40	3.6%	3.50 [1.26, 9.72]	2011
Alvares de Silva et al	2	28	1	35	0.8%	2.50 [0.24, 26.17]	2014
Sharma et al	21	31	9	30	7.7%	2.26 [1.24, 4.11]	2016
Sidhu et al	76	83	73	79	18.6%	0.99 [0.90, 1.09]	2018
Total (95% CI)		**424**		**419**	**100.0%**	**1.36 [1.01, 1.69]**	
Total events	302		226				

Heterogeneity: $Tau^2 = 0.06$; $Chi^2 = 48.38$, df = 8 ($P < 0.00001$); $I^2 = 83\%$
Test for overall effect: Z = 2.82 (P = 0.005)

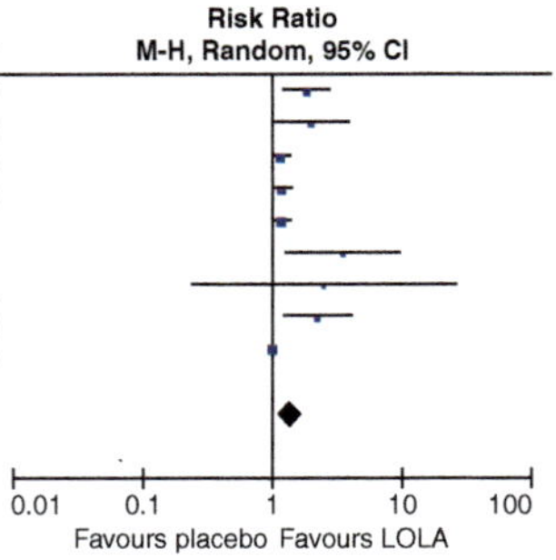

b

Study or subgroup	Control Events	Control Total	LOLA Events	LOLA Total	Weight	Risk Ratio M-H, Random, 95% CI	Year
Kircheis at al	28	37	14	36	8.4%	1.95 [1.24, 3.05]	1997
Stauch at al	16	23	8	20	1.5%	1.74 [0.95, 3.17]	1998
Chen et al	43	45	33	40	21.1%	1.16 [0.99, 1.35]	2005
Ahmad et al	37	40	31	40	19.3%	1.19 [0.99, 1.44]	2008
Abid et al	49	54	44	54	21.3%	1.11 [0.96, 1.30]	2011
Sidhu at al	76	83	73	79	24.4%	0.99 [0.90, 1.09]	2018
Total (95% CI)		**282**		**269**	**100.0%**	**1.19 [1.01, 1.39]**	
Total events	249		203				

Heterogeneity: $Tau^2 = 0.00$; $Chi^2 = 20.10$, df = 5 ($P = 0.001$); $I^2 = 75\%$
Test for overall effect: Z = 2.14 (P = 0.03)

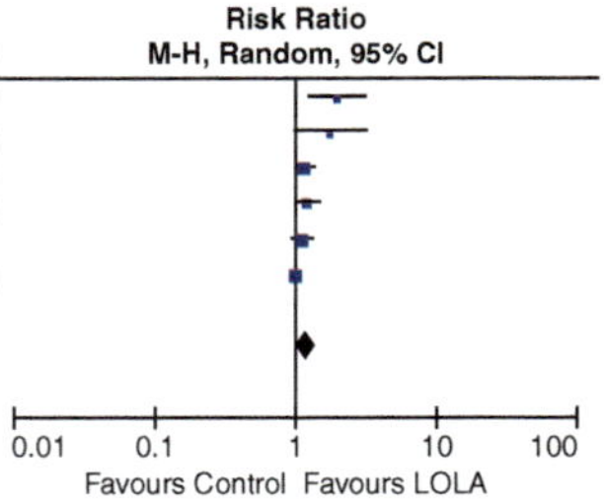

c

Study or subgroup	LOLA Events	LOLA Total	Control Events	Control Total	Weight	Risk Ratio M-H, Random, 95% CI	Year
Kircheis at al	9	26	6	27	18.3%	1.56 [0.65, 3.76]	1997
Stauch at al	1	11	0	12	1.5%	3.25 [0.15, 72.36]	1998
Abid et al	6	6	3	6	24.1%	1.86 [0.86, 4.01]	2011
Mittal et al	14	40	4	40	13.7%	3.50 [1.26, 9.72]	2011
Alvares de Silva et al	2	28	1	35	2.6%	2.50 [0.24, 26.17]	2014
Sharma at al	21	31	9	30	39.8%	2.26 [1.24, 4.11]	2016
Total (95% CI)		**142**		**150**	**100.0%**	**2.15 [1.48, 3.14]**	
Total events	53		23				

Heterogeneity: $Tau^2 = 0.00$; $Chi^2 = 1.70$, df = 5 ($P = 0.89$); $I^2 = 0\%$
Test for overall effect: Z = 3.98 ($P < 0.0001$)

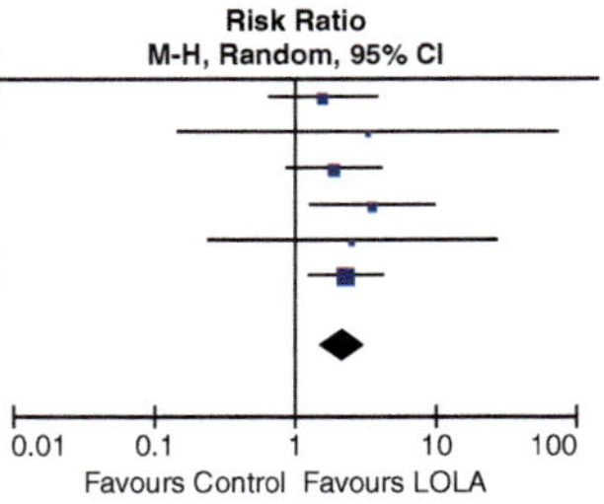

d

Study or subgroup	LOLA Events	LOLA Total	Control Events	Control Total	Weight	Risk Ratio M-H, Random, 95% CI	Year
Stauch at al	1	11	0	12	2.6%	3.25 [0.15, 72.36]	1998
Mittal et al	14	40	4	40	23.7%	3.25 [1.26, 9.72]	2011
Alvares de Silva et al	2	28	1	35	4.5%	2.50 [0.24, 26.17]	2014
Sharma et al	21	31	9	30	69.2%	2.26 [1.24, 4.11]	2016
Total (95% CI)		**110**		**117**	**100.0%**	**2.54 [1.54, 4.18]**	
Total events	38		14				

Heterogeneity: $Tau^2 = 0.00$; $Chi^2 = 0.58$, df = 3 ($P = 0.90$); $I^2 = 0\%$
Test for overall effect: Z = 3.67 (P = 0.0002)

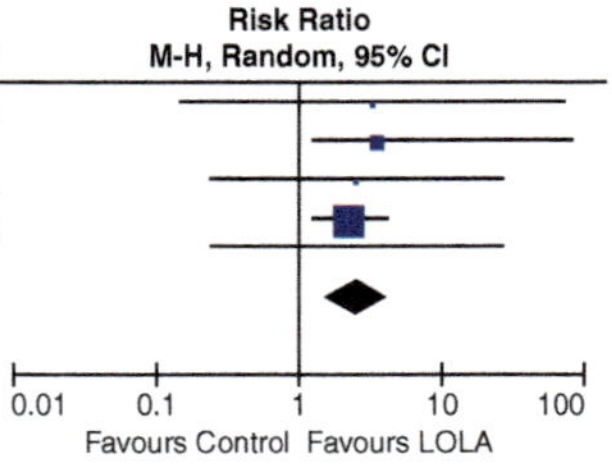

Fig. 13.6 (**a**) Effect of LOLA (iv or oral) versus placebo/no intervention for improvement of mental state in patients with HE regardless of type of HE. Trials are identified by the first author and year with full citation in reference list [3]. (**b**) Effect of LOLA (iv or oral) versus placebo/no intervention for improvement in mental state in patients with OHE. Identity of trials as in legend to (**a**). (**c**) Effect of LOLA (iv or oral) versus placebo/no intervention for improvement of mental state in patients with MHE. Identity of trials as in legend to (**a**). (**d**) Effect of LOLA (oral formulation) versus placebo/no intervention for improvement of mental state in patients with MHE. Identity of trials as in legend to (**a**)

Subgroup analysis revealed significant improvements in mental state in the 6 RCTs of 452 patients with cirrhosis and OHE who had been treated with LOLA (either formulation with RR: 1.19, 95% CI: 1.01–1.39, test for overall effect, $Z = 2.14$, $p < 0.03$) as shown in Fig. 13.6b.

Likewise, for the MHE subgroup of 292 patients included in 6 RCTs, beneficial effects of LOLA for mental state improvement were confirmed with RR: 2.15. 95% CI: 1.48–3.14, test for overall effect, $Z = 3.98$, $p < 0.0001$ as shown in Fig. 13.6c.

Of particular interest in this study was that the oral form of LOLA was superior to the intravenous one for MHE. In fact, in the subgroup of 227 patients with cirrhosis given the oral formulation of LOLA, mental state improvement was optimal with RR: 2.54, 95% CI: 1.54–4.18, test for overall effect $Z = 3.67$; $p = 0.0002$ as shown in Fig. 13.6d.

It is important to note that two additional systematic reviews with meta-analyses on the efficacy of LOLA for the treatment of HE in cirrhosis have been published.

In the first analysis, findings from 15 RCTs involving 1023 patients with cirrhosis showed that treatment with LOLA (either formulation) resulted in significant benefit in a subgroup of patients with acute episodes of chronic HE but no such benefit for patients with MHE [23]. This study was subsequently extended to include a further 21 RCTs for a grand total of 2377 patients with cirrhosis. Regrettably, most of the additional trials had been abandoned or incomplete, of very poor quality and lacking essential information required for the assessment of treatment outcome and/or risk of bias. Consequently, the investigators scored the results of their analysis "uncertain" [24].

The second systematic review with meta-analysis compared the efficacy of LOLA with placebo/no intervention and with other agents, including lactulose, rifaximin, probiotics with or without lactulose and BCAAs. Such a meta-analysis is generally referred to as a "network meta-analysis", which, in this case, examined only patients with MHE. In a subgroup of 59 patients in two RCTs, the efficacy of LOLA for mental state improvement was confirmed with odds ratio (OR): 0.11, 95% CI: 0.02–0.59, test for overall effect, $Z = 2.47$, $p = 0.01$ [25]. This result confirms the findings of the earlier meta-analysis [22].

13.6 Association Between Sarcopenia and MHE or OHE in Cirrhosis

Given that skeletal muscle is intimately involved in ammonia disposal in patients with all forms of HE, it is suggested that the presence of sarcopenia may present a predisposing factor for HE in these patients [26]. To investigate this possibility directly, a systematic review and meta-analysis involving five cross-sectional studies for a total of 1713 patients was undertaken. Diagnosis of sarcopenia was based on measurements of mid-arm muscle circumference or skeletal muscle index in patients with MHE or OHE by West-Haven criteria or psychometric testing for diagnosis of MHE. Significantly higher risks were encountered in patients with cirrhosis and sarcopenia compared to non-sarcopenic patients [27] thus:

For MHE: OR: 3.34, 95% CI: 1.68–6.67, test for overall effect: $Z = 3.43$, $p < 0.0006$.
For OHE: OR: 2.05, 95% CI: 1.28–3.29, test for overall effect: $Z = 2.99$, $p = 0.003$.

13.7 Efficacy of LOLA for the Prevention of OHE in Cirrhosis

OHE has a negative impact on health-related quality of life (HRQOL) and neurocognitive function both before [28] and after liver transplantation and survival of patients with cirrhosis. Moreover, each episode of OHE is associated with increased risk of further episodes [29]. Consequently, effective approaches aimed at the prevention of OHE are constantly under evaluation. A systematic review with meta-analysis was therefore undertaken to review the evidence in support of a beneficial effect of LOLA for the prevention/prophylaxis of OHE in 6 RCTs with a total of 384 such patients [3]. Trials were heterogeneous in nature including primary OHE prophylaxis, secondary OHE prophylaxis, post-TIPSS OHE prophylaxis, and the prevention of deterioration of MHE to OHE in patients with cirrhosis. The findings are shown in the form of forest plots in Fig. 13.7. Details related to each trial subgroup are provided in Sects. 13.7.1–13.7.4.

13.7.1 Efficacy of LOLA for Primary OHE Prophylaxis Following Acute Variceal Bleeding in Cirrhosis

A placebo-controlled RCT was initiated in 87 patients with cirrhosis and acute variceal bleeding in order to compare the efficacy of three standard agents (lactulose, rifaximin, and LOLA) for OHE prophylaxis compared to placebo [31]. The primary endpoint was the occurrence of OHE in the 7-day post-bleeding with secondary endpoints of the time in days for the first appearance of OHE and its occurrence in

	LOLA		Control			Risk Ratio	
Study or Subgroup	**Events**	**Total**	**Events**	**Total**	**Weight**	**M-H, Random, 95% CI**	**Year**
Mittal et al	2	40	4	40	8.7%	0.50 [0.10, 2.58]	2011
Abid et al	0	6	3	6	3.0%	0.14 [0.01, 2.28]	2011
Alvares de Silva et al	1	28	13	35	6.0%	0.10 [0.01, 0.69]	2014
Bai et al	1	21	3	19	4.9%	0.30 [0.03, 2.66]	2014
Higuera et al	5	22	12	22	31.7%	0.42 [0.18, 0.98]	2018
Varakanahalli et al	9	73	20	72	45.6%	0.44 [0.22, 0.91]	2018
Total (95% CI)		**190**		**194**	**100.0%**	**0.38 [0.23, 0.62]**	
Total events	18		55				

Heterogeneity: $Tau^2 = 0.00$; $Chi^2 = 2.92$, $df = 5$ ($P = 0.71$); $I^2 = 0\%$
Test for overall effect: $Z = 3.92$ ($P < 0.0001$)

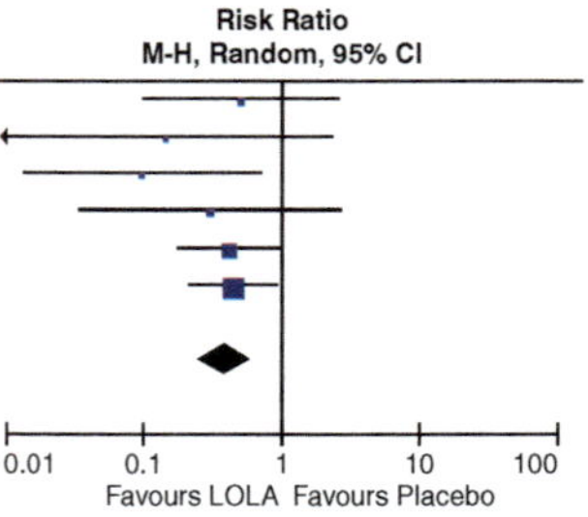

Fig. 13.7 Efficacy of LOLA versus placebo/no intervention for the prevention of OHE including primary, secondary, post-TIPSS prophylaxis and prevention of deterioration of MHE to OHE. Trials are identified by the first author and year with full citation in reference list [30]

the ensuing 28 days. LOLA was given as iv infusions (10 g/24 h for the 7-day period). Treatment with LOLA resulted in reduced frequency of OHE (22.7% compared to 54.5% in placebo with OR: 0.2, 95% CI: 0.06–0.88, $p < 0.03$), and the severity of OHE grade was significantly lower in the LOLA group. Treatment with rifaximin yielded protection similar in nature and magnitude to LOLA, but changes with lactulose failed to reach statistical significance.

13.7.2 Efficacy of LOLA for Secondary OHE Prophylaxis (Prevention of Recurrence) in Cirrhosis

In a double-blind RCT, the efficacy of LOLA (3 × 6 g/d) versus placebo for a 6-month period was compared to placebo in 150 patients with cirrhosis, all of whom had one or more previous episodes of OHE prior to treatment [32]. The primary objective was the assessment of the benefit of LOLA during a 6-month follow-up period. Secondary objectives included time to first OHE breakthrough, OHE grading, predictors of OHE recurrence, time to first OHE-related hospitalization, HRQOL, adverse events, and mortality. Results indicate that the frequency of development of OHE was significantly less with LOLA compared to placebo with $p < 0.022$ together with a 37% reduced probability of developing OHE (Fig. 13.8). At 6 months follow-up, patients in the LOLA group manifested significantly greater reductions in arterial ammonia with $p < 0.001$. Predictors of recurrence of OHE in these patients included baseline Child-Turcotte-Pugh, MELD, Psychometric Hepatic Encephalopathy Score (PHES), Critical Flicker Frequency (CFF) scores, and arterial ammonia.

Fig. 13.8 Secondary OHE prophylaxis in patients with cirrhosis indicating time to OHE breakthrough up to 6 months follow-up post-LOLA compared to placebo [32]

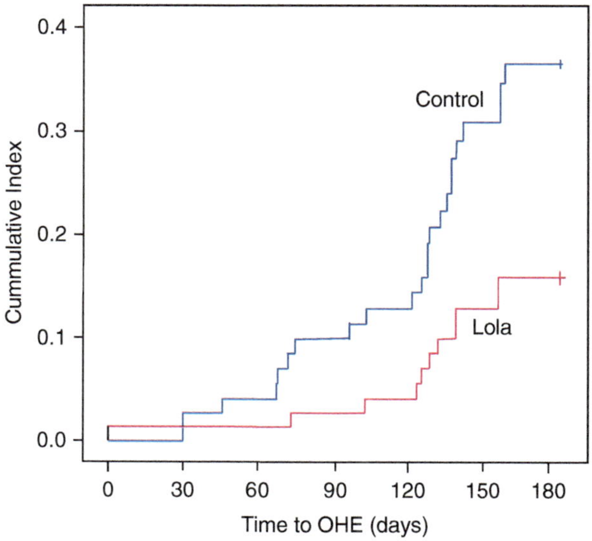

13.7.3 Efficacy of LOLA for Post-TIPSS OHE Prophylaxis in Cirrhosis

The TIPSS procedure for the treatment of the complications of portal hypertension results in new or worsening episodes of OHE in up to 50% of patients with cirrhosis [33]. Efforts have been made to develop agents to prevent OHE in these patients. Studies using lactitol or rifaximin were unsuccessful [34]. However, results of a subsequent RCT of 40 post-TIPSS patients given LOLA infusions (30 g/d for 7 consecutive days) demonstrated efficacy for the prevention of the deterioration of MHE to OHE in these patients with RR: 0.30, 95%CI: 0.03–2.66. The beneficial effect was accompanied by significant decreases in fasting and post-prandial ammonia [10].

13.7.4 Efficacy of LOLA for the Prevention of Deterioration of MHE to OHE in Cirrhosis

Three RCTs assessed the efficacy of LOLA compared to placebo/no intervention for the prevention of deterioration of MHE to OHE. Results in the form of forest plots are provided in Fig. 13.9.

In the first trial, 80 patients with cirrhosis and MHE were randomized to receive LOLA [18 g/d po] or no intervention for 3 months with a primary endpoint of progression to OHE. 4/40 patients in the no intervention group developed OHE compared to 2/40 patients in the LOLA treatment group with RR: 0.50, 95% CI: 0.10–2.58. Improvements in the LOLA group were accompanied by significant improvements in HRQOL. Efficacies comparable to that of LOLA were noted following treatment with lactulose or probiotics [35].

In the second trial, six patients with MHE were given LOLA (20 g/4 h p.o. for three consecutive days) or placebo. Deterioration of MHE and appearance of OHE occurred in 3/6 patients in the placebo group compared to 0/6 in the LOLA treatment group with RR: 0.14, 95% CI: 0.01–2.28 [8].

The third trial in the series comprised 64 patients with cirrhosis and MHE treated with LOLA (5 g p.o. tid for 60 days) or placebo. Five percent of 28 LOLA-treated patients experienced episodes of OHE at 6 months compared to 37.9% of 35 patients

Study or Subgroup	LOLA Events	LOLA Total	Control Events	Control Total	Weight	Risk Ratio M-H, Random, 95% CI	Year
Mittal et al	2	40	4	40	49.0%	0.50 [0.10, 2.58]	2011
Abid et al	0	6	3	6	17.1%	0.14 [0.01, 2.28]	2011
Alvares de Silva et al	1	28	13	35	33.9%	0.10 [0.01, 0.69]	2014
Total (95% CI)		**74**		**81**	**100.0%**	**0.23 [0.07, 0.73]**	
Total events	18		55				

Heterogeneity: Tau^2 = 0.00; Chi^2 = 1.84, df = 2 (P = 0.40); I^2 = 0%

Test for overall effect: Z = 2.50 (P = 0.01)

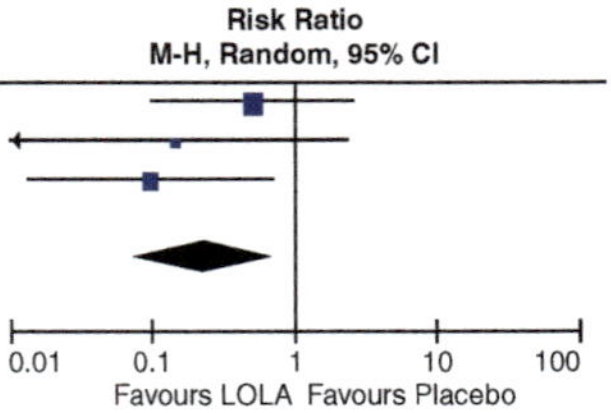

Fig. 13.9 Efficacy of LOLA versus placebo/no intervention for prevention of deterioration of MHE to OHE. Trials are identified by the first author and year with full citation in reference list. Identity of trials as in legend to Fig. 13.7

receiving placebo with RR: 0.10, 95% CI: 0.01–0.69, $p < 0.016$. Moreover, LOLA-treated patients in this trial also manifested evidence of improved liver function that included improvements in MELD and Child-Pugh scores [9].

All the above trials led to significant decreases of circulating ammonia following treatment with LOLA concomitant with the prevention of deterioration of MHE to OHE.

Significantly, a subsequent systematic review with network meta-analysis comparing efficacy of treatment options for MHE independently confirmed that LOLA was effective for preventing episodes of OHE compared to placebo or no intervention (OR: 0.19; 95% PrI: 0.04–0.91; SUCRA 75.1%: high moderate quality) [25].

13.8 Efficacy of LOLA for the Treatment of Episodic OHE in Cirrhosis

Episodes (bouts) of OHE occur in up to 40% of patients with cirrhosis so, given the lack of high-quality data on the effects of LOLA on episodic OHE, a prospective RCT was initiated to evaluate the efficacy of LOLA for the reversal of OHE in 193 patients with cirrhosis with bouts of OHE grades 2–4 by West-Haven criteria with or without precipitating factors [36]. Fasting venous ammonia, prothrombin time and liver function test were performed with primary outcome measure of mental state grade at day 5 of treatment. On days 1–4, the OHE grade was significantly lower in the LOLA-treated group compared to placebo and the mean time for recovery was less (1.92 +/– 0.93 versus 2.50 +/– 1.03 days with 95% CI: −0.852-0.202 and $p = 0.002$). By day 5, venous ammonia was lower on the LOLA group compared to placebo (39.63 +/– 33.47 ug/dL compared to 61.17 +/– 35.73 ug/dL for a difference of 22.44 ug/dL and 95%CI of 11.89–32.98 with $p < 0.0001$). Length of hospital stay was significantly shorter in the LOLA treatment group. There was no effect on cytokine levels between groups.

13.9 Efficacy of LOLA in Combination with Lactulose and Rifaximin for the Treatment of Severe (Grades 3 & 4) OHE in Cirrhosis

A double-blind, placebo-controlled trial was conducted in which 140 patients with cirrhosis with overt grades 3 or 4 HE according to West Haven criteria were randomized to either a combination of LOLA infusions (30 g/24 h for 5 days) plus lactulose plus rifaximin versus placebo plus lactulose plus rifaximin with primary outcome measure being reversal of HE or improvement of HE by 2 grades after 5 days of treatment. Secondary outcomes included blood ammonia and cytokines on days 0 and 5, rate of recovery from HE and length of hospitalization [37]. Randomization made use of blocks of computer-generated random numbers by an independent observer. Results indicate higher rates of improvement of HE severity at day 5 (92.5% versus 66%, $p < 0.001$) and lower times to complete recovery (2.70

+/− 0.46 versus 3.00 +/− 0.87 days, $p < 0.03$). It was concluded that the combination of LOLA with lactulose and rifaximin was more effective than the lactulose/rifaximin combination for improving HE grade and recovery time from OHE.

13.10 Reductions in Mortality by LOLA in Patients with Cirrhosis and OHE

Ranked as the eighth leading cause of death in the USA in 2010, liver cirrhosis renders the patient susceptible to a plethora of medical complications and ultimately reduced life expectancy. Such complications include gastrointestinal bleeding, infections, hepato-renal syndrome, ascites, and OHE, Mortality rates in patients with cirrhosis and OHE are estimated to be in the 40–50% range even in the first year, and OHE grades 3–4 at the time of wait-list inclusion significantly increases 90-day mortality independent of MELD scores.

Several RCTs have assessed the effects of LOLA (either as monotherapy or in combination with other agents) on mortality rates in patients with cirrhosis and HE and, in the case of LOLA monotherapy, more than 50% decreases in mortality rates were recorded over a range OHE grades from I to IV [8, 32, 38–40] and in cases of grade III-IV Episodic OHE [36]. Either intravenous or oral formulations of LOLA were found to be effective in these studies. The latter findings were confirmed in a prospective double-blind randomized placebo-controlled trials in 140 patients with cirrhosis and grades III-IV OHE who received LOLA (30 g/day over 24 h for 5 days) in which significant reductions of 28-day mortality from 41.8% (placebo) to 16.4% (LOLA) were recorded with $p = 0.001$ accompanied by significant reductions in blood ammonia [37].

13.11 Summary and Conclusions

Hyperammonemia is causally related to two important complications of cirrhosis namely sarcopenia and HE by virtue of ammonia's toxic effects on cellular communication systems leading to autophagy in skeletal muscle and impaired transmission in the brain. Muscle damage thus has the potential to result in the loss of an important ancillary system required for ammonia detoxification in cirrhosis.

Three international systematic reviews with meta-analyses are identified in the present chapter giving rise to new or confirmatory data based upon the published results of RCTs reporting that both intravenous and oral formulations of LOLA are effective for the lowering of blood ammonia in patients with cirrhosis. Network meta-analyses confirm that LOLA is equivalent or superior to other current treatments in this regard. Multiple mechanisms are involved in LOLA's ammonia-lowering action that includes activation of the urea cycle by both L-ornithine and L-aspartate in residual periportal hepatocytes and up-regulation of the glutamine synthetic pathway in both residual perivenous hepatocytes and skeletal muscle. In all cases, lowering of blood ammonia is accompanied by significant improvements in various HE subtypes, including OHE, MHE, and episodic OHE.

Interestingly, LOLA also has hepatoprotective properties indicated by improvements in liver enzymes, bilirubin, prothrombin time, Child-Pugh and MELD scores in patients with cirrhosis. Mechanisms proposed include increased production of the powerful antioxidant glutathione with the potential to reduce hepatic damage due to oxidative stress and increased nitric oxide resulting in improved hepatic microcirculation.

LOLA is particularly effective for OHE prevention/prophylaxis in a range of clinical presentations, including primary prophylaxis following a variceal bleed, secondary and post-TIPSS prophylaxis, and the prevention of progression to OHE in patients with MHE.

Results of a randomized placebo-controlled trial provide evidence for the efficacy of intravenous LOLA alone or in combination with lactulose and rifaximin for the treatment of acute severe (grades 3–4) OHE, in which the improvement of encephalopathy grade, time of recovery from HE and also mortality were significantly effective compared to the lactulose/rifaximin combination (control).

References

1. Kaiser S, Gerck W, Häussinger D. Ammonia and glutamine metabolism in human liver slices: new aspects on the pathogenesis of hyperammonaemia in chronic liver disease. Eur J Clin Invest. 1988;18:535–42.
2. Staedt U, Leweling H, Gladisch R, Kortsik C, Hagmüller E, Holm E. Effects of ornithine aspartate on plasma ammonia and plasma amino acids in patients with cirrhosis. A double-blind, randomized study using a four-fold crossover design. J Hepatol. 1993;19:424–30.
3. Butterworth RF, McPhail MJW. L-ornithine L-aspartate (LOLA) for hepatic encephalopathy in cirrhosis: results of randomized controlled trials and meta-analyses. Drugs. 2019;79:31–7.
4. Rose C, Michalak A, Pannunzio P, et al. L-ornithine-L-aspartate in experimental portal-systemic encephalopathy: therapeutic efficacy and mechanism of action. Metab Brain Dis. 1998;13:147–57.
5. Butterworth RF. Ammonia removal by metabolic scavengers for the prevention and treatment of hepatic encephalopathy in cirrhosis. Drugs R D. 2021;21:123–32.
6. Zacharias HD, Zacharias AP, Gluud LL, Morgan MY. Pharmacotherapies that specifically target ammonia for the prevention and treatment of hepatic encephalopathy in adults with cirrhosis. Cochrane Database Syst Rev. 2019;6:CD012334.
7. Grüngreiff K, Lambert-Baumann J. Efficacy of l-ornithine-l-aspartate granules in the treatment of chronic liver disease. Med Welt. 2001;52:219–26.
8. Abid S, Jafri W, Mumtaz K, et al. Efficacy of L-ornithine-L-aspartate as an adjuvant therapy in cirrhotic patients with hepatic encephalopathy. J Coll Physicians Surg Pak. 2011;21:666–71.
9. Alvares-da-Silva MR, de Araujo A, Vicenzi JR, et al. Oral l-ornithine-l-aspartate in minimal hepatic encephalopathy: a randomized, double-blind, placebo-controlled trial. Hepatol Res. 2014;44:956–63.
10. Bai M, He C, Yin Z, et al. Randomised clinical trial: L-ornithine-L-aspartate reduces significantly the increase of venous ammonia concentration after TIPSS. Aliment Pharmacol Ther. 2014;40:63–71.

11. Butterworth RF, Grüngreiff K. L-ornithine L-aspartate for the treatment of hepatic encephalopathy in cirrhosis: evidence for novel Hepatoprotective mechanisms. JSM Liver Clin Res. 2019;3:5.
12. Ganda OP, Ruderman NB. Muscle nitrogen metabolism in chronic hepatic insufficiency. Metabolism. 1976;25:427–35.
13. Lockwood AH, Weissenborn K, Butterworth RF. An image of the brain in patients with liver disease. Curr Opin Neurol. 1997;10:525–33.
14. Desjardins P, Rao KV, Michalak A, Rose C, Butterworth RF. Effect of portacaval anastomosis on glutamine synthetase protein and gene expression in brain, liver and skeletal muscle. Metab Brain Dis. 1999;14:273–80.
15. Periyalwar P, Dasarathy S. Malnutrition in cirrhosis: contribution and consequences of sarcopenia on metabolic and clinical responses. Clin Liver Dis. 2012;16:95–131.
16. Kumar A, Davuluri G, Silva RNE, et al. Ammonia lowering reverses sarcopenia of cirrhosis by restoring skeletal muscle proteostasis. Hepatology. 2017;65:2045–58.
17. Qiu J, Tsien C, Thapalaya S, et al. Hyperammonemia-mediated autophagy in skeletal muscle contributes to sarcopenia of cirrhosis. Am J Physiol Endocrinol Metab. 2012;303:E983–93.
18. Butterworth RF. L-ornithine L-aspartate for the treatment of sarcopenia in chronic liver disease: the taming of a vicious cycle. Can J Gastroenterol Hepatol. 2019a;2019:8182195.
19. Reynolds N, Downie K, Smith K, Kircheis G, Rennie MJ. Treatment with L-ornithine L-aspartate (LOLA) infusion restores muscle protein synthesis responsiveness to feeding in patients with cirrhosis. J Hepatol. 1999;30:3.
20. Pasha Y, Taylor-Robinson S, Leech R, et al. PWE-091 L-ornithine L-aspartate in minimal hepatic encephalopathy: possible effects on the brain-muscle axis? Gut. 2018;67:A117–8.
21. Butterworth RF. L-ornithine L-aspartate for the treatment of sarcopenia in cirrhosis: potential impact on the outcome of liver transplantation. Ann Gastroenterol Dig Dis. 2019b;2:006–9.
22. Butterworth RF, Kircheis G, Hilger N, McPhail MJW. Efficacy of l-ornithine l-aspartate for the treatment of hepatic encephalopathy and Hyperammonemia in cirrhosis: systematic review and meta-analysis of randomized controlled trials. J Clin Exp Hepatol. 2018;8:301–13.
23. Goh ET, Stokes CS, Vilstrup H, Gluud LL, Morgan MY. L-ornithine L-aspartate for hepatic encephalopathy: a systematic review with meta-analyses of randomised controlled trials. J Clin Experiment Hepatol. 2017;7:S65–6.
24. Goh ET, Stokes CS, Sidhu SS, Vilstrup H, Gluud LL, Morgan MY. L-ornithine L-aspartate for prevention and treatment of hepatic encephalopathy in people with cirrhosis. Cochrane Database Syst Rev. 2018;5:CD012410.
25. Dhiman RK, Thumburu KK, Verma N, Chopra M, Rathi S, Dutta U, Singal AK, Taneja S, Duseja A, Singh M. Comparative efficacy of treatment options for minimal hepatic encephalopathy: a systematic review and network meta-analysis. Clin Gastroenterol Hepatol 2020;18:800–12.e25.
26. Lattanzi B, D'Ambrosio D, Merli M. Hepatic encephalopathy and sarcopenia: two faces of the same metabolic alteration. J Clin Exp Hepatol. 2019;9:125–30.
27. Wijarnpreecha K, Werlang M, Panjawatanan P, et al. Association between sarcopenia and hepatic encephalopathy: a systematic review and meta-analysis. Ann Hepatol. 2020;19:245–50.
28. Wong RJ, Gish RG, Ahmed A. Hepatic encephalopathy is associated with significantly increased mortality among patients awaiting liver transplantation. Liver Transpl. 2014;20:1454–61.
29. Weissenborn K. Hepatic encephalopathy: definition, clinical grading and diagnostic principles. Drugs. 2019;79:5–9.
30. Butterworth RF. Beneficial effects of L-ornithine L-aspartate for prevention of overt hepatic encephalopathy in patients with cirrhosis: a systematic review with meta-analysis. Metab Brain Dis. 2020;35:75–81.
31. Higuera-de-la-Tijera F, Servín-Caamaño AI, Salas-Gordillo F, et al. Primary prophylaxis to prevent the development of hepatic encephalopathy in cirrhotic patients with acute variceal bleeding. Can J Gastroenterol Hepatol. 2018;2018:3015891.

32. Varakanahalli S, Sharma BC, Srivastava S, Sachdeva S, Dahale AS. Secondary prophylaxis of hepatic encephalopathy in cirrhosis of liver: a double-blind randomized controlled trial of L-ornithine L-aspartate versus placebo. Eur J Gastroenterol Hepatol. 2018;30:951–8.
33. Rössle M, Haag K, Ochs A, et al. The transjugular intrahepatic portosystemic stent-shunt procedure for variceal bleeding. N Engl J Med. 1994;330:165–71.
34. Riggio O, Masini A, Efrati C, Nicolao F, Angeloni S, Salvatori FM, Bezzi M, Adolfo F, Attili AF, Merli M. Pharmacological prophylaxis of hepatic encephalopathy after transjugular intrahepatic portosystemic shunt: a randomized controlled study. J Hepatol 2005;42:674–679
35. Mittal VV, Sharma BC, Sharma P, Sarin SK. A randomized controlled trial comparing lactulose, probiotics, and L-ornithine L-aspartate in treatment of minimal hepatic encephalopathy. Eur J Gastroenterol Hepatol. 2011;23:725–32.
36. Sidhu SS, Sharma BC, Goyal O, Kishore H, Kaur N. L-ornithine L-aspartate in bouts of overt hepatic encephalopathy. Hepatology. 2018;67:700–10.
37. Jain A, Sharma BC, Mahajan B, Srivastava S, Kumar A, Sachdeva S, Sonika U, Dalal A. L-ornithine L-aspartate in acute treatment of severe hepatic encephalopathy: a double-blind randomized controlled trial. Hepatology. 2022;75:1194–203.
38. Ahmad I, Khan AA, Alam A, Dilshad A, Butt AK, Shafqat F, Malik K. Sarwar S.L-ornithine L-aspartate infusion efficacy in hepatic encephalopathy. J Coll Phys Surg Pakistan. 2008;18:684–7.
39. Chen M, Rucheng LI, Chen C, Gao X. Observation of clinical effect of L-ornithine L-aspartate therapy on liver cirrhosis complicated by hepatic encephalopathy. Chin Libr Classification # R575.2. 2005.
40. Sharma K, Pant S, Misra S, Dwivendi M, Misra A, Narang S, et al. Effect of rifaximin, probiotics and L-ornithine L-aspartate on minimal hepatic encephalopathy: a randomized controlled trial. Saudi. J Gastroenterol. 2014;20:225–32.

Lactulose in Liver Cirrhosis

14

Jessica Faccioli, Stefania Gioia, Silvia Nardelli,
Oliviero Riggio, and Lorenzo Ridola

Abstract

Cirrhosis represents the final stage of any chronic liver disease. Some studies have demonstrated that intestinal microbiota can be responsible for some cirrhosis-related complications due to alterations in this system. In fact, its composition is different from that of healthy people, because there is a lower bacterial diversity with an increase in Gram-negatives and species of oral origin and shortage of native and beneficial families. Lactulose is a non-absorbable disaccharide widely used in clinical practice among cirrhotic patients which can modify intestinal microbiota. In particular, it represents the standard-of-care for hepatic encephalopathy (HE) treatment due to its cathartic effect and its ability to acidify the intestinal content. These properties are fundamental for the reduction of blood ammonium level, considered a key element in the pathogenesis of HE, through different mechanisms, such as the laxative effect, the ammonium ionization, the reduction of intestinal ammonium production, and finally the beneficial effect on intestinal microbiota. Several studies have demonstrated the role of this substance in the treatment of acute episodes of HE, secondary prophylaxis of HE, and treatment of minimal HE (MHE). However, some concern exists about the evaluation of the target to be reached, which up to now has been based on number of daily evacuations, and the indication for MHE treatment.

Keywords

Lactulose · Hepatic encephalopathy · Ammoniemia · Intestinal microbiota

J. Faccioli · S. Gioia · S. Nardelli · O. Riggio · L. Ridola (✉)
Department of Translational and Precision Medicine, "Sapienza" University of Rome, Rome, Italy
e-mail: jessica.faccioli@uniroma1.it; stefania.gioia@uniroma1.it; oliviero.riggio@uniroma1.it; lorenzo.ridola@uniroma1.it

X. Qi, Y. Yang (eds.), *Pharmacotherapy for Liver Cirrhosis and Its Complications*, https://doi.org/10.1007/978-981-19-2615-0_14

14.1 Intestinal Microbiota in Liver Cirrhosis and Lactulose Therapy

Cirrhosis represents the final stage of any chronic liver disease and results from different mechanisms of liver damage that cause necroinflammation and fibrogenesis [1]. From an epidemiological point of view, it represents a growing cause of morbidity and mortality in developed countries, being the 14th cause of death worldwide and the fourth in central Europe [1]. The natural history of cirrhosis is characterized by an asymptomatic compensatory phase, followed by a rapidly progressive phase of decompensation due to the presence of clinically significant portal hypertension in which evident clinical signs of disease appear. Esophageal varices are the first relevant clinical consequence of portal hypertension, while ascites is often the first sign of decompensation to appear [1, 2]. The transition from compensated to decompensated phase occurs at a rate of approximately 5% to 7% per year, and once it occurs, cirrhosis becomes a systemic condition associated with multiorgan dysfunction [3]. This step represents a turning point as it affects the quality of life, probability of hospitalization, and risk of mortality [4].

During the development and progression of cirrhosis, the whole organism adapts to this condition [5]. Recent evidences suggest that intestinal microbiota is responsible for some of the cirrhosis complications. This role emerged in the middle of the last century after the evidences regarding the relationship between hepatic encephalopathy (HE) and intestinal absorption of nitrogenous substances [6]. In line with this concept, some researchers support that in indeterminate cases of decompensation, in which it is not possible to identify a true precipitating factor, microbiota and related metabolites can be primarily involved [4]. Human intestine of healthy subjects is physiologically inhabited by different microorganisms, whose number is equal to approximately 10^{14}-10^{15} CFU/ml. Therefore, we can consider man as a superorganism containing human and bacterial cells and whose genome is the sum of human and microbial ones [6]. There is some degree of inter-individual diversity in the bacterial species constituting the microbiota [7]. However, in about 90% of subjects, intestinal bacteria come from two main phyla which are Bacteroidetes and Firmicutes; the rest come from Proteobacteria, Actinobacteria, Verrucomicrobia, and Fusobacteria one [7]. These bacteria constitute a real organ because they play a primary role in the regulation and maintenance of metabolism and immune functions. In particular, they perform various fundamental activities, such as digestion of complex carbohydrates, synthesis of vitamins (i.e. vitamin K), fermentation of simple sugars, synthesis of short-chain fatty acids, such as butyrate, propionate, and acetate [8], and modulation of intestinal and systemic immune response [7].

Cirrhotic patients may have some alterations of this system. First of all, liver acts as a barrier against the passage of bacteria and their products from intestine to systemic circulation [7]. So, loss of this function as seen in liver cirrhosis can be responsible for infectious complications, such as sepsis, spontaneous bacterial peritonitis (SBP), and hepatorenal syndrome [7]. In addition to the loss of liver filter, it is known that microbiota changes during the development and progression of cirrhosis [5] and that these changes in turn contribute to the progression of liver disease [9]. For this reason, it constitutes an attractive therapeutic target [9].

In cirrhotic patients, many intrinsic and extrinsic factors can affect the composition and function of intestinal microbiota [9]. These factors include age, ethnicity, alcohol consumption, comorbidities and drug use, etiology of cirrhosis and its stage [9]. Even taking antibiotics, for example, during hospitalization, can alter the intestinal flora. The study by Pérez-Cobas et al. showed that during the first day of antibiotic therapy in cirrhotic patients most of the microbiota includes species from Firmicutes phylum, while after a week of treatment the predominant taxa are members of Streptococcaceae, Clostridiaceae, and Bacteroidaceae, which are considered non-autochronous bacteria [10]. In addition to these factors, changes in motility, permeability, and intestinal barrier function, as well as alteration of enterohepatic circulation of bile salts, would also appear to be responsible for dysbiosis.

In fact, cirrhosis causes a reduction in intestinal primary bile acid secretion and this would seem to favor the overgrowth of pathogenic and pro-inflammatory bacteria, such as Porphyromonadaceae and Enterobacteriaceae [11]. This reduction also determines a lower absorption of fats and fat-soluble vitamins, a lower production of secondary bile acids which have antimicrobial activities (especially deoxycholic acid) [5], and a lower activation of intestinal bile acid receptor called Farnesoid X receptor (FXR) which participates in maintaining the integrity of intestinal epithelial and vascular barrier and preventing bacterial translocation [5]. In addition, intestinal microbiota of cirrhotic patients is characterized by a lower bacterial diversity and richness and a bacterial overgrowth in the small intestine (SIBO). Regarding this last point, it is reasonable that this is partly related to alterations in intestinal motility, changes in gastric pH, and reduction of intestinal bile acids concentration which causes poor control of bacterial overgrowth [10]. Furthermore, it would seem that the composition of intestinal microbiota is different from that of healthy subjects [7] and these alterations are found even when the etiological agent is not in direct contact with intestinal microbiota [5]. In particular, there is an increase in Gram-negatives and species of oral origin [9] and a reduction in native families [6]. For these reasons, it was introduced the cirrhosis-dysbiosis ratio (CDR), defined as the ratio between autocronous and non-autocronous taxa; a low ratio is indicative of intestinal dysbiosis [12].

Among the gram-negatives, the members of the Enterobacteriaceae family prevail and they are the main organisms responsible for SBP; bacteria of oral origin derive mainly from Streptococcaceae and Porphyromonadaceae, whose increase can be modulated by proton pump inhibitors use [13, 14]. On the contrary, Firmicutes and in particular Lachnospiraceae and Ruminococcaceae families, are lacking [15]. The study published by Chen et al. in 2011 first demonstrated the presence of intestinal dysbiosis in patients with liver cirrhosis, after having analyzed fecal microbiota using 16S ribosomal PCR sequencing [15]; compared to healthy subjects, the study demonstrated a reduction in Bacteroidetes and an increase in Proteobacteria and Fusobacteria, which was also confirmed in 2014 by Quin et al. [13], but also in Enterobacteriaceae, Veillonellaceae, and Streptococcaceae [15]. This study also found a correlation between some microbial species and stage of cirrhosis measured with Child–Pugh class; this correlation was positive for Streptococcaceae and negative for Lachnospiraceae [15]. In conclusion, the prevalence of potentially pathogenic bacteria, such as Enterobacteriaceae and Streptococcaceae, and the lack of beneficial populations, such as Lachnospiraceae, can affect the cirrhotic patients' prognosis [15].

Lactulose is a drug widely used in clinical practice among cirrhotic patients which can modify intestinal microbiota. It is a non-absorbable disaccharide composed of galactose and fructose, used in clinical practice since 1957 for chronic constipation and HE [16]. After oral ingestion, intestinal absorption is almost negligible because it is not digested by human gastrointestinal enzymes. In this way, it can reach into the colon where it can be fermented by resident bacteria [16]. In healthy subjects, lactulose is metabolized in the proximal colon by saccharolytic bacteria, such as Bifidobacteria, Lactobacilli, and Streptococci [17]. In particular, once the cecum is reached, it is converted into short-chain fatty acids (mainly lactic and acetic acid), methane and hydrogen causing a reduction of intestinal pH and a modification of composition and activities of resident flora [18]. Some studies have shown that the effect of lactulose is dose and patient-dependent and that not all subjects have the same beneficial response with the same dosage, probably depending on intestinal flora composition before consumption [18]. A recent in vitro study documented this dose-dependent relationship on a computer model of human intestine; at a low dose (2–3 g/day), there was a low production of SCFA and an increase in bifidobacteria, but not in lactobacilli; at a dosage of 5 g/day, the correct balance was reached between microbial population (Bifidobacteria, Lactobacilli and Anaerostipes) and SCFA production; further increasing the dosage up to 10 g/day, the authors observed a significant reduction in butyrate production and an increase in that of acetate, probably as a consequence of the growth of bifidobacteria that usually produce acetate from their metabolism [19]. In line with this pre-clinical evidence, it has been demonstrated that lactulose in healthy subjects can increase the frequency of defecation and number of fecal Bifidobacteria, and improve the consistency of feces [20]. For this reason, lactulose is considered a prebiotic that is an indigestible element with beneficial potential as it is able to selectively stimulate the growth and/or activity of favorable colon bacteria, such as Bifidobacteria [18], suppress the growth of potential pathogens, such as Clostridium and Escherichia Coli, and reduce intestinal transit time [21].

14.2 Lactulose in Hepatic Encephalopathy: Mechanism of Action

HE is one of the most frequent and disabling complications of liver cirrhosis and marks the transition from compensated to decompensated form [22]. Guidelines from the European Association for the Study of the Liver (EASL) and the American Association for the Study of Liver Diseases (AASLD) define this condition as a "brain dysfunction associated with liver insufficiency or portal-systemic shunting".

The severity of this condition is variable and includes a subclinical form called minimal HE (MHE) and a more severe form characterized by complete alteration of consciousness called overt HE (OHE). MHE is clinically silent, in fact it can only be found through psychometric evaluations or electrophysiological tests that investigate attention, psychomotor speed, and visuospatial skills. Despite this, it has a significant clinical impact on a patient's life since it is related to risk of falls and road accidents, work ability, sarcopenia, quality of life, and ultimately prognosis. It also constitutes a risk factor for developing OHE. On the contrary, OHE is characterized by personality changes, such as apathy, irritability, disinhibition, and alterations in state of consciousness. There may also be alterations in sleep–wake cycle with daytime sleepiness and nocturnal insomnia, disorientation in time and space, and finally coma.

Based on etiology, HE is classified into three types: type A results from acute liver failure (ALF), type B due to the presence of portosystemic shunts, and type C due to cirrhosis. Severity of clinical manifestations is assessed with the West Heaven scale. Based on its course, HE is classified into episodic if precipitated, recurrent if there are at least two episodes within six months, and persistent if neurological alterations are persistent and interspersed with relapse episodes. Typically, the latter patients have large spontaneous or iatrogenic portosystemic shunts [2]. Based on triggered factors, HE is classified as non-precipitated and precipitated. The most common precipitating factors that should be sought in patient with OHE are infections, constipation, dehydration, hypokalaemia and/or hyponatremia, digestive bleeding, and use of psychoactive drugs, such as opioids or benzodiazepines [22]. In 50% of cases, a precipitating cause is not identified [23].

Clinical manifestations of HE depend on systemic factors that affect permeability or integrity of blood-brain barrier [24]. Specifically, factors that are normally excluded from cerebral circulation are able to cross the barrier, while others that normally cross it, such as ammonium, enter the nervous system and cause damage [24]. Cerebral hyperammonemia in patients with cirrhosis and HE represents a key pathogenetic element and results primarily from an increase in circulating ammonium [25]. Ammonium derives from intestine as the final product of protein digestion, amino acid deamination and bacterial urease activity [24]. In healthy subjects with a normally functioning urea cycle, ammonium is detoxified and partly used in various biochemical reactions [24]. In liver cirrhosis, ammonium metabolism is altered and in this way, this substance can cause brain damage through various mechanisms, such as cell swelling, inflammation, oxidative stress, mitochondrial dysfunction, alteration of cellular energy systems, change of cell pH and in membrane potential [24].

Not only cirrhosis, as previously mentioned, but also HE would be associated with changes in intestinal microbiota [12]. In the study by Bajaj et al., the microbiota of cirrhotic patients with HE was compared with those without HE and with controls [26]. High levels of Alcaligenaceae, Enterobacteriaceae, and Fusobacteriaceae and low levels of Ruminococcaceae and Lachnospiraceae were found in HE patients compared to controls and patients without HE [26].

Furthermore, high concentrations of Veillonellaceae, endotoxin, and inflammatory markers (Interleukine 6, Tumor necrosis factor-α, Interleukin-2, and Interleukin-13) were found in patients with HE and cognitive impairment. Alcaligenaceae and Porphyromonadaceae were positively correlated with cognitive decline [26]. Therefore, alterations of intestinal microbiota in patients with HE constitute an important therapeutic target and for this reason, many studies focused on the use of prebiotics, such as lactulose.

Lactulose is considered the standard-of-care for HE treatment and prevention of recurrent episodes. The rationale for lactulose use in clinical practice is based on the fact that this substance is able to reduce systemic ammonium levels through various mechanisms [23]:

- Laxative effect: one of the main mechanisms of action is the creation of a hyperosmolar intestinal environment which, acting as a laxative, prevents effective ammonium absorption [27].
- Ammonium ionization: acidification of the intestinal contents determines the ionization of ammonium, which cannot diffuse freely through cellular membranes [28].
- Bacterial ammonium uptake: changes in endoluminal pH favor the leaching of ammonia from circulation to the colon; moreover, the volatile fatty acids released after lactulose metabolism are used by bacteria as a substrate for proliferation. In this way, they can use the ammonia trapped in the colon as a source of nitrogen for protein synthesis. Moreover, bacterial growth also increases the fecal mass, and this further favors the cathartic effect of this substance.
- Reduction of intestinal ammonium production: lactulose inhibits the activity of glutaminase enzyme and interferes with glutamine intestinal uptake and its subsequent conversion into ammonium.
- Beneficial effect on intestinal microbiota [23] having both prebiotic and probiotic effects.

On the latter point, it should be considered that the first published studies on lactulose effect in cirrhotic patients showed a facilitating effect on the growth of acidophilic bacteria with urease deficiency [29]. However, these studies were conducted on fecal cultures, which have limitations. Most gut bacteria cannot be grown or reliably differentiated from other associated bacteria. Furthermore, these techniques are qualitative or semi-quantitative and therefore do not allow to define the relative abundance of a bacterium in a mixture of bacteria [29]. However, more recent evidences from work, in which the 16S rRNA sequencing technique has been used, have shown neither changes in microbiota after lactulose administration, nor changes in bacterial diversity or in the amount of ammonia-producing bacteria [7]. So, it would seem that the beneficial effect of lactulose on HE is linked to mechanisms other than intestinal microbiota modification.

14.3 Lactulose in Hepatic Encephalopathy: Indication for Treatment

About HE treatment, three different situations should be considered: the management of hospitalized patients with episodic HE, secondary prophylaxis after an acute episode of HE, and management of patients with MHE.

For the first situation, management of a cirrhotic patient with an altered state of consciousness involves hospitalization, which should occur in an intensive setting for airways protection if grade III HE occurs. It is essential to undertake therapies to reduce circulating ammonium levels, this being an undoubted pathogenetic mechanism of HE. The most widely used empirical pharmacology is that of orally or rectally non-absorbable disaccharides, used in clinical practice for this purpose since the 1960s. Since 1966, when lactulose was introduced into clinical practice, several controlled trials and observational studies have evaluated its role in HE treatment versus placebo or no intervention [23]. The review by Gluudd et al. included randomized controlled clinical trials that focused on the evaluation of non-absorbable disaccharides for the prevention and treatment of HE. From this analysis emerged that non-absorbable disaccharides have positive effects on HE treatment (RR: 0.58) and on risk of major adverse events associated with cirrhosis (RR: 0.47), such as liver failure, variceal bleeding, infections, and hepato-renal syndrome. Their use also confers a reduction of liver and non-liver-related death (RR: 0.59) [23]. When HE is precipitantly induced, the patient can benefit from the prompt recognition and elimination of the trigger agent, although these are not identified in 50% of cases. Other agents, such as branched-chain amino acids, probiotics, antibiotics, or L-ornithine L-aspartate [30], are available, but the evidence supporting their efficacy, especially their effect on patient survival, is weak [31].

In literature, there are also trials comparing lactulose with other substances or in association with other drugs, such as rifaximin and albumin. Rifaximin is a semi-synthetic non-absorbable antibiotic effective against gram +, gram −, aerobic, and anaerobic enterobacteria; it does not change the composition of microbiota, but it has beneficial effects on its functionality because it reduces secondary bile acids production. In a randomized controlled trial, Sharma et al. showed that the association of lactulose with rifaximin resulted in a significantly higher resolution of HE than lactulose alone, a shorter hospital stay, and greater survival due to a reduction of deaths related to sepsis [32]. A similar result was found by the same group in 2017, using the association of lactulose with intravenous albumin compared with lactulose alone [33]. As mentioned previously, several controlled trials have been conducted on the treatment of acute HE episodes using drugs other than lactulose. Among these, Polyethylene glycol 3350-electrolyte solution (PEG) has aroused the interest of several researchers who have compared it to standard of care. Shehata et al., in a randomized controlled trial conducted on hospitalized patients with overt HE, showed that the number of patients with improvement in HE was greater in the PEG group than in the lactulose group, and that response time and hospitalization period were significantly minor, with no differences in adverse events [34]. About lactulose therapy, the American guidelines for HE indicate the initial dosage to be 25 ml every 1–2 hours. This therapy is not without risks; in fact, in the first days of therapy, adverse effects, such as abdominal pain, bloating, and diarrhea, may appear. In this regard, lactulose overdose can worsen the patient's clinical picture, as it can cause dehydration and electrolyte imbalance, both of which are known triggers for HE episodes [22]. Both American and European guidelines also claim to titrate the dosage to achieve at least two bowel movements per day of soft stools [22, 24].

However, there are currently doubts on the evaluation of the efficacy of lactulose based on the number of evacuations obtained. In fact, Duong et al., in a recently published study, disapproved of the dogma of the number of daily evacuations as a target for lactulose therapy in HE treatment [35]. It is unlikely that the effect of lactulose is linked only to its laxative effect, but also to the trapping of ammonium in an acidic environment [36]. However, stool acidification, which occurs mainly in the right colon, does not necessarily lead to an increase in the number of bowel movements; conversely, an increase in the number of bowel movements may not be associated with stool acidification [35]. In conclusion, the efficacy of lactulose in the treatment of HE is mainly linked to the increase in intestinal transit and the acidification of fecal pH, rather than to the modification of the intestinal flora [24]. In this way, the production and absorption of ammonium are reduced, while fecal excretion is increased [24]. In particular, the acidification of colic content derives from organic acids, especially lactic acid, which are formed following the intestinal bacterial hydrolysis of lactulose; it has been shown that this process is associated with a free ammonium concentration reduction [37] and that there is a direct positive correlation between lactulose dosage, fecal pH and ammonium levels [38].

The second indication for lactulose therapy is secondary HE prophylaxis; this is a real therapeutic challenge as patients who recover from an acute episode are at high risk of recurrence [2]. Secondary prophylaxis should begin with the administration of non-absorbable disaccharides [24, 39]. The study by Sharma et al. in 2009 demonstrated that lactulose significantly reduced the risk of relapse compared to placebo, without differences in mortality and rate of hospitalization for different causes [40]. If recurrent HE, lactulose can be administered in combination with rifaximin, because in these patients the combination therapy reduces the risk of new episodes and hospitalization [41], without increasing the rate of long-term adverse events [42]. There are no data on primary HE prophylaxis. This is generally not recommended, although patients with advanced cirrhosis (Child–Pugh class B or C) are at high risk of developing this complication.

A separate case is made up of patients with upper digestive bleeding. In a randomized controlled trial, Sharma et al. showed that the number of patients with variceal bleeding who developed HE was larger in the placebo group than in the lactulose group, and in multivariate analysis, lactulose therapy was one of the predictors of HE development [43].

Finally, MHE, although not clinically evident, has an important impact on daily life of patients and caregivers. This is especially important if we consider that HE is not a completely reversible condition and that after the resolution of an episode of HE, a certain degree of cognitive decline may persist [44]. Despite the higher risk of OHE development, current guidelines affirm that MHE treatment is not routinely recommended, but that the decision should be made on a case-by-case basis, because of doubts about the available data and design of controlled clinical trials [23, 39]. Several randomized controlled clinical trials have been produced on this topic using different therapies, such as lactulose, rifaximin, probiotics, L-ornithine L-aspartate, and branched chain amino acids, evaluating the performance in psychometric and driving tests, quality of life, and risk of developing OHE after therapy.

Studies focusing on lactulose use in this category of patients, published as early as the late 1990s, have actually demonstrated the achievement of significant endpoints [45–50]. For example, the study by Watanabe et al. showed that the administration of lactulose to patients with MHE resulted in an improvement in psychometric tests at 4 and 8 weeks and disappearance in half of the patients treated at 8 weeks, but the persistence of signs of MHE in 85% of untreated patients [45]. Similar results have been reported in the studies by Horsmans et al. and Dhiman et al. [49]. Prasad et al. also demonstrated that lactulose caused not only a significant improvement in cognitive function but also in the quality of life [51]. Despite this, the treatment of MHE still remains an unresolved issue. Table 14.1 [32–34, 52], Table 14.2 [40, 53, 54], and Table 14.3 [45–47, 51, 55–57] summarize the published studies on lactulose treatment for acute episodic HE, secondary prophylaxis of HE, and treatment of MHE, respectively.

14.4 Final Consideration

Lactulose is widely used in daily clinical practice for HE treatment, in light of its cathartic effect and its ability to acidify the intestinal contents following its own metabolism. In particular, it represents the standard-of-care for acute episodes of OHE and for the prevention of recurrence of patients with previous episodes, possibly in association with rifaximin. A first criticism regarding lactulose therapy concerns the evaluation of the target to be reached, which up to now has been based on the number of daily evacuations. The classic 2–3 daily bowel movements probably represent an unreliable target and therefore further data on fixed dose and lactulose dosage based on fecal pH and cognitive response are needed. Randomized controlled trials on the management of episodic HE are extremely complex to design and carry on, primarily because the only management of the precipitating factor(s) may be sufficient to resolve HE. Generally, most of studies are based on these "therapeutic approaches" as resolution/amelioration of HE symptoms. However, in patients with episodic, precipitant-induced HE, the effect of the active treatment and that of stopping the precipitant and of general care can be hardly

Table 14.1 Published studies on episodic hepatic encephalopathy treatment with lactulose

First author	Year	Study type	Active treatment (s)	Patients treated	Period of treatment	Objectives	Main results
Sharma et al. "A randomized, double-blind, controlled trial comparing rifaximin plus lactulose with lactulose alone in treatment of overt hepatic encephalopathy" *Am J Gastroenterol*	2013	Randomized controlled trial	Lactulose + rifaximin	63 (57)	Hospitalization	Amelioration/ resolution of HE	76% of patients compared with 50.8% had complete reversal of HE ($P < 0.004$). There was a significant decrease in mortality after treatment with lactulose plus rifaximin vs. lactulose and placebo (23.8% vs. 49.1%, $P < 0.05$).
Rahimi et al. "Lactulose vs polyethylene glycol 3350--electrolyte solution for treatment of overt hepatic encephalopathy: the HELP randomized clinical trial" *JAMA Intern Med*	2014	Randomized controlled trial	Polyethylene glycol 3350-electrolyte solution (PEG)	25 (25)	Hospitalization	Amelioration of HE	21 vs 13 patients had an improvement of 1 or more in HESA score ($P < 0.01$)
Sharma et al. "randomized controlled trial comparing lactulose plus albumin versus lactulose alone for treatment of hepatic encephalopathy" *Hepatology*	2017	Randomized controlled trial	Lactulose + albumin	60 (60)	10 days	Amelioration/ resolution of HE	Resolution within 10 days: 75% with lactulose plus albumin 53% in control group ($P = 0.03$)
Shehata et al. "randomized controlled trial of polyethylene glycol versus lactulose for the treatment of overt hepatic encephalopathy" *European Journal of Gastroenterology & Hepatology*	2018	Randomized controlled trial	Polyethylene glycol 3350-electrolyte solution (PEG)	50 (50)	Hospitalization	At least one scale improvement in HESA score	36/50 (72%) patients improved one grade or more in HE scoring algorithm score after 24 h of lactulose therapy versus 47/50 (94%) of those on PEG therapy ($P < 0.05$). The time needed for resolution of HE and length of hospital stay were significantly lower in PEG group versus lactulose group ($P < 0.001$). Both therapies were tolerated, and no significant adverse events were reported.

Table 14.2 Published studies on secondary prophylaxis of hepatic encephalopathy with lactulose

First author	Year	Study type	Active treatment (s)	Patients treated	Period of Treatment	Objectives	Main results
Riggio et al. "Pharmacological prophylaxis of hepatic encephalopathy after transjugular intrahepatic portosystemic shunt: a randomized controlled study" *J Hepatol*	2005	Randomized controlled trial	Lactitol/ Rifaximin	50 (25)	30 days	Efficacy of a pharmacological prophylaxis on the incidence of post-TIPS HE	25 pts. developed hepatic encephalopathy (33%, CI 95% = 22–45%). One-month incidence was similar in the three groups ($P = 0.97$). Previous hepatic encephalopathy (relative Hazard = 3.79;1.27–11.31) and basal-TMT-A Z-score > 1.5 (RH = 3.55;1.24–10.2) were predictors of post-TIPS encephalopathy at multivariate analysis.
Sharma et al. "Secondary prophylaxis of hepatic encephalopathy: an open-label randomized controlled trial of lactulose versus placebo" *Gastroenterology*	2009	Randomized controlled trial	Lactulose	61 (64)	Minimum of 6 months after enrollment	Recurrence of HE	12 (19.6%) of 61 patients in the HE-L group and 30 (46.8%) of 64 in the HE-NL group ($P = 0.001$) developed HE.
Agrawal et al. "Secondary prophylaxis of hepatic encephalopathy in cirrhosis: an open-label, randomized controlled trial of lactulose, probiotics, and no therapy" *Am J Gastroenterol*	2012	Randomized controlled trial	Lactulose/ probiotics	80/77 (78)	12 months	Recurrence of HE	77 patients developed HE (L, $n = 18$; P, $n = 22$; and N, $n = 37$). There was a significant difference between L and N ($P = 0.001$) and between P and N ($P = 0.02$), but no difference between the L and P groups ($P = 0.349$).

Table 14.3 Published studies on MHE treatment with lactulose

First author	Year	Study type	MHE/CHE diagnosis	Active treatment(s)	Patients treated	Weeks of Treatment	Objectives	Main results
Watanabe et al. "Clinical efficacy of lactulose in cirrhotic patients with and without subclinical hepatic encephalopathy" m*Hepatology*	1997	Original, randomized	NCT A, symbol digit test, BDT	Lactulose	22 out of 36	8	Psychometry	MHE had disappeared in 10 (50%) of the 20 treated patients at week 8, but it persisted in 11 (85%) of the 13 untreated patients
Horsmans et al. "Lactulose improves psychometric testing in cirrhotic patients with subclinical encephalopathy" *Aliment Pharmacol Ther*	1997	Original, randomized	NCT, RTT, sinusoid test, psychomotor performance tests	Lactulose	7 out of 14	2	Psychometry, ammonia	NCT improved respectively in 5/7 vs. 1/7; RRT in 6/7 vs. 4/7 and ammonia levels in 5/7 vs. 1/7
Dhiman et al. "Efficacy of lactulose in cirrhotic patients with subclinical hepatic encephalopathy" *Dig Dis Sci*	2000	Original, randomized	NCT A, NCT B, FCT A, FCT B, PC, BDT	Lactulose	10 out of 18	12	Psychometry	Psychometry improvement in 8/10 vs. 0/8
Prasad et al. "Lactulose improves cognitive functions and health-related quality of life in patients with cirrhosis who have minimal hepatic encephalopathy" *Hepatology*	2007	Original, randomized	NCT A, NCT B, FCT A, FCT B, PC, BDT	Lactulose	45 (25)	12	Psychometry, QoL	Significant improvement in psychometry: $P < 0001$; and QoL: $P < 0.002$. Improvement in HRQoL was related to the improvement in psychometry

Sharma et al. "An open-label randomized controlled trial of lactulose and probiotics in the treatment of minimal hepatic encephalopathy" *Eur J Gastroenterol Hepatol*	2008	Original, randomized controlled trial	NCT A, NCT B or FCT A and FCTB, CEP	Lactulose or probiotic or lactulose+probiotic	92 (31/31)	4	Psychometry, CEP, ammonia	Normalization of all parameters in half of treated patients (17/31, 16/31 and 17/30 respectively)
Mittal et al. "A randomized controlled trial comparing lactulose, probiotics, and L-ornithine L-aspartate in treatment of minimal hepatic encephalopathy" *Eur J Gastroenterol Hepatol.*	2011	Original, randomized	NCT A, NCT B, FCT A, FCT B, PC, BDT	Lactulose or probiotics or LOLA	160 (40/40/40)	12	Psychometry, ammonia, QoL	MHE reversal in 19/40 vs. 14/40 vs. 14/40 vs. 4/40. Improvement in QoL
Sidhu et al. "Rifaximin vs. lactulose in treatment of minimal hepatic encephalopathy" *Liver Int*	2016	Original, randomized	NCT A, FCT A, digit symbol test, BDT, PC	Lactulose vs. rifaximin	112 (55/57)	12	MHE reversal, QoL	MHE reversal in 38/55 and in 42/57; HRQoL was significantly improved in both groups

(maybe never) distinguished. To avoid the confounding role following the resolution of precipitating factors, maintaining a standard treatment in both groups, and adding the treatment under evaluation in the study group only and the placebo in the control group could be useful. On the contrary, in case of a positive result, what is working could be considered as the effect of a combined treatment's approach, and there is no possibility to suggest the use of the new one alone instead of the old one. Moreover, robust clinical outcomes, such as in-hospital stay and survival, liver-related and total deaths, completeness, and speed of recovery from HE, number of days in intensive care, quality-of-life evaluations, and costs for the healthcare services, should be considered. Large multicenter randomized controlled trials are therefore strongly needed to assess the role of any treatment for episodic precipitant-induced HE. Therapeutic strategies aimed to prevent the development of HE in cirrhotic patients are also considered of strong clinical and social importance. Most of the papers published on secondary prophylaxis of HE considered a "preventive approach" in both patients who recovered from HE and patients with recurrent HE. A large series of studies have been published following this aim and the main results have been reported in Tables 14.1, 14.2, and 14.3. It was unanimously agreed that trials for secondary prophylaxis for HE should be randomized and placebo-controlled, enrolling out-patients stabilized after one or more episodes of HE and absence of HE at inclusion. Trans-jugular Intrahepatic Portosystemic Shunt (TIPS) carriers should be excluded or enrolled in different randomized controlled trials aimed at this specific setting. The sample size could be estimated from the incidence of HE in the population at risk. The inclusion of a "no-treatment" or a "placebo" group should be considered mandatory. Regarding end-points, the development of one or more episodes of overt HE (Grade II or more) represents the most robust primary end-point, whereas secondary end-point should be considered, hospitalization, survival, socio-economic burden analysis, and Health-Related Quality of Life, because a prophylactic treatment should be prolonged lifelong, and the ideal therapy should be extremely safe and well tolerated. Another critical issue concerns MHE therapy. European and American guidelines do not recommend routine treatment. This is because there are some concerns about the studies published so far on this topic. Specifically, these focus the effectiveness of the therapy on non-clinical outcomes, such as reduction of ammonia or performance of psychometric tests. It is therefore essential to focus attention on solid endpoints, such as improvement of quality of life or development of OHE in the context of large randomized controlled trials. Therefore, large multicentre studies should be designed and considered in parallel with a placebo or a no-treatment arm. These represent important focuses on which to concentrate forces in the future.

References

1. European Association for the Study of the Liver. EASL clinical practice guidelines for the management of patients with decompensated cirrhosis. J Hepatol. 2018;69:406–60.
2. Ridola L, Faccioli J, Nardelli S, Gioia S, Riggio O. Hepatic encephalopathy: diagnosis and management. J Transl Int Med. 2020;8:210–9.
3. Mansour D, McPherson S. Management of decompensated cirrhosis. Clin Med (Lond). 2018;18:s60–5.
4. Ruszkowski J, Witkowski JM. Lactulose: patient- and dose-dependent prebiotic properties in humans. Anaerobe. 2019;59:100–6.
5. Trebicka J, Macnaughtan J, Schnabl B, Shawcross DL, Bajaj JS. The microbiota in cirrhosis and its role in hepatic decompensation. J Hepatol. 2021;75:S67–81.
6. Giannelli V, Di Gregorio V, Iebba V, Giusto M, Schippa S, Merli M, Thalheimer U. Microbiota and the gut-liver axis: bacterial translocation, inflammation and infection in cirrhosis. World J Gastroenterol. 2014;20:16795–810.
7. Sarangi AN, Goel A, Singh A, Sasi A, Aggarwal R. Faecal bacterial microbiota in patients with cirrhosis and the effect of lactulose administration. BMC Gastroenterol. 2017;17:125.
8. Acharya C, Sahingur SE, Bajaj JS. Microbiota, cirrhosis, and the emerging oral-gut-liver axis. JCI Insight. 2017;2:e94416.
9. Bajaj JS, Khoruts A. Microbiota changes and intestinal microbiota transplantation in liver diseases and cirrhosis. J Hepatol. 2020;72:1003–27.
10. Pérez-Cobas AE, Gosalbes MJ, Friedrichs A, Knecht H, Artacho A, Eismann K, Otto W, Rojo D, Bargiela R, von Bergen M, Neulinger SC, Däumer C, Heinsen FA, Latorre A, Barbas C, Seifert J, dos Santos VM, Ott SJ, Ferrer M, Moya A. Gut microbiota disturbance during antibiotic therapy: a multi-omic approach. Gut. 2013;62:1591–601.
11. Ridlon JM, Alves JM, Hylemon PB, Bajaj JS. Cirrhosis, bile acids and gut microbiota: unraveling a complex relationship. Gut Microbes. 2013;4:382–7.
12. Davis BC, Bajaj JS. The human gut microbiome in liver diseases. Semin Liver Dis. 2017;37:128–40.
13. Qin N, YanF LA, Prifti E, Chen Y, Shao L, Guo J, Le Chatelier E, Yao J, Wu L, Zhou J, Ni S, Liu L, Pons N, Batto JM, Kennedy SP, Leonard P, Yuan C, Ding W, Chen Y, Hu X, Zheng B, Qian G, Xu W, Ehrlich SD, Zheng S, Li L. Alterations of the human gut microbiome in liver cirrhosis. Nature. 2014;513:59–64.
14. Bajaj JS, Acharya C, FaganA WMB, Gavis E, Heuman DM, Hylemon PB, Fuchs M, Puri P, Schubert ML, Sanyal AJ, Sterling RK, Stravitz TR, Siddiqui MS, Luketic V, Lee H, Sikaroodi M, Gillevet PM. Proton pump inhibitor initiation and withdrawal affects gut microbiota and readmission risk in cirrhosis. Am J Gastroenterol. 2018;113:1177–86.
15. Chen Y, Yang F, Lu H, Wang B, Chen Y, Lei D, Wang Y, Zhu B, Li L. Characterization of fecal microbial communities in patients with liver cirrhosis. Hepatology. 2011;54:562–72.
16. Gustot T, Stadlbauer V, Laleman W, Alessandria C, Thursz M. Transition to decompensation and acute-on-chronic liver failure: role of predisposing factors and precipitating events. J Hepatol. 2021;75:S36–48.
17. Bouhnik Y, Attar A, Joly FA, Riottot M, Dyard F, Flourié B. Lactulose ingestion increases faecal bifidobacterial counts: a randomised double-blind study in healthy humans. Eur J Clin Nutr. 2004;58:462–6.
18. Guarino MPL, Altomare A, Emerenziani S, Di Rosa C, Ribolsi M, Balestrieri P, Iovino P, Rocchi G, Cicala M. Mechanisms of action of prebiotics and their effects on gastro-intestinal disorders in adults. Nutrients. 2020;12:1037.
19. Sakai Y, Seki N, Hamano H, Ochi H, Abe F, Shimizu F, Masuda K, Iino H. A study of the prebiotic effect of lactulose at low dosages in healthy Japanese women. Biosci microbiota food. Health. 2019;38:69–72.

20. Bothe MK, Maathuis AJH, Bellmann S, van der Vossen JMBM, Berressem D, Koehler A, Schwejda-Guettes S, Gaigg B, Kuchinka-Koch A, Stover JF. Dose-dependent prebiotic effect of lactulose in a computer-controlled in vitro model of the human large intestine. Nutrients. 2017;9:767.
21. Sitanggang AB, Drews A, Kraume M. Recent advances on prebiotic lactulose production. World J Microbiol Biotechnol. 2016;32:154.
22. Vilstrup H, Amodio P, Bajaj J, Cordoba J, Ferenci P, Mullen KD, Weissenborn K, Wong P. Hepatic encephalopathy in chronic liver disease: 2014 practice guideline by the American Association for the Study of Liver Diseases and the European Association for the Study of the liver. Hepatology. 2014;60:715–35.
23. Lotte Gluud L, Vilstrup H, Morgan MY. Non-absorbable disaccharides versus placebo/no intervention and lactulose versus lactitol for the prevention and treatment of hepatic encephalopathy in people with cirrhosis. Cochrane Database Syst Rev. 2016;2016:CD003044.
24. Rose CF, Amodio P, Bajaj JS, Dhiman RK, Montagnese S, Taylor-Robinson SD, Vilstrup H, Jalan R. Hepatic encephalopathy: novel insights into classification, pathophysiology and therapy. J Hepatol. 2020;73:1526–47.
25. Keiding S, Sørensen M, Bender D, Munk OL, Ott P, Vilstrup H. Brain metabolism of 13N-ammonia during acute hepatic encephalopathy in cirrhosis measured by positron emission tomography. Hepatology. 2006;43:42–50.
26. Bajaj JS, Ridlon JM, Hylemon PB, Thacker LR, Heuman DM, Smith S, Sikaroodi M, Gillevet PM. Linkage of gut microbiome with cognition in hepatic encephalopathy. Am J Physiol Gastrointest Liver Physiol. 2012;302:G168–75.
27. Hadjihambi A, Arias N, Sheikh M, Jalan R. Hepatic encephalopathy: a critical current review. Hepatol Int. 2018;12:135–47.
28. Zeegen R, Drinkwater JE, Fenton JC, Vince A, Dawson AM. Some observations on the effects of treatment with lactulose on patients with chronic hepatic encephalopathy. Q J Med. 1970;39:245–63.
29. Riggio O, Varriale M, Testore GP, Di Rosa R, Di Rosa E, Merli M, Romiti A, Candiani C, Capocaccia L. Effect of lactitol and lactulose administration on the fecal flora in cirrhotic patients. J Clin Gastroenterol. 1990;12:433–6.
30. Montes-Cortés DH, Novelo-Del Valle JL, Olivares-Corichi IM, Rosas-Barrientos JV, Jara LJ, Cruz-Domínguez MP. Impact of intestinal mannitol on hyperammonemia, oxidative stress and severity of hepatic encephalopathy in the ED. Am J Emerg Med. 2018;36:1570–6.
31. Ridola L, Riggio O, Gioia S, Faccioli J, Nardelli S. Clinical management of type C hepatic encephalopathy. United European Gastroenterol J. 2020;8:536–43.
32. Sharma BC, Sharma P, Lunia MK, Srivastava S, Goyal R, Sarin SK. A randomized, double-blind, controlled trial comparing rifaximin plus lactulose with lactulose alone in treatment of overt hepatic encephalopathy. Am J Gastroenterol. 2013;108:1458–63.
33. Sharma BC, Singh J, Srivastava S, Sangam A, Mantri AK, Trehanpati N, Sarin SK. Randomized controlled trial comparing lactulose plus albumin versus lactulose alone for treatment of hepatic encephalopathy. J Gastroenterol Hepatol. 2017;32:1234–9.
34. Shehata HH, Elfert AA, Abdin AA, Soliman SM, Elkhouly RA, Hawash NI, Soliman HH. Randomized controlled trial of polyethylene glycol versus lactulose for the treatment of overt hepatic encephalopathy. Eur J Gastroenterol Hepatol. 2018;30:1476–81.
35. Duong N, Reuter B, Saraireh H, Nadhem O, Acharya C, Fagan A, Hassouneh R, Bajaj JS. Bowel movement frequency is not linked with cognitive function in cirrhosis. Clin Gastroenterol Hepatol. 2021;S1542-3565:00517–6.
36. Agostini L, Down PF, Murison J, Wrong OM. Faecal ammonia and pH during lactulose administration in man: comparison with other cathartics. Gut. 1972;13:859–66.
37. Avery GS, Davies EF, Brogden RN. Lactulose: a review of its therapeutic and pharmacological properties with particular reference to ammonia metabolism and its mode of action of portal systemic encephalopathy. Drugs. 1972;4:7–48.

38. Elkington SG, Floch MH, Conn HO. Lactulose in the treatment of chronic portal-systemic encephalopathy. A double-blind clinical trial. N Engl J Med. 1969;281:408–12.
39. Montagnese S, Russo FP, Amodio P, Burra P, Gasbarrini A, Loguercio C, Marchesini G, Merli M, Ponziani FR, Riggio O, Scarpignato C. Hepatic encephalopathy 2018: a clinical practice guideline by the Italian Association for the Study of the liver (AISF). Dig Liver Dis. 2019;51:190–205.
40. Sharma BC, Sharma P, Agrawal A, Sarin SK. Secondary prophylaxis of hepatic encephalopathy: an open-label randomized controlled trial of lactulose versus placebo. Gastroenterology 2009;137:885–91.e1.
41. Bass NM, Mullen KD, Sanyal A, Poordad F, Neff G, Leevy CB, Sigal S, Sheikh MY, Beavers K, Frederick T, Teperman L, Hillebrand D, Huang S, Merchant K, Shaw A, Bortey E, Forbes WP. Rifaximin treatment in hepatic encephalopathy. N Engl J Med. 2010;362:1071–81.
42. Mullen KD, Sanyal AJ, Bass NM, Poordad FF, Sheikh MY, Frederick RT, Bortey E, Forbes WP. Rifaximin is safe and well tolerated for long-term maintenance of remission from overt hepatic encephalopathy. Clin Gastroenterol Hepatol. 2014;12:1390–7.e2.
43. Sharma P, Agrawal A, Sharma BC, Sarin SK. Prophylaxis of hepatic encephalopathy in acute variceal bleed: a randomized controlled trial of lactulose versus no lactulose. J Gastroenterol Hepatol. 2011;26:996–1003.
44. Riggio O, Ridola L, Pasquale C, Nardelli S, Pentassuglio I, Moscucci F, Merli M. Evidence of persistent cognitive impairment after resolution of overt hepatic encephalopathy. Clin Gastroenterol Hepatol. 2011;9:181–3.
45. Watanabe A, Sakai T, Sato S, Imai F, Ohto M, Arakawa Y, Toda G, Kobayashi K, Muto Y, Tsujii T, Kawasaki H, Okita K, Tanikawa K, Fujiyama S, Shimada S. Clinical efficacy of lactulose in cirrhotic patients with and without subclinical hepatic encephalopathy. Hepatology. 1997;26:1410–4.
46. Horsmans Y, Solbreux PM, Daenens CM, Desager JP, Geubel AP. Lactulose improves psychometric testing in cirrhotic patients with subclinical encephalopathy. Aliment Pharmacol Ther. 1997;11:165–70.
47. Dhiman RK, Sawhney MS, Chawla YK, Das G, Ram S, Dilawari JB. Efficacy of lactulose in cirrhotic patients with subclinical hepatic encephalopathy. Dig Dis Sci. 2000;45:1549–52.
48. Bajaj JS, Saeian KS, Christensen KM, Hafeezullah M, Varma RR, Franco J, Pleuss JA, Krakower G, Hoffmann RG, Binion DG. Probiotic yogurt for the treatment of minimal hepatic encephalopathy. Am J Gastroenterol. 2008;103:1707–15.
49. Sidhu SS, Goyal O, Mishra BP, Sood A, Chhina RS, Soni RK. Rifaximin improves psychometric performance and health-related quality of life in patients with minimal hepatic encephalopathy (the RIME trial). Am J Gastroenterol. 2011;106:307–16.
50. Bajaj JS, Heuman DM, Wade JB, Gibson DP, Saeian K, Wegelin JA, Hafeezullah M, Bell DE, Sterling RK, Stravitz RT, Fuchs M, Luketic V, Sanyal AJ. Rifaximin improves driving simulator performance in a randomized trial of patients with minimal hepatic encephalopathy. Gastroenterology. 2011;140:478–87.e1.
51. Prasad S, Dhiman RK, Duseja A, Chawla JK, Sharma A, Agarwal R. Lactulose improves cognitive functions and health-related quality of life in patients with cirrhosis who have minimal hepatic encephalopathy. Hepatology. 2007;45:549–59.
52. Rahimi RS, Singal AG, Cuthbert JA, Rockey DC. Lactulose vs polyethylene glycol 3350--electrolyte solution for treatment of overt hepatic encephalopathy: the HELP randomized clinical trial. JAMA Intern Med. 2014;174:1727–33.
53. Riggio O, Masini A, Efrati C, Nicolao F, Angeloni S, Salvatori FM, Bezzi M, Attili AF, Merli M. Pharmacological prophylaxis of hepatic encephalopathy after transjugular intrahepatic portosystemic shunt: a randomized controlled study. J Hepatol. 2005;42:674–9.
54. Agrawal A, Sharma BC, Sharma P, Sarin SK. Secondary prophylaxis of hepatic encephalopathy in cirrhosis: an open-label, randomized controlled trial of lactulose, probiotics, and no therapy. Am J Gastroenterol. 2012;107:1043–50.

55. Sharma P, Sharma BC, Puri V, Sarin SK. An open-label randomized controlled trial of lactulose and probiotics in the treatment of minimal hepatic encephalopathy. Eur J Gastroenterol Hepatol. 2008;20:506–11.
56. Mittal VV, Sharma BC, Sharma P, Sarin SK. A randomized controlled trial comparing lactulose, probiotics, and L-ornithine L-aspartate in treatment of minimal hepatic encephalopathy. Eur J Gastroenterol Hepatol. 2011;23:725–32.
57. Sidhu SS, Goyal O, Parker RA, Kishore H, Sood A. Rifaximin vs. lactulose in treatment of minimal hepatic encephalopathy. Liver Int. 2016;36:378–85.

GPSR Compliance

The European Union's (EU) General Product Safety Regulation (GPSR) is a set of rules that requires consumer products to be safe and our obligations to ensure this.

If you have any concerns about our products, you can contact us on ProductSafety@springernature.com

In case Publisher is established outside the EU, the EU authorized representative is:

Springer Nature Customer Service Center GmbH
Europaplatz 3
69115 Heidelberg, Germany

Batch number: 10726060

Printed by Printforce, the Netherlands